THE LIVING WELL
WITH CANCER COOKBOOK

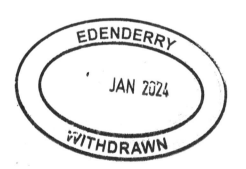

Fran Warde's career has been fuelled by a passion for food. Trained as a chef, she worked at the Café Royal, on an Australian prawn trawler, ran her own cookery school and then moved into food styling and food writing. She was food editor at *Red* magazine and has written and co-authored several bestselling cookery books, including *Ginger Pig Meat Book, Ginger Pig Farmhouse Cookbook, The French Kitchen* and *The French Market*. She has also written for the *Sunday Times* magazine, *Waitrose Food Illustrated, Olive* magazine and BBC Good Food. She lives in West London with her husband and two boys.

Catherine Zabilowicz, BSc (Hons), PG Cert, MBANT, CNHC, was inspired to embark on a Nutritional Therapy degree and a Masters in Nutritional Medicine at Surrey University after researching the link between nutrition and cancer during her son's treatment for leukaemia. She works as the Nutrition Advisor at Maggie's Cancer Caring Centre at Charing Cross Hospital and with patients with brain cancer who wish to implement the Ketogenic Diet through the charity Matthew's Friends. She also works in private practice through Body Soul Nutrition. In the past she has run healthy-eating programmes in schools and the community and has been Nutrition Advisor for a food company. She lives in Surrey and has four boys.

THE
LIVING WELL
WITH CANCER
COOKBOOK

An essential guide to nutrition,
lifestyle and health

FRAN WARDE &
CATHERINE ZABILOWICZ

IN SUPPORT OF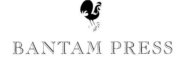

BANTAM PRESS

LONDON · NEW YORK · TORONTO · SYDNEY · AUCKLAND

TRANSWORLD PUBLISHERS
61–63 Uxbridge Road, London W5 5SA
www.transworldbooks.co.uk

Transworld is part of the Penguin Random House group of companies
whose addresses can be found at global.penguinrandomhouse.com

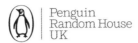

Penguin
Random House
UK

First published in Great Britain in 2016 by Bantam Press an imprint of Transworld Publishers

A CIP catalogue record for this book is available from the British Library.

ISBN 9780593075753

Typeset in ITC Stone Serif
Printed and bound in China

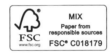

MIX
Paper from
responsible sources
FSC
www.fsc.org   FSC® C018179

1 3 5 7 9 10 8 6 4 2

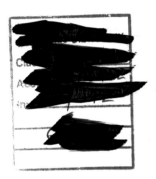

All photographs by Kristen Perers except:

Maggie's Centres: photographs of Maggie's West London on pp. 9, 34/5, 107, 126/7, 131;
Shutterstock: p.50 (all); Depositphotos: p.42

Illustrations by Kristen Perers except:

Shutterstock: pp.140/1, 166/7, 216/17, 236/7, 248/9; Depositphotos: pp.140/1 (b/ground), p.198/9

Dedication

This book is dedicated to anyone affected by cancer and to all who are striving to bring about an integrative approach to mainstream cancer care.

Acknowledgements

We are extremely grateful to Maggie's and all those working and associated with the charity who have made our involvement and this book possible.

Many thanks to our families who for many months endured our being either chained to a computer, writing, or disrupting the kitchen creating and testing recipes. Also to those friends and family who, having been affected by cancer themselves, offered their thoughts on the content of the book and were happy to be a part of our photography day at Maggie's, West London.

We are very grateful for the patience and kindness shown by our wonderful editor, Brenda Kimber, and the rest of the talented team at Transworld, particularly Leah Feltham, Phil Lord and Katrina Whone. Thank you to our agent, Anna Power, to Kristin Perers for her inspiring photography and canvas artworks, Iris Bromet for the tasteful props, Brenda Updegraff for her detailed editing skills and Lisa Horton for the beautiful design.

Last but not least, thank you to our contributors for their expert knowledge, including clinical oncologist Dr Brian Haylock, who gave invaluable guidance during the writing of this book.

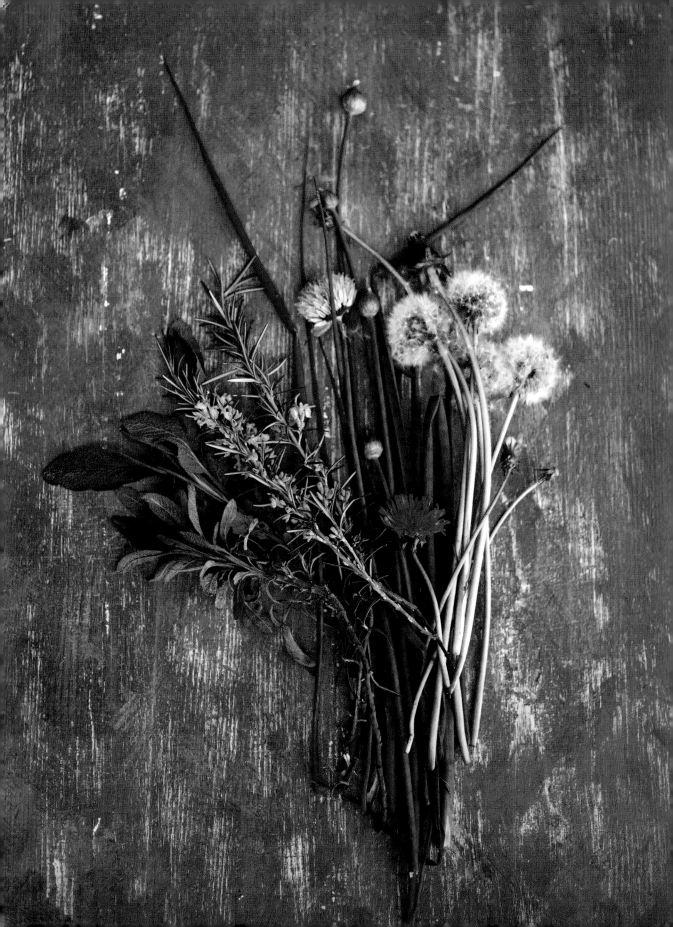

Contents

Introduction: Becoming an Active Partner 8

PART ONE Cancer, Nutrition and Lifestyle

1 Why Food Matters 16
2 The Science Behind Cancer 22
3 Nourishing Your Body 36
4 Coping with Common Side-effects of Cancer and Its Treatment 94
5 'Outside the Box' Approaches to Cancer 106
6 Life After Treatment 126

PART TWO The Nutritional Kitchen

Preparing Your Kitchen for a Healthy Diet 134
Starting the Day 140
Energizing Snacks 152
A Vegetarian Rainbow 166
Fabulous Fish 198
Satisfying Meat 216
Something Sweet 236
Super Staples 248

Food Diary 270
Glossary 271
Bibliography 273
Useful websites and resources 278
Index 279
Maggie's Centres 287

Introduction

Becoming an Active Partner

THIS IS A POSITIVE BOOK, and we hope it will lift your spirits by reassuring you that, as someone affected by cancer, there is plenty that you can do through diet and lifestyle to improve your quality of life and, possibly, the outcome. It covers all you need to know about cancer, nutrition and way of life when you embark on a cancer journey, whether you are the person diagnosed or a carer; and it provides a range of delicious, easy-to-prepare recipes to kick-start your healthy eating habits.

By using this book and our suggested resources you can arm yourself with a great deal of information that will help to reduce the feelings of helplessness and anxiety you will inevitably be experiencing as you are swept along in a fog of hospital visits and unfamiliar language about protocols (treatment plans) and procedures. It aims to give you an understanding of how food, lifestyle and treatment choices fit into the development of cancer cells and tumours, showing you that by creating a healthy environment within your body in which your normal cells can flourish, you will also create a hostile environment in which cancer cells will struggle to survive or thrive.

A new era is dawning in the understanding of cancer and its treatment, and we hope to bring you a voice of fact, honesty and reason that will inspire you to become an 'active partner' in your cancer journey, just as Maggie's Centres (see pages 287–8) are designed to do. It is never too late to make meaningful changes to your diet and lifestyle, whether you suspect you have cancer, you've just been diagnosed, or you are well down the path and want to reduce the risk of recurrence.

A major inspiration for this book has been Maggie Keswick Jencks's *A View from the Frontline*, which can be found on the Maggie's website (see page 288) and I certainly encourage you to read it. Through working with cancer patients, I have come to realize that being proactive is one of the most important steps you can take. Each person is 'in charge' of their own disease, just as they are of their own life. Taking on the role of 'active partner' during illness can be extremely empowering: it can help you through periods of rollercoaster emotions.

A range of approaches may be open to you in treating your cancer. If you are being rushed into decisions, remember that a few more days or even weeks (depending on the diagnosis) is unlikely to change the outcome in any major way, and it may give you the space to get your head around treatment choices

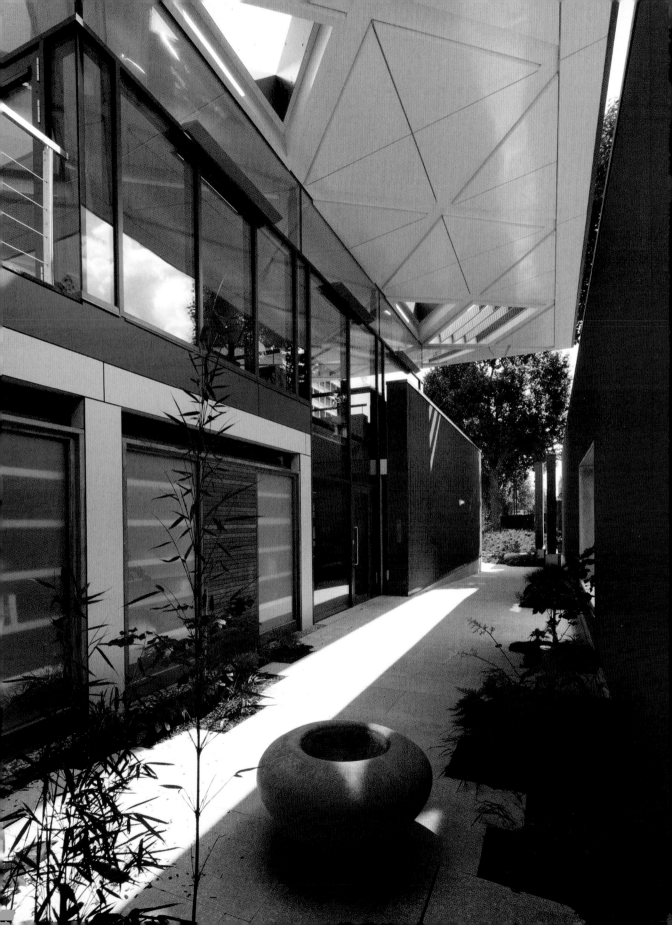

and what is right for you. It can be helpful to have time to prepare your body and mind. It is understandable that many people panic and are driven by fear to begin treatment as quickly as possible. Of course, in the case of some high-grade tumours or in certain acute situations radical surgery or immediate and aggressive treatment may be a lifesaver. Be guided by your oncologist and medical team, but remember they are working for you and you do have the right to choose the path that best reflects your preferences and beliefs.

We hope to encourage you to ask questions and explore all pathways, but we do appreciate being proactive is not always easy and there will probably be times when a passive role can seem the easier option. Use this book to guide and motivate yourself, and the resource section to help you gain further accurate and balanced information. This will serve you far better than trawling the internet, which often throws up confusing or conflicting advice and can lead to additional anxiety. Maintaining or gaining quality of life after a cancer diagnosis and especially during treatment can be one of the main goals for many people, as is keeping the cancer at bay for longer. This is something that nutrition, amongst other things, can help with immensely.

In her book *Radical Remission*, Kelly Turner interviewed many people across the world who had achieved spontaneous remission from cancer. She discovered that there were nine key factors, two of which were radically changing your diet and taking herbs and supplements, but the other factors all involved the mind. It may be a combination of several approaches that works in the end, but the importance of mindset cannot be over-estimated. We believe that no one should be left without hope. This book is about achieving it.

Fran

Catherine

FRAN'S STORY

AFTER THE SUDDEN LOSS OF MY MOTHER to cancer I wanted to try to comprehend this disease in a positive manner. My first port of call was Maggie's West London, as I live in the area. I knew very little about the charity, apart from having raised some money for it many years ago by hosting a supper. Following a visit and then a few meetings there I began helping as a volunteer. I had never done anything like this before; nor had I met many people with cancer. I was honoured to be given this opportunity.

On my first day – once I had stopped gawping in awe at the wonderful architecture of the place – I slowly settled into domestic chores in the kitchen, generally helped out where I could, and started to meet the visitors to the Centre. My emotions were somewhat chaotic as I was still grieving for my mother, but I kept telling myself off in my head: 'Stop it, Fran – it's about others, not about you.' As the weeks went by I started to get to know the most amazing mix of people, suffering with various stages of cancer, and I also met their families. I was astounded at their ability to be so serene and practical in such difficult circumstances. I strongly believe that the Maggie's Centres are havens that nurture such positivity.

Working in this favourable environment is the most fantastic team, willing to help and offer advice to anyone who walks through the front door. It was in the kitchen that I met Catherine, the Centre's Nutrition Advisor, who gives workshops on the connection between diet and cancer, and I started sitting in on her discussions and talks with people she was helping or had helped. They loved her so much that they just came back for more.

Catherine was a fount of easily understood, practical dietary knowledge. I was fascinated. We chatted endlessly about food and quickly realized that we shared a keen appetite for good, nutritious meals cooked from scratch. I already knew a lot about food, but now I was learning so much more about seeds, nuts, oils, turmeric, the rainbow diet, looking after our gut – it was endless, and I was excited by everything Catherine said. Having written numerous cookery books, I suggested that we should work on one together, offering super-tasty but also healthy recipes and nutritional advice for cancer sufferers.

I have learned so many new nutritious tips from Catherine: how to make my own 'easy-peasy' almond milk; grind a small quantity of seeds into a casserole to thicken it; place mushrooms in the sun so that they produce vitamin D; eat as much turmeric as possible; replace sugar and flour with more nutritious alternatives; always buy raw honey . . . The tips are endless, and they are all here in this book, worked into my tasty recipes.

So get cooking and embrace the *Living Well With Cancer* diet – it will benefit your health in a multitude of ways.

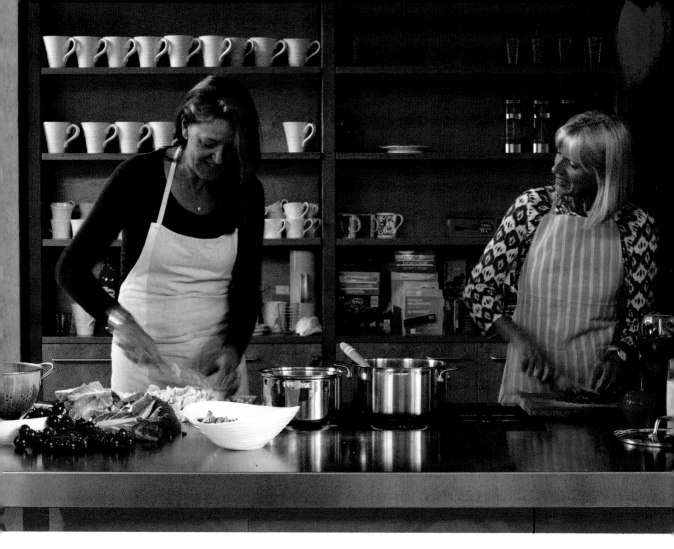

CATHERINE'S STORY

MY CULINARY JOURNEY THROUGH CANCER began when I became a carer for my son Sebastian, who was diagnosed with acute lymphoblastic leukaemia aged seven. Even though I felt we generally ate healthily and cooked from scratch, I could see that there was room for change. We switched to eating mainly organic, enjoying the delights of our weekly organic veg box delivery; we tried a gluten-free diet (which ended in tears); and we juiced regularly.

I also spent the three and a half years of my son's successful treatment trawling research papers and the internet to find any evidence I could about the impact of nutrition and lifestyle on cancer cells. This fuelled my desire to learn more, so I embarked on four years of study, then further postgraduate studies in Nutritional

Medicine, leading to my special interest in diet and oncology. That was fifteen years ago and Sebastian now has a biochemistry degree and is hoping to work in the field of cancer research in the future.

My undergraduate research included a very small pilot study looking at the effects of chemotherapy on gut function and its possible long-term consequences. On the back of this I was lucky enough to be offered the position of Nutritional Advisor at Maggie's West London, where I have been running regular nutrition workshops since it opened in 2008. I feel passionately that preserving and restoring gut function throughout cancer and beyond is of vital importance to wellbeing and future health; it is an important feature of all my workshops and of this book (see pages 82–84).

I also work privately for Body Soul Nutrition, alongside some very experienced practitioners, and am involved with the charity Matthew's Friends, which started out helping children with epilepsy through the Ketogenic Diet (see page 106) but has also moved into oncology. Research into ketogenic therapy and cancer has been gaining pace in the US, while here in the UK we are accumulating comprehensive case studies and designing a clinical trial on its use for brain tumour patients.

I believe the wealth of experience I've gathered over the years has given me a broad understanding of the needs of anyone affected by cancer and of the challenges they face, and it has taught me how to help them find their way through the maze. I remember how helpless I felt on my son's diagnosis. My hope is that this book will pull together the information that I would have been so grateful to have had back then.

SEBASTIAN'S STORY

I still remember as a young child going out to tea with various friends and getting very excited at the prospect of eating 'normal' food, as I perceived it – probably chicken nuggets and chips. It was not until a few years later that I really appreciated the delicious and highly nutritious meals my parents cooked at home. I am very grateful for having been brought up to appreciate the importance of diet and nutrition, especially its effects on an individual's mental state and happiness, and of course the cancer-prevention aspects too. As I grew older, I got less excited about the idea of biscuits, crisps and sweets, and although the financial strains of university tested my commitment to healthy eating, I still feel more delight in a hearty, healthy home-cooked meal than in any ready meal. Having studied biochemistry, I further realize the significance of what you put in your body and I believe any reader, cancer patient or not, can learn from this book.

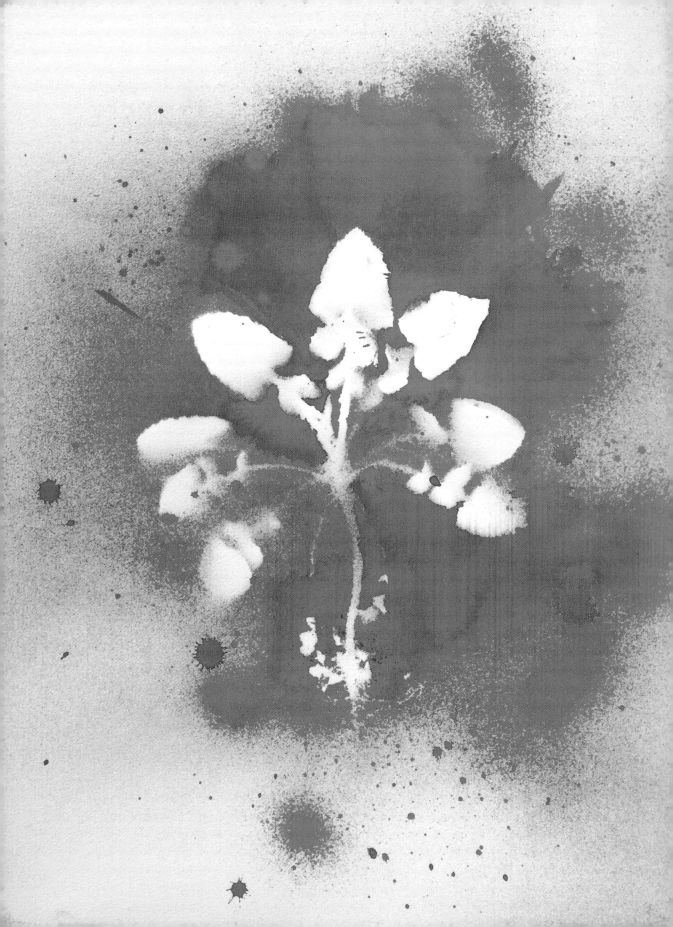

PART ONE

Cancer, Nutrition and Lifestyle

1 Why Food Matters

PEOPLE OFTEN SAY TO ME, 'Well I had a healthy diet and lifestyle and still I got cancer.' I empathize, because I felt like that when my son was diagnosed with leukaemia. I had always had a strong interest in food and nutrition, and as a family I thought we were doing well on the healthy-food front. Then when cancer struck, like many people I wondered whether my dedication to a healthy diet had been worth it. But then a friend pointed out that if we had been eating junk maybe my son's prognosis would not have been so positive. I took heart from that and now, having worked with so many people undergoing cancer treatment, I can see that those who start off better nourished often fare better and have fewer side-effects from treatment.

However, anyone reading this and now beating themselves up about an unhealthy diet should understand that it doesn't take too much to turn things around, build up nutrient levels and control blood sugar, and it is certainly never too late. It should also sound an alert to us all: we never know what is around the corner healthwise, so we should all be nurturing our bodies to give ourselves the best chance whatever happens.

Cancer is not just one condition – there are many different types. Equally, we are very individual beings, so the experience of the disease will be different for every one of us. A whole-person approach needs to be taken, looking at underlying causes and what may be driving the cancer growth. The conditions surrounding and within our cells, often referred to as the 'internal terrain', may be ripe for cancer to thrive. We need to make this environment as inhospitable as possible for cancer cells and as favourable as possible for the maintenance of our healthy cells. What we put into our body is without doubt going to influence this terrain.

The biochemistry of the body is governed to a large extent by how it is fuelled. Just like a car, put in the wrong fuel and it will splutter and grind to a halt; put the right fuel in, oil it well, care for it and it should purr along. With sufficient nurture and nourishment the body can be helped to heal itself. 'We are what we eat' might sound very clichéd and is somewhat simplistic – we also have to ensure that nutrients are absorbed and utilized efficiently – but holding that thought in your mind is a great starting point in managing such a multi-dimensional disease.

Since planning this book I have been asking visitors to Maggie's what they would like to get out of such a publication. Invariably the answer is clarification where there is confusion about what they should and shouldn't eat. I know that worry. Just when you have decided to fill your cupboard with food you have read has anti-cancer properties, you then read that too much of that particular food may actually cause cancer, or that you should only eat it in a certain form. No one really seems to know what is best. You despair and worry, then you feel like giving up.

Food, diet and nutrition are some of the most contentious subjects around and cause many a heated debate. It can seem that everyone has an opinion they want to share with you, especially after you have been given a cancer diagnosis. There are so many different dietary fads and some debatable dietary claims, and the media is always full of revolutionary cures and foods that stop cancer in its tracks. But this information is often misguided and inaccurate, gleaned from one-off studies which probably haven't made it to human trials. (You can read more on such controversies in the section on evidence-based medicine on page 18.)

The problem is that nutrition is a young science. It cannot promise all the answers because scientific research is constantly moving on and information is changing along with scientists' understanding of the behaviour of cancer cells. But research into foods and their anti-cancer and healing properties is coming on in leaps and bounds, and in 2007 the World Cancer Research Fund (WCRF) reported on a systematic review of research on the links between diet, physical activity, weight and cancer which is now continuously updated. It has consistently found that a diet rich in plant foods is beneficial in reducing cancer risk.

No one can any longer deny that food can definitely be a medicine too, and nowadays most people also realize that a lot of what we eat bears no resemblance to food in its natural form. We now know it is imperative to eat a balance of fresh, natural, nutrient-dense produce, with minimal tampering from manufacturing processes, so that nature can work as intended. There are anti-cancer diets that advocate a vegan approach; others that are based on a high intake of fat and are low in carbohydrates; and some that take a more individualized approach. But all of them advocate that plant foods, especially green leafy vegetables, should be consumed without question.

This book aims to empower you with an intuition for those foods that can help you to be as strong and as healthy as possible throughout your cancer and beyond. If we can understand the power and importance of nutritious food and where it fits into the lifecycle of a cancer cell, we can start seeing foods in a new light. 'Nourishing' is one of my favourite words, along with 'delicious' and 'nutritious': they sum up what food should be to us. Once you start regarding food as a beautiful and wondrous thing which has the potential to heal the body, I believe you start to understand the power and control you can have over your body, your health and, subsequently, your life.

Relationships with food can be extremely complex but the body's amazing healing powers will always aim for health when given the right nudge and being in tune with your body and listening to what it is telling you helps to achieve this. Foods that are well digested and tolerated by one person may not be by another, so treat your body gently. Recording your intake in a food and symptom diary (see page 270) or journal can be a helpful way of recognizing possible intolerances or problem foods and is certainly something I advocate when you are first making changes to your diet.

With the power of the mind being so important, it is imperative that you feel happy with the dietary and lifestyle changes you implement and that you believe they will make a difference. We all know the power of the placebo effect: if you think something will do you good, it can have a profoundly positive influence on your health.

I feel it is important that we learn at least a little about what is happening in our bodies when we have cancer in order to realize that we can take positive steps and make a difference; for that reason, Chapter 2 outlines the basic science underlying the disease. Beyond that, however, maybe we should take the science bit out of the equation and develop our innate understanding that chemically laden, processed foods are not what our body was designed to be fuelled by. Eating a balance and variety of fresh, mainly plant-based, whole, natural foods that are organic or of high provenance is the best we can do for our bodies, and we surely don't need a scientific study to prove this!

If you think there is a touch of the zealot in me, let me reassure you that I do believe that too much of anything – even fantastically healthy things – could be detrimental, as it can tip the body's biochemistry out of kilter. Balance is key. Also, in my opinion the *odd* treat may do no harm and may even perk us up, but this is provided it is in combination with a predominately nutrient-dense diet that is positively supporting all our body systems. Our bodies should then be able to cope with any detrimental effects from less desirable foods and lifestyle. So if you feel the need for the occasional glass of alcohol, or a sweet treat on someone's birthday, or a less-than-healthy meal out, there is no need to beat yourself up about it – enjoy it, move on and don't feel guilty! The important thing is to keep everything as simple as possible, as I also believe that getting too stressed about your diet is possibly even more detrimental than an unhealthy diet. If you worry too much about every little thing, feeding yourself can become a source of anxiety or a chore, and you risk losing the joy of eating.

Evidence-based Medicine (EBM)

This is another area of healthcare fraught with controversy. Before I provoke the wrath of some individuals, scientists and medics, I would like to make it clear that I am extremely grateful for sound evidence-based medicine, which has been such a success story in improving the outcome of blood cancers. My son Sebastian would not be here if it wasn't for chemotherapy. But we have to put it in perspective and make sure that reliance on EBM doesn't rule out other treatment choices. An integrated and open approach must be the best policy, allowing patients to make some decisions for themselves without being chastised in the process.

The randomized control trial (RCT) has always been viewed as the gold standard evidence base for any health-related therapy. In an ideal world we would all love to be able to base our decisions about treatments on flawless, unbiased and honest scientific evidence, but this is somewhat unrealistic. Because of both the range of complementary and alternative medicines (CAM) and their highly individual approaches, research into these treatments is often extremely complex and there is rarely enough money for large enough trials. As a result, what research is carried out tends to come to the general conclusion that more investigation is needed on larger population bases. This is all very well, but many patients do not have the luxury of being able to wait years for such studies to be completed, and besides, funding for larger-scale trials is very hard to secure.

Research into food and dietary approaches is even more problematic, because it is difficult to measure consumption adequately – dietary recall or food diaries can be notoriously inaccurate.

Naturally, in any treatment safety should be the prime concern and any potential toxicity issues need to be thoroughly investigated. Many CAM therapies – such as massage, reiki, reflexology, mindfulness and counselling – are now offered at most oncology centres, often through charities such as Maggie's, as they are deemed very safe. But diet, supplements and herbs are areas where sensible advice can be hard to access because research is of mixed quality and safety may be questionable. All too often a natural food or herbal compound may have demonstrated anti-cancer properties in a test tube and have proven beneficial effects when tested on animals, but there is unlikely to be any solid evidence of its benefit to humans. Unfortunately this type of evidence cannot be considered robust, even if many people have taken certain compounds, seen improvements in their health and, what's more, lived to tell the tale. Such foods, treatments and dietary approaches are generally dismissed in orthodox medicine circles as unproven, worthless and possibly dangerous.

So the big question is, if some inconclusive research exists showing that a certain type of food, diet or drug inhibits cancer progression, sufficient safety has been established and no harmful effects have been observed, should we wait for a strong scientific evidence base which could take years, if it happens at all? Or should we follow our instincts and go with the best studies available and maybe a touch of anecdotal evidence too?

Of course this suggestion is going to cause uproar in some circles, as it is not the scientific way. But the truth is that many people try other therapies without revealing the fact to their medical team for fear of disapproval. It would be so much safer if patients felt that they could share this information with an open-minded team so that results could be monitored and recorded in a systematic way, leading to useful case studies which could then inform future treatment protocols. For instance, many natural compounds or therapies may increase the power of chemotherapy and radiotherapy, and prior experience and knowledge of this could allow doses to be adjusted accordingly.

Cancer is so complex, with so many genes and mechanisms involved, that I do wonder whether we will ever narrow treatment to just a handful of protocols. A personalized approach in medicine is already being touted as the way forward, but we need to broaden this by listening to patients rather than dismissing their wishes, and by being prepared to think 'outside the box'. Every person is unique, both in the course their cancer takes and in how they respond to treatments. This is why a patient should work alongside a health professional who can assess their individual responses to therapy and adapt their protocol accordingly. Unfortunately, therapies considered alternative are often used as a last resort when it may well have been very helpful to have integrated them from the start.

The arguments against such a personalized approach are often money, doctor's lack of knowledge of CAM, and the time required to address the disease with a more individualized strategy. However, I am confident that if patients saw a multidisciplinary team, including nutrition experts, as soon as they were diagnosed, healthcare costs could be reduced and outcomes improved.

'EBM – WOULDN'T IT BE A GOOD IDEA?'

Jerome Burne, health journalist

What could be more important in medicine than knowing if a treatment works and that it is safe, or at least that its side-effects aren't worse than the condition it is being used to treat?

That's the admirable idea behind EBM, which emerged in the mid-1990s in the wake of such embarrassing revelations as the finding that a drug regularly given to patients after a heart attack to cut the chances that the heart would develop a dangerous irregular rhythm was killing one in twenty of them. The point being that only by running trials can you see the big picture that won't emerge if you rely on personal clinical experience.

The hope was that with RCTs that compared any new drug with a placebo before giving a licence, such disasters could be avoided. However such well-intentioned initiatives frequently have 'unintended consequences' or it turns out that the 'devil is in the details'. In the case of EBM both of these applied.

Unintended, for instance, is the consequence that despite nearly thirty large-scale randomized trials of cholesterol-lowering statins, there is still no general agreement about whether the benefits of these drugs do actually outweigh the side-effects.

The trials have all been run by the companies, no one else can see the full results and side-effect data is often not gathered. If EBM can't provide a clear answer to such a basic question about one of the most widely used and most profitable drugs ever, what chance that it is a useful (as opposed to, say, convenient or acceptable) tool for assessing others?

The 'detail' failure has been that drug companies have proved far more ready to twist and distort the results of trials until they yield up the required answer than, presumably, anyone expected. The variety of imaginative ways to fudge results, from excluding patients who responded too strongly to a placebo (makes it harder to produce a result showing the drug to be effective) to simply hiding, or not publishing, an unfavourable one, has been recorded in exhaustive detail in Ben Goldacre's book *Bad Pharma*.

And he's not the only one. Recently *Lancet* editor Richard Horton wrote an editorial about a symposium held in London on the 'reproducibility and reliability of biomedical research'.

'The case against science is straightforward,' writes Horton. 'Much of the scientific literature, perhaps half, may simply be untrue. Afflicted by studies with small sample sizes, tiny effects, invalid exploratory analyses, and flagrant conflicts of interest . . . it has taken a turn towards darkness.'

Ben Goldacre's exposé of drug companies' ability to play fast and loose with the data was written in 2012 and three years on there is still a major problem. In June 2015 he wrote in top medical journal the *BMJ*: 'Well documented problems exist in the funding and prioritisation of research, the conduct of trials, the withholding of results, the dissemination of evidence, and its implementation with patients.' Even so he is optimistic that the system can be fixed.

Despite these severe failures of the EBM project, it has proved very effective at making a distinction between supposedly scientifically tested drug medicine and unscientific non-drug treatments such as acupuncture, herbs or clinical nutrition. The result is that they can then be dismissed as 'quackery which relies on anecdote and the placebo for any apparent effects'.

And nowhere is the EBM/quackery boundary policed more vigorously than in the field of cancer where, at 30 million-plus, RCTs provide the stamp of scientific respectability for a new drug. However, a recent article in the *BMJ* suggests that this EBM fig-leaf has become dreadfully tattered.

The *BMJ* article – 'Why do cancer drugs get such an easy ride?' – shows that, far from occupying the scientific high ground, testing of cancer drugs is actually far less rigorous than the standard required for licensing in other fields.

For instance, a review that looked at nearly 9,000 trials of cancer drugs, run between 2007 and 2010, found that compared with drugs for other conditions, they were nearly 3 times more likely not to be randomized, 2.6 times more likely not to be compared with any other treatment and 1.8 times more likely not to be blinded.

Now of course showing that drugs benefit hugely from light-touch regulation does not show that cancer treatments without an RCT are not effective and safe. But what it does suggest is that dividing cancer treatments into scientific and non-scientific is misleading and not beneficial to patients.

2 The Science Behind Cancer

WHEN MY SON WAS DIAGNOSED with leukaemia I was desperate to understand what exactly was going on so that I could make sense of the treatment and dietary and lifestyle influences. I wanted to be armed with as much information as possible so that I could make informed choices and have some level of control over the situation. I know not everyone necessarily feels the same way, and maybe there is a different sense of responsibility when it is your child who is ill. However, I do believe that a basic understanding of cellular activity within the body can enable us to see why certain diet and lifestyle choices may influence outcomes; and this in turn may help to spark motivation for changing how we take care of ourselves.

Keeping the science simple is not always easy. If you read the following and feel you need further explanation, there are some great animated videos online which may help make things clearer. Also, see the table on page 30 for a simplified version of mechanisms and where food fits in.

This chapter is designed so that, once you have read it, you can refer back to it as you read other parts of the book. There is also a Glossary on page 272 to clarify any unfamiliar terms.

What Caused My Cancer?

Cancer is the name we give to diseases stemming from the uncontrolled division of abnormal cells in the body. One of the first questions people tend to ask is what could have caused this to happen? Radiation, chemicals – especially those produced by smoking – and infectious organisms are well-documented causes, but the fact is that cancer is a complex and diverse disease, at the heart of which is damage to our DNA (deoxyribonucleic acid). DNA contains the instructions that dictate how our cells behave and damage to it can lead to mutations making our cells defective. This is something that is happening continually and generally our bodies are primed to nip these mutations in the bud, but sometimes the mechanisms go awry.

One such mechanism is 'cell apoptosis' or 'programmed' cell death. Our cells constantly reproduce themselves by division, which is essential for tissue maintenance and repair. The rate at which this happens varies widely between different cell types and slows down as we get older. Adult 'stem cells' are our back-up as we age: these are cells that are able to 'differentiate' – that is, change themselves into any specialized cell type that is needed and therefore perform the vital function of repairing damaged tissue within our bodies.

The rates of cell death and cell division in adults must remain in balance if body tissues are to stay the same size. When everything is working properly, damaged or old cells die and are removed in a managed, orderly fashion by the mechanism of apoptosis. Cancer cells, however, manage to override this mechanism of programmed death, leading to unruly and disordered division, and hence cell immortality and the growth of an abnormal mass or tumour. Cancer cells that are dividing very quickly don't have time to mature and tend to be more unruly and poorly differentiated. The extent of this differentiation, or how alike the cells are to our normal tissue, is the basis for the grading of tumours. Grade 1 bears the closest resemblance to the normal tissue and is generally the slowest-growing type.

Once cancer cells have taken hold, we need to create both an environment that is hostile to them and a strong immune system. We often need to take a multi-pronged approach to treatment, maybe even changing some of our tactics regularly in order to outsmart the cancer cells before they can build up a resistance.

The ideal solution is to kill the cancer cells gently either by making them more recognizable to the immune system so that they are killed and ingested by the immune cells, or by triggering normal apoptosis so that they die in an ordered manner and are recycled naturally. This approach does not stress the body and eliminates the need for the liver to work hard to break down the dead cells. Chemotherapy and radiotherapy (see page 33) give a more vicious attack and cause 'necrosis' or 'unprogrammed' death of not only cancer cells but healthy cells too. This in turn causes inflammation (see page 27) and stress on the body.

Many foods and herbs have been shown to target cancer cells gently. For instance curcumin, a substance present in turmeric, has been shown to block a whole raft of mechanisms which cancer cells use to proliferate. Unfortunately there is no scientific evidence that natural compounds can work alone to treat cancer, but, used in conjunction with other treatments, some have been shown to have a powerful effect (see page 112).

One in two people will develop cancer during their lifetime, but recent research suggests that although around 30 per cent of cancers can be explained by diet, lifestyle and genetics, the rest is down to plain bad luck. Many researchers would question this, as it does not explain the dramatic increase in cancer rates over the last hundred years, which may well be down to recent environmental influences.

Cancer Research UK states that an estimated 600,000 cancer cases could have been avoided over the last five years if the UK population had been healthier. Of course we all know people who have smoked and eaten an unhealthy diet throughout their lives and have managed to avoid cancer. Who knows what has contributed to their resilience. Cancer is like a jigsaw puzzle with a whole lot of contributing factors which need to come together to make a whole. However, the bottom line is that the body has failed to maintain equilibrium and this more than likely comes down to changes in its biochemistry, possibly caused by toxicity and nutrient deficiencies. These changes have allowed the terrain (see page 24) to be tipped out of balance, thus creating the right conditions for cancer cells to thrive.

Genes and Epigenetics

You may have thought that cancer is primarily a genetic disease and that if we have a certain type of cancer within our immediate family we are more likely to get that cancer ourselves.

This is true to a certain extent and, although it takes more than one mutation in a cell to make a cancer cell, when a person inherits an abnormal copy of a gene such as BRAC1, which is linked to breast cancer, they basically have a head start. However, we need to understand that our genetic make-up is not set in stone.

The genes within our cells are responsible for making proteins. Proteins are the building blocks of our cells and hundreds can be made from the thousands of genes in the human body, but when a mutation occurs in a gene then the result may be a defective or missing protein. If the affected protein is responsible for how and when the cell divides or dies, then the cell may continue to divide uncontrollably, leading to a tumour.

Some proteins also act as the switches for turning our genes on ('expressing') or turning them off. For instance, we have certain genes that are referred to as 'oncogenes' or cancer-inducing genes, and others known as tumour-suppressor genes. Problems occur when these become mutated. However, whether these genes get expressed or not, or whether they trigger the cell to produce tumours, appears to be heavily influenced by the micro-environment (see below) inside our bodies.

The ability to control gene activity by biochemical reactions is known as 'epigenetics'. It is this knowledge that has changed the way we view disease and aging and has enabled us to understand the important 'epigenetic' role diet and lifestyle have to play. So in a nutshell, what we put into our body, plus our activity levels, can influence which genes are expressed – genes load the gun and lifestyle pulls the trigger!

The following are important factors to consider in order to increase our understanding of where food compounds and lifestyle factors fit into helping us to reduce our risk of cancer and its proliferation.

The terrain or micro-environment

I have already mentioned how the terrain within our body can be hostile or welcoming to cancer-cell production. For the most part, the terrain we are talking about is the milieu surrounding and bathing our cells, known in scientific terms as the 'extracellular matrix' (ECM) or the micro-environment. This micro-environment keeps the cells tightly packed together so that they can interact via chemical signalling and behave in an ordered, healthy manner. A healthy micro-environment is nutrient- and oxygen-rich, well hydrated, and effectively eliminates stressors such as toxins via the circulatory system.

When this micro-environment is out of balance, the signalling between the cells becomes disordered and chaotic, leading to cells behaving abnormally, becoming damaged and possibly cancerous. Investigation into certain cells has shown that even if an oncogene is activated, that cell does not become cancerous until the conditions surrounding it are favourable – namely until a dysfunctional micro-environment has been created. The elements to which we are exposed, the air we breathe, the food we eat and the water we drink all infiltrate our body and influence the way our cells behave.

Cancer stem cells

Cancer stem cells have been the subject of extensive research in the last few decades. Adult stem cells have the ability to self-renew and regenerate damaged tissue. Some cancers have been found to have rare cancer stem cells within them and these have this same capability to self-renew. They can drive the growth of the cancer and researchers believe they may be responsible for treatment resistance and cancer relapses.

Unfortunately, cancer stem cells are not recognized by the immune system, but much of the research points to the micro-environment (see above) as having a significant impact on their proliferation and possibly on drug resistance too. In cell-culture studies some bioactive food compounds – such as vitamin A (carotenoids), catechins (green tea), theanine (tea), sulforaphane (cruciferous veg), vitamin D, turmeric, genistein (soya), and choline (mainly animal foods) – have been shown to have the ability to modify or suppress the chaotic self-renewal of cancer stem cells. It is thought that this may be due to the modulation of the micro-environment. All these compounds can be gained from a healthy, balanced diet (see page 42).

The pivotal role of mitochondria in cancer protection

Metabolism is the breaking down of food into energy within the body, and most of this happens in the mitochondria. Mitochondria are akin to an energy factory within a cell. We have billions of them in our body and they break down the chemical bonds of the food molecules we eat and turn it into energy in the form of ATP. This process is known as 'aerobic cellular respiration'. A healthy diet and lifestyle is important to keep our mitochondria functioning optimally and to increase their presence within our cells, particularly as they appear to play a pivotal role in cancer protection.

It has been firmly established that exercise stimulates the production of mitochondria in skeletal muscle, but the same has now been seen in other tissues and organs throughout the body, including the brain. This corresponds with the fact that exercise is known to reduce the risk of cancer.

Many nutrients have been shown to enhance mitochondrial function and production, demonstrating the need to eat a balanced diet rich in a variety of vitamins and minerals. But we should not consume more food than we need, and should perhaps consider short-term fasting (see page 108), as calorie restriction has also been shown to stimulate the production of mitochondria. Calorie restriction also appears to induce 'autophagy', which is the clean-up operation within cells whereby damaged proteins and mitochondria are broken down and eliminated – a process that is vital to normal cellular health.

Finally, mitochondria are also vulnerable to environmental pollutants, which can damage their DNA. It is thought that damaged mitochondrial DNA may be pivotal in cells becoming cancerous (see below).

Cellular respiration and the Warburg effect

When cells respire to produce energy in the presence of oxygen, they manufacture hydrogen as a by-product and this is bound to oxygen to form harmless water. If there is a lack of oxygen, normal cellular respiration is impaired and a process called 'fermentation' takes place outside the mitochondrion but within the cell body. This produces a very limited amount of energy, with lactic acid as the by-product. This is what happens after a hard workout when our muscles do not get sufficient oxygen. The lactic acid build-up makes our muscles ache and reduces stamina. We pant to get more oxygen back into our body to alleviate this.

Cancer cells do not necessarily rely on mitochondria for producing energy. Instead, whether there is a supply of oxygen or not, they consume increased amounts of glucose – far greater than normal cells – to produce energy via fermentation. This similarly results in a build-up of lactic acid, which produces a very acidic environment and appears to contribute to tumour growth and progression. This phenomenon formed the basis of the Warburg hypothesis, named after Otto Warburg, the Nobel Prize-winning biochemist who, in 1924, proposed that cancer forms from cells with disordered metabolism. This is illustrated in PET (positron emission tomography) scans which can be used to detect cancer. The patient is given a radioactively labelled glucose molecule and this accumulates in a cancerous area where the cancer cells consume the glucose at a much faster rate than healthy cells and thus light up on a scan.

It appears that cancer cells may reprogram their own metabolism in order to fuel their rapid proliferation even when oxygen levels are low. This may be a survival mechanism because their disordered environment struggles to deliver enough oxygen and glucose via blood vessels. To ensure an abundance of fuel, they increase their uptake of glucose by increasing the number of glucose transporters on their cell membranes.

Another explanation is that cancer is a metabolic disease, whereby the changes to the way the cell fuels itself happen due to damaged mitochondria within the cell and it is this altered metabolism that induces a cell to become cancerous. It is thought that an unhealthy diet and lifestyle – such as excessive calories, an abundance of sugar and a lack of exercise which starves the cells of oxygen – play a role in inflicting this damage on the mitochondria. In hypoxic conditions (lack of oxygen) the mitochondria leak high levels of free radicals (see below) and this gives rise to a vicious circle of events that damage the cell further.

It is not yet clearly understood why cancer cells behave in this way, but there are two schools of thought – basically a chicken or egg situation. Is it the expression of cancer-inducing oncogenes that leads to cell mutations and a disordered micro-environment? Or is it an already disordered micro-environment that is the catalyst for a potentially cancerous cell to progress to malignancy and reproduce uncontrollably? The micro-environment is now an emerging area of research and, although we can draw no definitive conclusions yet, I feel it is fair to say that our diet, lifestyle, stress levels and the environment in which we live are a major influence on how cancer-hostile our micro-environment or terrain is.

Interest in the Warburg effect was renewed when it was found that the anti-diabetic drug Metformin reduced the risk and mortality of some cancers. Metformin lowers blood-glucose levels, therefore it can be surmised that high blood-glucose levels provide the perfect environment for some malignancies.

Free Radicals

Free radicals are rogue molecules whose electrons have become unbalanced by numerous environmental factors (smoking, junk food, chemicals, toxins, stress), body inflammation (see page 27) and by the body's natural chemical processes, such as cell aging. Free radicals impinge on our immune system and cause tissue damage. They are also thought to contribute to aging (through tissue damage) and to the development of heart disease and cancers (through interaction with DNA).

Although some free-radical action in the body is unavoidable, and in fact necessary to prime our cells to function well, an excessive amount is harmful. This chemical reaction is termed 'oxidation' and the result is 'oxidative stress'. An intake of 'antioxidants' in the right proportion can literally rebalance this reaction, reducing oxidative stress damage. Antioxidants are key vitamins, minerals and phytonutrients found in many fruits, vegetables and whole grains.

Chemotherapy and radiation also cause oxidative stress in the body, but this is necessary to kill the cancer cells. This was one of the reasons behind the hesitation in recommending antioxidants during treatment (see page 114) because they may mop up the free radicals and negate the efficacy of the treatment. However, research is beginning to show that antioxidants, certainly through foods, may be beneficial rather than detrimental.

Inflammation

There are many conditions that we associate with inflammation, such as arthritis, colitis, mastitis (-itis means inflammation), but we don't often think of a disease such as cancer being inflammatory. However, at the heart of many chronic diseases is chronic inflammation. This is different from the acute inflammation experienced when your body responds to injury by activating an array of immune cells to cause temporary swelling and redness. Acute inflammation is crucial to sustaining life and should be inactivated when the emergency is over. However, when cellular messages get confused and inflammation persists in the body it can become chronic and long-term damage can ensue. Much of the damage is caused by inflammatory

molecules called 'cytokines' which trigger the production of biochemicals that can act as tumour promoters. This can happen by damaging DNA, stimulating cell division and reducing cell death (see page 23). Inflammation also promotes 'angiogenesis' (see page 29) and generally causes a disordered micro-environment (see page 24). Unfortunately, persistent inflammation within the body is something of which we are often unaware until the damaging effects have become detrimental.

In addition, inflammation can also initiate 'cachexia' (muscle wasting and weight loss, see page 95) by reducing appetite and causing abnormalities in metabolism. This is why weight loss often accompanies a cancer diagnosis. It is therefore clear that reducing inflammation is vital.

Processed foods, particularly those that are high in sugar, unhealthy fats and additives, can promote inflammation in the body, whereas vegetables, fruit and healthy fats are known to ameliorate it. It is thought that this may be due to the acid-inducing properties of processed foods, whilst vegetables and fruits are alkalizing, leading to the reasoning that we should be aiming to help our body tissues remain more alkaline and so less inflammatory. A diet high in sugars also stimulates the release of high levels of insulin, and insulin has been shown to prevent our regulatory immune cells from suppressing inflammation.

Body-fat cells are also inflammation inducers as they secrete an array of inflammatory chemicals, thus promoting tumour growth. This is why obesity is one of the leading causes of cancer and maintaining a healthy weight is the first step to cancer prevention.

Cancer itself causes an acid environment, which in turn promotes inflammation. Added to that, many cancer treatments induce inflammation and as cancer cells die off they increase acidity and in turn inflammation. Therefore a diet high in anti-inflammatory foods is important throughout treatment (see the table on page 98).

The Immune System

Cancer to some extent is the result of a dysfunctional immune system which has failed in its job of killing mutated cells, although some fast-growing cancer cells can become very wily and develop ways of evading our patrolling immune cells. Nevertheless, a strong immune system can play a pivotal role in reducing cancer progression. It is unfortunate, then, that there are so many aspects of our diet and lifestyle that take their toll on it. However, on a positive note, there are also many things we can do to enhance it.

The immune system uses inflammation to regulate health, but when inflammatory responses take hold in our body (see page 27), then our immune system suffers. Heavy metals, pesticides, a high sugar intake, loss of blood-sugar control, many toxins and stress can all induce inflammation and reduce the number of immune cells. Alcohol can also take its toll. Recent research has found that binge-drinking alcohol suppresses the immune system.

To optimize the immune system we need to remove these triggers and feed the immune system with the nutrients it needs.

Gut immunity

If we understand that our immune system is vital to overcoming cancer, we need to also understand that in order to have a healthily functioning immune system we need to take great care of the gut, as 80 per cent of our immune system is in the mucosal layer of the gut lining. It is also our first point of detoxification, as it is responsible for eliminating those things we do not want to be absorbed into our body. When the integrity of our gut barrier is impeded (see leaky gut, page 82) and damaging molecules get through into our bloodstream, they then challenge the immune system, thus diverting it from its job of policing for cancer cells. If the immune system is constantly challenged by this kind of extra burden, then it is more likely to fail us.

Hormones, Insulin and Insulin-like Growth Factor (IGF-1)

Some types of cancers, such as breast, prostate and ovarian, are hormonally driven by oestrogen, progesterone, testosterone and androgens, but the link between cancer in general and all our hormones is well documented. All cells, including cancer cells, have hormone receptors on their surface on to which our hormones can lock and influence the activity of that cell, including stimulating growth. Hormones such as the stress hormone cortisol can suppress our immune system, whilst others can increase inflammatory chemicals.

Insulin is a hormone, and there is plenty of evidence that points to it playing a significant role in cancer risk and progression. When a high amount of insulin is circulating in the bloodstream it is desperately searching for cells to latch on to. A high amount may be due to excess simple sugars and refined carbohydrates in the diet, or to the person's normal cells having become insulin-resistant. Cancer cells have an increased number of insulin receptors and are more than happy to have insulin latch on to them and exert its influences. This can be by dumping its cargo of glucose into the cell or by stimulating growth. Insulin stimulates the release of the hormone insulin-like growth factor (IGF-1), which regulates cell behaviour and appears to have a potent effect on the growth of cancer cells and development of tumours.

Unlike most other growth factors, IGF-1 occurs in large concentrations in the circulation, where under normal conditions it binds to a protein to form a complex that inhibits its action. Nutrient deficiencies, unhealthy foods, excess weight and excessive levels of circulating insulin can decrease concentrations of this IGF-1 binding protein, resulting in increased circulating levels of 'bioavailable' or free IGF-1. This may create changes in the cellular environment and increase the risk of tumour growth.

Luckily, diet and lifestyle can play a significant role in dampening down the deleterious effects of hormones. Following the advice in this book and adjusting your diet, taking exercise, eating certain hormone-modulating foods, along with looking after your gut and liver, can have a very positive influence.

Angiogenesis

Robust tumour growth requires the formation of a local blood-vessel network that supplies both oxygen and nutrients to the tumour cells. In normal tissue this is tightly regulated. However, as always, cancer cells are very crafty and find their way around all sorts of challenging scenarios. When oxygen supplies diminish, normal cells eventually die, but cancer cells can function fairly adequately.

With high levels of stress, low levels of oxygen, and gene alterations, cancer cells start producing a chemical called hypoxia-inducible factor (HIF-1). HIF-1 stimulates an increase in glucose transporters on the surface of cancer cells, allowing the cells to utilize more glucose. It also influences the release of other chemicals, such as the growth factor VEGF which stimulates the formation of a rather disordered network of blood vessels to feed the tumour and allow it to grow further. This formation of new blood vessels is known as 'angiogenesis' and, whilst there are some drugs which target the phenomenon, equally there are compounds in foods such as green tea and mushrooms which appear to inhibit angiogenesis too (see the table on page 30).

Increasing the oxygen to cancer cells may help to keep them in order and reduce the need for them to form vascular networks. Exercise and some nutrients can increase the oxygen levels in the blood, as can hyperbaric oxygen therapy (see page 122).

Metastasis

Metastasis is a very inefficient process and involves the tumour cells breaking away from the primary site into the blood and lymph to be carried around the body. At this point they are open to assault by the immune system and often do not survive. Those cells that do survive tend to accumulate in areas of sluggish circulation, such as the liver or lungs, which can result in secondary malignant growths. Therefore increasing circulation of the blood and lymph may be a weapon against metastasis. My contention is that we can aid our circulatory and lymph system by exercise, skin brushing (see page 123) and foods to support immune cells (see the table on page 30).

HALLMARKS OF CANCER AND FOOD AS MEDICINE

Hallmark of Cancer	Food & Lifestyle Medicine	Effects
Genetic instability	Low glycaemic load diet (see page 74)	Lowers insulin response and inflammation
	Anti-inflammatory foods – flaxseeds, pumpkin and hemp seeds, walnuts, oily fish, berries, turmeric	Anti-inflammatory effects
	Beans, brown rice and sesame seeds contain inositol hexaphosphate (IP6)	IP6 increases tumour-suppressor gene activity
	Budwig Protocol (see page 109)	Oxygenates cells/ enhances cellular function
Disordered and chaotic micro-environment	Anti-inflammatory foods, especially turmeric	Anti-inflammatory effects
	Plant-based diet	Alkalizing effects
	Exercise/rebounding/dry skin brushing (see page 123)	Increased oxygen levels. Helps circulatory and lymph system clear away toxic waste products
Proliferation of cancer stem cells	Polyphenols – green tea, cruciferous vegetables, turmeric, oily fish, carotenoids, soya	Suppresses renewal capabilities of cancer stem cells
	Eggs, fish, poultry, green leafy vegetables	Choline suppresses cancer stem cells in cell culture
	Quercetin – onions, apples, capers, cranberries, plums, blueberries, cherries, red-leaf lettuce, kale, asparagus	Works in conjunction with green tea (EGCG) to inhibit the self-renewal properties of prostate cancer stem cells
Lack of apoptosis (programmed cell death)	Turmeric, saffron, green tea, berries (ellagic acid and resveratrol), cruciferous vegetables, ginger root, pineapple (bromelain), apples (pectin), tomatoes, beans and lentils, mushrooms, brown rice, sesame seeds	Slow cancer growth by inducing apoptosis of damaged cells
	Calorie restriction/ketogenic diet	Starve the cells to death

Hallmark of Cancer	Food & Lifestyle Medicine	Effects
Mitochondrial damage	Calorie restriction	Induces autophagy – the cleaning process within cells
	Balanced diet – protein, healthy fats and carbohydrates, turmeric	Enhance mitochondrial production
	Exercise/Budwig Protocol (see page 109)	Stimulates mitochondrial production
	Reduce intake of toxins	To reduce damaging toxins
	Cruciferous vegetables, ellagic acid, green tea	Enhance detoxification
Cellular respiration and the Warburg effect	Low glycaemic load/ketogenic diet (see pages 74 and 109)	Lower levels of glucose available to cancer cells
	Exercise/Budwig Protocol (see page 109)	Supply of oxygen to cells
Free radicals and oxidative stress	Diet rich in important phytonutrients	Antioxidants to balance free radicals
	Enhance detoxification, organic food	Increased levels of phytonutrients and less toxicity
Inflammation	Anti-inflammatory diet, especially turmeric, omega-3, ginger, pineapple (bromelain), onions	
	Avoid excess sugars and trans-fats/low glycaemic diet	Reduce inflammatory chemicals
	Eliminate potential toxicity	
	Weight management	
The immune system	Mushrooms (beta-glucans)	Increase numbers of white cells, especially macrophages which clear cancer cells
	Foods rich in vitamins A, Bs, C, D, E, folate, zinc, iron, selenium	Antioxidants, liver support, oxygenate blood, control inflammation

Hallmark of Cancer	Food & Lifestyle Medicine	Effects
Gut immunity	Pre- and probiotic foods	Encourage beneficial gut bacteria
	Vitamin A	Fuels and heals gut cells
	Turmeric	Anti-inflammatory
Hormones	Phytoestrogen foods, especially flaxseeds, soya, sesame seeds, alfalfa, oats, barley, fenugreek, beans and lentils	Reduce the effects of natural more potent hormones; mild oestrogenic effects which are considered beneficial and may reduce the risk of hormonally related cancers
	Weight management	Reduce oestrogenic effects of fat cells
	Quercetin foods (see above)	Shown to inhibit human breast-cancer cells
Insulin and IGF-1	Low glycaemic load diet (see page 74)	Reduce and control glucose levels
	Spices – cinnamon, fenugreek, ginger	Slow release of glucose, increase insulin sensitivity
	Reduce or avoid dairy consumption	Reduce levels of ingested IGF-1
	Weight management	
Angiogenesis	Foods rich in polyphenols, especially green tea, mushrooms, liquorice, herbs, spices (especially turmeric)	Anti-inflammatory
Metastasis	Foods that support the immune system	Deal with any circulating cancer cells
	Exercise/rebounding, dry skin brushing (see page 123)	Encourage circulation. Cancer cells accumulate and metastasize in areas of sluggish circulation, i.e. lungs, liver, brain

Standard Treatments and Procedures

Here is a brief summary of some of the procedures and treatments you may encounter after a cancer diagnosis. It is a good idea to arm yourself with as much information as possible. Sometimes you will be told that you have a 'watch and wait' situation whereby the cancer will be monitored closely but no immediate treatment is proposed. In this situation you have an ideal window of opportunity to ensure you are doing all you can to discourage the cancer cells from thriving and multiplying.

Biopsy

A biopsy is generally used initially to extract some cells for diagnosis. It is the only way to make a definitive diagnosis although there is often concern from patients that a biopsy may allow cancer cells to break away and spread. This is unlikely, but you can help the situation by supporting your immune system through diet during this time to optimize immune surveillance for any circulating cancer cells.

Surgery

Surgery may be used initially to diagnose a cancer but generally it is used to remove many types of tumours and surrounding tissue.

Chemotherapy

This is the use of drugs to treat cancer. These are generally administered intravenously (IV) but some can be taken in orally depending on the drug and whether it is broken down in the bowel. It is destructive to both cancer cells and healthy cells, but once chemotherapy ceases most acute symptoms will cease too, as the body replaces the damaged normal cells. Chemo most commonly affects the rapidly growing cells such as the hair and gut-lining cells.

Radiation therapy

This is the use of beams of high-energy radiation which travel like light waves and are usually focused on a localized area of tumour, or tumour bed if the tumour has been surgically removed. It is usually delivered each day in small doses called 'fractions'; normal tissues then have the maximum time to repair between fractions. However, side-effects are cumulative and hence are worse at the end of a course of treatment; they may continue to increase for a couple of weeks after treatment ceases. Modern treatments are now very focused – conformal therapy or volume modulated ablative therapy (VMAT) – thanks to computer software. This enables the maximum dose of radiation to the tumour whilst minimizing the dose received by normal tissue.

It is important to inform your oncologist about any CAM treatments you may be using which may alter the therapeutic ratio – i.e. the balance of the effects on the tumour to that on your normal cells. Some treatments may sensitize the body to the effects of radiation and this needs to be taken into account.

Biologic or targeted therapy

Many newer precision drugs are being investigated which consider the genes and proteins involved, plus other factors, to give a more personalized approach. They are therapies that interfere with cancer-cell growth. They may: inhibit angiogenesis (see page 29); block certain chemical signals within the cancer cell, thus inhibiting growth; take the form of a vaccine which primes the immune system to recognize the cancer cells and kill them; or take the form of monoclonal antibodies which target proteins on the cell surface, either triggering an immune attack or delivering a drug or radioactive substance to destroy the cancer cell.

Hormone therapy

Hormone therapies are used to treat hormone-related cancers such as prostate and breast cancer. They act by blocking either the production or the effects of testosterone or oestrogen and may be given before surgery to shrink a tumour, but are more commonly prescribed after surgery and treatment as maintenance therapy.

Learning More

Relevant scientific research is often hard to find, difficult to access and may not be easy to understand; however, if you want to learn more, some scientific journals will allow access to patients at a reduced cost. Pubmed is a free search engine which can be useful for finding medical and health-related studies and articles. Therefore you may be able to check out the science yourself and establish how relevant it is to you.

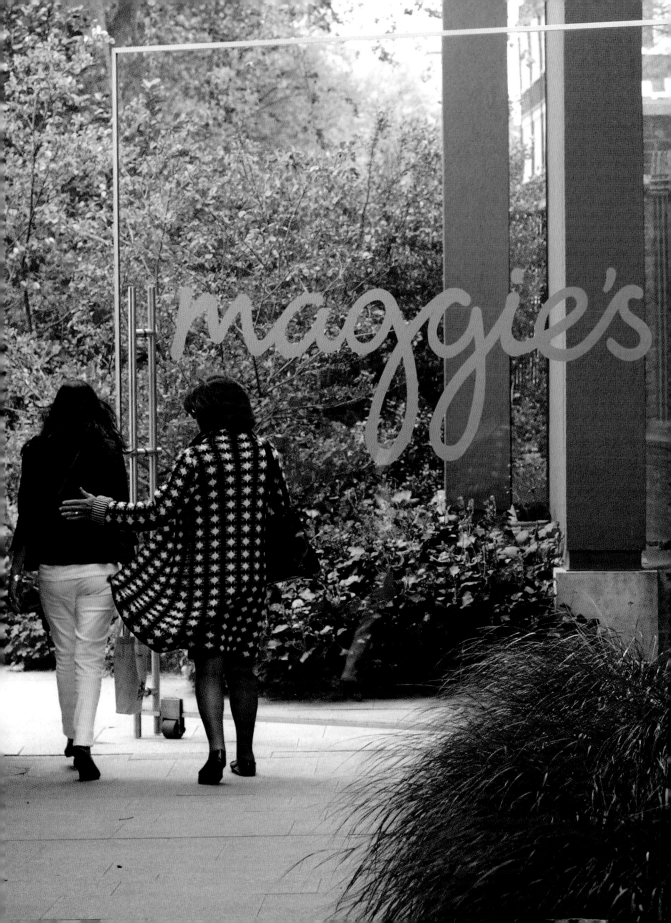

3 Nourishing Your Body

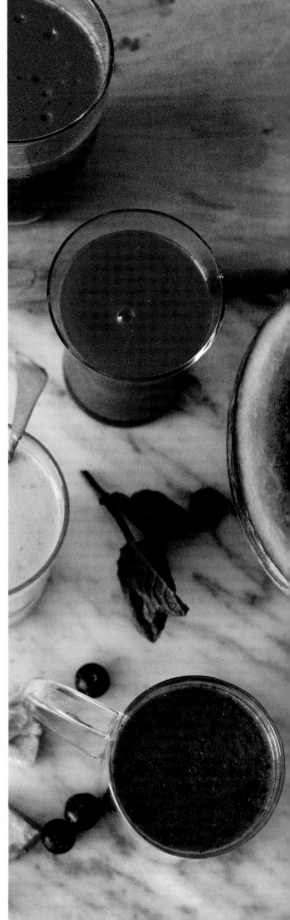

IN CONTRAST TO WHEN I FIRST STARTED running nutrition workshops at Maggie's, I now find that on being given a cancer diagnosis almost everyone begins to give some thought to their diet. There is so much more research and information out there these days and many cancer charities now prioritize this area. The WCRF has a website and resources packed with information on diet, lifestyle and cancer, along with the research links.

Patients often bemoan the fact that their oncologist has dismissed the idea that nutrition plays an important role, but this is mainly due to the fact that there is not much focus on nutrition during medical training. However, attitudes are changing, with many more medics now embracing the idea and encouraging their patients to seek out support. Indeed, on pages 114–15 you can read about the work of Dr Robert Thomas and his research into the food supplement Pomi-T. He is a great proponent of the positive effects of diet and lifestyle on cancer outcome. There are dietitians who offer advice within the hospital setting, but their remit here is generally acute care where there is a very specific diet-related issue. Often the only free personalized advice is from networks such as Maggie's.

This book will provide you with a good grounding for making those very important dietary and lifestyle changes, but for added support and motivation do find your nearest Maggie's Centre and enquire about a nutrition workshop. For a personalized and holistic nutrition plan, consulting a qualified nutrition expert – such as a nutritional therapist who has experience in the oncology field – can be extremely helpful. Nutritional therapists consider each individual to be unique and recommend personalized nutrition and lifestyle programmes rather than a 'one size fits all' approach.

Practitioners never recommend nutritional therapy as a replacement for medical advice and frequently work alongside medical and other healthcare professionals to create a therapeutic partnership between the patient and their medical team. You can find a listing of practitioners through the charity 'Yes to Life' and BANT (British Association for Applied Nutrition & Nutritional Therapy) – see 'Useful websites and resources', page 278. It will be money wisely spent.

Nutritional tests

If you feel your diet has been less than healthy, ask your oncologist or GP if they could run some tests for nutrient levels. Private laboratories offer many more tests not covered on the NHS, including those to assess certain cellular functions, hormone levels and gut function, but these are costly. A nutritional therapist or nutritional doctor would take a whole-person approach when supporting someone with cancer and, if deemed necessary, would be able to refer to a lab for these additional tests (see the resources section, page 278). Assessing nutrient levels and other biochemical pathways at the time of diagnosis is ideal, as the results would be used by a holistic practitioner to assess all the body systems and address any underlying causes of disease. It is only after careful assessment that any high-dose vitamins or mineral supplementation would be considered. However, in the absence of any lab tests, a good overview of dietary intake can be obtained from a food diary; along with assessing certain symptoms, this will often give an indication of possible deficiencies.

One important test is for vitamin D levels (see page 62), as it appears to have an abundance of anti-cancer properties and much of the British population is thought to be deficient. Many GPs and oncologists are happy to recommend a test for this and you would be given supplementation if found to be deficient.

Dietary advice

Most research points towards a plant-based Mediterranean-style diet as being the healthiest way to eat. The emphasis should be on vegetables, fruit, legumes, olive oil, nuts and seeds, along with good-quality animal produce. However, to add to the confusion there are many diets that have been advocated as anti-cancer diets. Some of these are explored in Chapter 5, but in summary it would be true to say that no one diet has been proven as a standalone cure for cancer, although many seem to have been helpful to some people.

When you read about them you will see that these diets can contradict each other. The decision to follow a specific regime has to come from the individual, based on what they feel they can cope with and what suits them. Without support, many special diets are very hard to adhere to and you may feel you would prefer to take just some components of a particular diet that seem to make sense to you and work those into your lifestyle.

In choosing to follow any diet, though, do be careful that you are getting adequate essential nutrients and that you are not losing weight unless you are keen to do so. A certain diet may suit you, leaving you feeling energetic and thriving; but if it doesn't – and certainly if it makes you miserable – don't do it! The most important advice is to listen to your own body and get a feeling for what is helping and what is hindering. Use your food diary and symptom diary (see page 270) as a tool and seek advice from a health professional if necessary.

A QUICK GUIDE TO PREPARING YOURSELF FOR TREATMENT

• Buy a notebook and start a journal with notes on information, feelings/emotions, symptoms and questions to ask. Keep it in a folder with your medical notes and test results.

• Read about nutrition (pages 42–51). Cast a critical eye over the present contents of your kitchen cupboards and fridge and get rid of the items on the 'Empty your kitchen cupboard and fridge of' list (see page 136).

• Start a food diary – this can be a useful tool for motivating healthy changes to your diet (see page 270).

• Start a healthy-living shopping list (see our ideas on the 'Fill your kitchen cupboard and fridge with' list, pages 134–6). Online shopping can make life easier, especially if your energy levels are low or you find that on entering a shop you are in danger of filling your basket with undesirable items.

• Stock up on healthy kitchen staples (see our list, page 134) which you can easily cook up into nutritious dishes or snacks. Making double portions when you feel you have the energy and freezing the extra one can be a good way of ensuring you have a ready supply of homemade convenience foods for those days when energy is low. Do bear in mind, however, that your taste in food may change during some treatments.

• Reduce or eliminate alcohol (see page 81).

• Stay hydrated with plenty of water.

• Speak to a nutrition and cancer expert who can supply you with invaluable information on diet and possible fortifying supplements, as well as getting you motivated to make any necessary changes.

• Seek advice if you need to address any excessively unhealthy vices such as smoking, alcohol, lack of exercise, etc. You may feel motivated enough to give up or rectify any detrimental lifestyle choices, or you may feel this just isn't the time to cope with big changes. If the latter is the case, then even just preparing to change can be a beneficial step. Take a look at our section on behaviour change (page 129) and begin by taking small steps towards making these changes.

Support your immune system

• Ensure your diet is nutrient-dense.

• Consider immune-enhancing supplements (see the table on page 113).

• Take a critical look at your stress

levels. Of course a cancer diagnosis itself will cause stress, but look at any long-term issues that may be stressing you or making you unhappy and think about ways to reduce or override them.

• Learn some relaxation and breathing techniques (see 'Mindfulness', page 125).

• Try to take some daily exercise, such as a walk. Start an exercise routine that you may be able to continue throughout treatment. Exercise has been shown to reduce anxiety and depression along with physically preparing you for treatment (see 'Exercise', page 93).

• Get sufficient sleep each night. The body uses the time we are asleep to heal and repair. The average person needs 7–8 hours' sleep a night. Do not fall asleep watching TV and don't use your computer or iPad before sleeping. It is best to allow at least an hour's relaxation before going to sleep and the use of electronic devices in this time is not generally conducive to a good night's rest.

Build a support network

• Friends and family can be a tremendous support at this time, but so often in meaning to do the right thing and give you guidance they can actually derail you. Well-meaning people will no doubt offer you all sorts of advice; some of it may be very useful, but some may just be confusing and disempowering.

Dietary, supplement and lifestyle advice is often the main culprit here. Everyone seems to have read about something you should be eating, taking, doing, and at this stage it can be information overload.

• Rally friends and family in a way that works best for you. You may want to talk over your thoughts and feelings with them or have them visit often; or you may not. Tell them what you want! If you are getting them to support you by helping with meals, set up a rota and give ideas on foods you would like to eat. Generally people really want to help constructively and find it much easier if they have some guidelines. Loved ones often feel at a complete loss as to what to say and how to help, and are feeling extremely anxious too.

• If necessary, sort out a rota with lifts to hospital appointments or someone to sit with you through treatment.

• Many hospitals have a buddy system where someone who has been through a similar diagnosis to you can become your mentor. Do ask the oncology department if they offer this service.

• Find out about support groups in your area and contact them.

• Faith of any kind can be a tremendous support at this time.

Choosing the right food

Good nourishment starts with choosing the right food and this means 'real food'. Being able to afford to eat a healthy diet is not beyond the reach of any of us. It may require a bit more thought and time than buying a ready meal, but this is your health you are playing with. Often it is just a case of changing old habits and mindset (see page 128).

A great deal of the food on offer in supermarkets and shops is processed, or laden with chemicals and sugar. But if we shun cheap synthetic food, manufacturers will need to change. Thankfully there are already positive global movements to change agricultural and food-industry practices, but there is still a long way to go. Vote with your pound to support natural practices and products to bring about meaningful change for our wellbeing now and in the future. Be vigilant about food labelling and continue to fight for transparency so that we know exactly what we are eating. Feeling connected to the food we eat and caring about where it comes from can take the joy of eating to another level. Eating factory-made food with an additive list as long as your arm will never sit well with our psyche, even if we think it tastes quite delicious.

Food actually accounts for very little of many people's household spending (approximately 12 per cent now, compared with around 30 per cent in the 1950s), but we have to understand the need to prioritize it over other consumables in life. Cheap food will use cheap ingredients which often need to be dressed up and disguised with additives, salt, sugar and unhealthy fats. The rise in chronic disease, including obesity, does appear to have gone hand in hand with the rise in the consumption of cheap, chemical-laden, processed food.

Organic produce is often referred to as 'clean' food and is certainly the ideal way to eat, but for a lot of us it is beyond our food budget and is not always easily available. Many people are also quite distrusting of the authenticity of organic food, but there are ways of ensuring a reliable source (see page 69).

If you enjoy cooking, that will assist you immensely in eating healthily, but the recipes in this book are here to help you gain the confidence and know-how to produce some tasty meals with minimum fuss and ingredients. It really doesn't need to be complicated or time-consuming. One of the keys to making it work is to have only the right ingredients in your cupboard and none of the wrong ones that may tempt you to stray into junk-food territory. Quite simply, if it is not in your cupboards or fridge, you cannot eat it when you are at home. See the lists of foods to have in your house and those to reject, pages 134–6. (When you are out it is a different story – then you have to exercise restraint.)

It's also important to consider the packaging food is wrapped in. Wherever possible, try to steer clear of buying pre-wrapped food, although this is easier said than done. When you are wrapping food yourself at home, try to avoid wrapping fatty foods such as cheese in cling film, because anything fatty will absorb some of the toxins, plasticizers and oestrogens in the material (see page 85). Use glass containers and bottles to store food where possible.

You should also avoid heating food in plastic containers or using cling film to cover food in a microwave. This goes for ready meals too: if you choose to heat them in the microwave, decant the food into a china or glass bowl and use another plate to cover it, as the high heat generated by the microwaves may enable chemicals to leach into the food from the plastic containers. Research has shown that chemicals from plastics are seen in high amounts in the urine samples of people who eat a lot of packaged food. When they switch to eating non-packaged foods there is a significant reduction in these levels.

EATING AND LIVING HEALTHILY ON A BUDGET

- If you can, shop on a daily basis, or as frequently as you can, so that you can make the most of reductions on fresh produce with expiring use-by dates.

- Buy the cheaper root vegetables and make batches of soup – great for freezing in portions and using for a convenient lunch or supper.

- Avoid unhealthy, expensive items such as gimmicky, refined cereal products and alcohol.

- Cut down on unhealthy snacks such as crisps, biscuits, cakes and pastries and so save money. We do not need them and it doesn't take much effort to form good habits by swapping them for healthy alternatives.

- Eat a predominantly plant-based or vegetarian diet to keep costs down. Beans and lentils are cheap and can be used to pad out a meat dish: for example, less *carne* in the chilli – more beans.

- Go for quality over quantity, particularly in animal products. We do not need a large portion of meat to give us sufficient protein (see page 43). Think of meat as the accompaniment to your vegetables.

- Get to know your local butcher and ask him for cheaper offcuts of meat. These usually need to be cooked for longer to tenderize them, but slow-cooked casseroles are much healthier for us (see 'Cooking Methods', page 91).

- Make friends with your fishmonger and ask him to save ends of fish for you. With luck he will let you have them very cheaply and they are perfect for a healthy fish pie or stock for soups (see our recipe for Super Stocks, page 256).

- Avoid wasting food: plan ahead and use up leftovers.

- Make use of everything you buy. Make stocks, soups and smoothies from excess veg – you will find plenty of suggestions in the recipe section of this book. If you cut off the thick stalks of broccoli, use them to make soup. Save the green parts of leeks and spring onions to put into soups and stock.

- If you use olive oil for cooking you do not need to spend extra on cold-pressed extra-virgin. Use cheaper varieties for heating and save the best for drizzling and dressings.

- Ask your butcher for any bones and make bone broth, which can then be used in a variety of ways (see page 256).

- Shopping online can sometimes make it easier to find offers and can help you stick to your shopping list rather than being tempted down the unhealthy supermarket aisles.

- Most of us consume more than enough food. Slim down your food bill and your body by slimming down the amount you eat.

- Buy produce direct from suppliers – for example from farm shops and veg-box schemes.

- Freeze leftovers for use as a handy and healthy ready meal when time is short. Make sure you clearly label the container with contents and date, because things are pretty hard to recognize once frozen.

- Vinegar and bicarbonate of soda are cheap, natural alternatives to many cleaning products.

The Important Components of a Healthy Diet

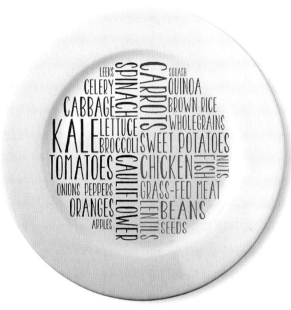

A balanced diet consists of protein, fat and carbohydrate, which includes fruit and vegetables.

Protein

We all need a consistent supply of protein in our diet. It is responsible for many important functions, including building and repairing our body tissues, cells, muscles, organs and skin, along with making hormones, enzymes, neurotransmitters, antibodies and haemoglobin, to name a few. When digested, proteins are broken down into amino acids, which are required for the proper functioning of our bodies. Some are essential as they cannot be made in our body, therefore it is important to gain them from our diet.

Any extra stress on the body, such as surgery or illness, requires an increase in protein intake from around 0.8g per kg body weight per day to around 1.5g per kg to meet the demands of healing. An average sedentary person requires a total of around 45–55g of protein per day, but after surgery or treatment the need would increase to an approximate average of 80–120g per day.

The WCRF guide to portion sizes shows that 80g of red meat or oily fish will meet average needs – that's a portion about the size of a deck of cards. That is probably less than you may have thought, and it is very easy to eat more than we need; most meat or fish eaters probably consume larger portion sizes.

The best sources of protein are those from animals (see the table opposite), because they contain all the essential amino acids. It is important to ensure that the protein you are eating is of high quality. Many manufactured foods, such as ready meals, pies and sausages, rely on fillers and additives, making them less healthy. This is where eating on a budget can be made viable. Eat less in quantity but of a higher quality and you will spend the same amount of money.

It is a little more challenging for a vegetarian to obtain all their protein needs and essential amino acids from their diet. Most vegetarian sources of protein lack one or more essential amino acid. Variety is the key, because the amino acid that is missing from one vegetarian source of protein will be supplied by another. As you can see from the table opposite, soya beans are the vegetarian source with the highest amount of protein, but do read the section on soya (page 80) before you indulge.

In general, vegetarians can gain their protein requirements from beans, lentils, nuts, seeds, grains and, if lacto-ovo vegetarian, dairy and eggs.

Beware of supplementing with high levels of protein such as protein shakes if you have abnormal kidney function, as this can lead to renal failure.

ANIMAL PROTEIN

Source	Amount of protein
100g chicken breast (no skin)	30.9g
100g turkey breast (no skin)	29.9g
100g beef fillet (lean)	29g
100g pork fillet (lean)	21.4g
100g salmon	20.2g
80g prawns	19.6g
2 eggs	16g
100g cottage cheese	14g
200ml whole milk or yoghurt	8g

VEGETARIAN PROTEIN

Source	Amount of protein
50g soya beans (dry weight)	18g
100g quinoa	13g
50g red kidney beans (dry weight)	11g
50g almonds	10.6g
50g pumpkin seeds	9.5g
2 tbsp peanut butter	9g
50g cashews	8.9g
100g tofu	8.1g
100g cooked lentils	7.6g

Fat – a bad reputation?

In the last few decades there has been a very negative message about fat in the diet and this is still hard to shake off. It stems from a study in the US in the 1950s that supported the fact that fat consumption causes heart disease. It was proved to be a flawed piece of research, but it was picked up by the government and the food industry, who ran with it and basically created the fat phobia we have even now.

Large-scale industrial farming, which began towards the end of the nineteenth century and intensified further with the Agriculture Act of 1947, has a lot to answer for when it comes to the quality of dietary fats and the health of Western nations. Demonizing saturated fats as bad for our health was, in this case, probably justified, because the fat content of intensively farmed animals is very different from that of free-range animals that eat a diet natural to them.

Pasture-fed cattle, which spend much of the year cavorting around a field, have much higher ratios of the desirable omega-3 to omega-6 fats (see pages 43–6) and 25–50 per cent less saturated fat than intensively farmed animals. They also have higher levels of protein, vitamin E and beta-carotene. Intensively farmed cattle generally eat a diet high in corn and soy – feed that is not natural to them and certainly not right for their digestive systems. Along with stressful living conditions, it is thought that this increases the levels of unhealthy, inflammatory stress chemicals in their bodies. As we are next in the food chain, we are eating meat from a less than healthy animal with higher levels of inflammatory fats. This goes for all intensively farmed animals, be they lamb, pork or poultry, along with dairy. Lamb is probably the safest bet if you are deciding on non-free-range meat, as it is mostly reared on open pastureland.

The other debacle in the story of fats is the use of hydrogenated fats in food manufacturing, which also happens to correlate with a rise in heart disease and possibly cancers. Hydrogenated fats, also known as trans-fats, are unsaturated fats that have hydrogen added to them, turning them into partially or completely saturated fats. It is a way of making liquid oils solid at room temperature, just like saturated fats such as butter. The process of hydrogenation was patented in 1902 and Proctor & Gamble acquired the rights in 1909, launching their first hydrogenated shortening very soon afterwards. What appealed to manufacturers further was the fact that hydrogenated vegetable oils, although solid, were actually soft enough to spread when taken straight from the fridge, and thus spreadable margarine was born. The product gained in popularity, especially as it was a way to make use of the soya oil by-product in soy-protein production, and it had enhanced shelf-life and taste. It was marketed as good for the heart, even though some scientists had reservations. In fact, as early as the 1940s research was pointing to the possible carcinogenic properties of hydrogenated fats. Since then, correlations have been found between trans-fat consumption and many chronic diseases.

Trans-fats are banned in some countries and in some states in the US due to these extremely damaging effects on our health. (See also section on trans-fats, page 47.)

Why we need fat

So as we have seen, the story of fats is a chequered one. But despite its bad press, we do need fat in our diet. What is important is that we understand which fats are good and which are bad, as the bad ones are involved in fuelling inflammation and damaging our DNA, which may lead to cells becoming cancerous.

Healthy fats are essential for cell-membrane structure, keeping them lubricated and flexible, which increases their ability to stay hydrated, hold on to nutrients and electrolytes, and to communicate with each other. In turn, this ensures a healthy terrain around the cells. Fat is crucial for our brain cells too, as 60 per cent of the brain is fat and without healthy dietary fat its performance will be impaired. A fat deficiency in children and adults can lead to problems with concentration, behaviour and mood.

Fats are also vital for hormone production, nerve transmission, blood clotting, organ function and healthy eyes, and they can lower cholesterol. The omega fats also have an anti-inflammatory effect. Other functions of fats are supplying the body with energy, aiding the absorption of the fat-soluble vitamins A, D, E and K, protecting the vital organs and keeping the body insulated.

Foods which contain high levels of fats, such as nuts, are best kept in the fridge to avoid them going rancid. Ground seeds, such as flaxseeds (linseeds), should be used when fresh and any leftover should be kept in the fridge and used within a few days. This is because, once ground, they are open to oxidation and easily spoiled. Rancid fats are damaging to our cells.

Saturated fats

All fatty foods will have a mixture of different types of fats, but those that are solid or waxy at room temperature contain a higher proportion of saturated fats. They are generally derived from meat products and dairy products that contain whole milk (butter, cream, cheese, lard). They are extremely stable fats, which can be heated without damage. Some studies have linked a diet high in animal saturated fat to certain cancers, but this is not conclusive. I suspect that any link is due to the unhealthier fats of low-welfare animal products and the pesticides and hormones they have been exposed to through grain feed. Toxins and hormones from animals accumulate in fat cells, so if we eat excessive amounts of animal fat we will be ingesting a higher proportion of these. To limit this exposure, eat higher-welfare animal products and less of them.

Coconut and palm oil are vegetarian sources of saturated fat and contain no cholesterol, although they can increase our healthy HDL cholesterol levels. Coconut oil is thought to be very beneficial to health and is an excellent choice for cooking, as its chemical structure is very stable, making it suitable for cooking at high temperatures.

Polyunsaturated fats

These remain liquid at room temperature. The polyunsaturated fats to avoid are vegetable oils such as corn oil and refined sunflower oil – generally all the cheaper oils sold in abundance in plastic bottles. Chemicals may leach from the plastic into the oil, and many of these cheaper vegetable oils have been highly processed and are already damaged. It is best to buy good-quality oils and be frugal in how much you use. Choose types sold in dark glass bottles as these will not have been damaged so easily by light.

The polyunsaturates to include in your diet are the essential fatty acids (EFAs) omega-3 and omega-6.

Omega-3 (alpha-linolenic acid) This is an essential fat, meaning we cannot make it ourselves and so we need to obtain it from our diet. Omega fatty acids, especially omega-3, are important for the healthy functioning of our cells. They are incorporated into the cell wall, making it flexible. This allows our cellular processes to work optimally, letting nutrients in and waste materials out. Omega-3 is important for its anti-inflammatory effects (see 'Inflammation', page 27), but unfortunately many of us are deficient in it.

Foods that contain omega-3 are oily fish such as salmon, mackerel, anchovies, sardines, herring, fresh tuna, trout and pilchards, as well as grass-fed meat and dairy. Vegetarian sources are flaxseeds (linseeds), walnuts and pumpkin seeds. However, in general our body finds it much easier to utilize beneficially the omega-3 from oily fish than from nuts and seeds.

Unfortunately, oily fish contain pollutants from the ocean such as mercury; therefore there are recommendations on safe levels to eat. UK government guidelines for adults and children recommend eating at least one and up to four portions of oily fish a week; but women and girls who are currently pregnant or breastfeeding, or who may become pregnant in the future, are advised to consume no more than two portions a week. The larger varieties such as tuna or swordfish have greater levels of toxins due to being higher up the food chain and swimming in the ocean for longer, so should not be eaten more than once a week. Tinned tuna does not count as an oily fish, as the canning process reduces the fats, but other canned varieties of fish – such as sardines – are fine.

In 2013 a human study linked high levels of omega-3 fatty acids in the body to an increased risk of prostate cancer. The researchers looked at circulating levels of omega-3 in men with and without prostate cancer and found that those with prostate cancer tended to have a higher concentration in their blood. There could be many reasons for this, however, and the researchers do admit to weaknesses in the study. It is also inconsistent with other studies, which point to omega-3 having a protective element. One difficulty in recommending levels of intake is that within a population there may be considerable genetic variation in how efficiently the omega fats are metabolized. Laboratory testing to monitor cell-membrane fatty acids is ideal but, in the absence of this, dietary intake should be varied to include oily fish, nuts, seeds and their oils.

The consumption of high amounts of dietary omega-3 has been found to improve the outcomes of breast cancer. A systematic review of research on omega-3, cancer and cachexia (weight loss or muscle wasting) found that administering a dose of 1.5g per day for a prolonged period of time to those with advanced cancer improved their quality of life, in some cases increasing appetite and weight.

Omega-6 (linoleic acid) Omega-6 is another essential fat, but we don't tend to be as deficient in omega-6 because it is easier to obtain from our diet. Good sources are peanuts (try to eat these unsalted!), most other nuts, particularly walnuts, almonds and Brazils, seeds such as sunflower, sesame and hemp, and soya beans.

Although omega-6 is important, we need to ensure we consume a balance of omega-3 to omega-6 in a ratio of around 1:4. In a Western diet the intake of omega-6 to omega-3 has typically been much higher, in part due to our excessive consumption of seed oils such as sunflower and corn oil, and also because in general animal fats are higher in omega-6 due to their being fed on corn and soya containing omega-6. Excessive omega-6 intake can block the uptake of omega-3 and it can also lead to a high level of pro-inflammatory compounds being formed in the body, which is not desirable. It's therefore important to consume the good forms of omega fats by eating a variety of the plant foods which have a natural balance of omega-6 to omega-3 along with animal fats from grass-fed animals. This will help to maintain a healthy ratio of these fats and ensure we are not subjected to the detrimental effects of damaged fats that have been implicated in some cancers.

Conjugated linoleic acid This is similar to omega-6 and naturally occurs in meat and dairy products from grass-fed cows. It appears to have anti-cancer properties by reducing cancer-cell proliferation. It also has a possible role in ameliorating inflammatory bowel disease and therefore may be of particular importance in reducing bowel-cancer risk.

Monounsaturated fats

These healthy fats sit between saturated and polyunsaturated fats and are liquid at room temperature but solid when chilled. They are found in a wide variety of oils, with the highest levels being in olive oil. Olive oil is a key component of the Mediterranean diet and contains omega-9. It is known for its many health benefits. Other good sources are avocados and nuts. A study in Sweden that tracked 60,000 women found that those who consumed more monounsaturated fat than polyunsaturated had a reduced risk of breast cancer.

Trans-fats

These are naturally found in the milk and fat of cows, sheep and other ruminant animals, but only in trace amounts of around 2–5 per cent, which is very easy for the body to process. However, manufactured hydrogenated fats (see page 44) may be found in meat products, vegetable shortening, some margarines, some processed foods, biscuits, cakes, sweets and fried foods such as doughnuts and French fries. In manufactured goods the amount of trans-fat may be as high as 40 per cent, and with the body unable to handle these levels it is thought that they may remain in the bloodstream, causing raised LDL or 'bad' cholesterol, increased atherosclerosis (hardening of the arteries) and increased inflammation (see page 27). They can block the very important omega-3 and omega-6 (see pages 45–6) pathways and are definitely not part of a healthy diet. Consumption of trans-fats has been linked to cancer, so it is important that we reduce our intake.

When we cook and bake from scratch we know exactly what the ingredients of that recipe are. This is the best way to eliminate the worry of consuming these toxic fats in large amounts, plus you don't have to spend time scouring food labels for hidden nasties. Trans-fats may be shown on a food label as hydrogenated, partially or semi-hydrogenated, or as shortening. A label which states '0g trans-fats' does not necessarily mean there are none, as manufacturers can include up to 0.5g without declaring it.

Carbohydrates

Carbs can be divided into starches and sugars. Starchy carbohydrates consist of grains, cereals and potatoes, along with some vegetables such as corn and legumes which have high levels of starch. Sugars include not only the refined added sugar we know to be unhealthy (see page 72 on sugars), but also the natural sugar present in fruits and vegetables. Both starches and sugars break down into glucose when digested and this is used for energy. Bear in mind that many cancer cells have a voracious appetite for glucose to help fuel their growth and survival (see 'Cellular respiration and the Warburg effect', page 25).

Starchy carbs

These can be divided again into refined and unrefined. Refined carbs are generally grains that have been stripped of their fibrous outer husk – all white flour products, such as white bread, pasta, biscuits and cakes; white rice; and the zillion refined cereals we unfortunately see in abundance on our supermarket shelves. Not only have these lost their fibre content, but also their natural nutrient value because most of the vitamins in grain are in the outer layers. (See page 72 on sugars.)

Unrefined or 'complex' carbs, as they are often known, are our wholegrain products such as wholemeal bread, wholewheat pasta and wholegrain cereals. These are the grains we should be aiming to eat, because they provide us with healthy fibre (see below) and are nutrient-dense. However, we should be careful not to rely on them too much as part of our diet, as they still break down to sugars, which we want to keep in check (see page 72).

Facts on fibre

Fibre is an essential part of our daily diet. It is found in the walls of plant cells and is resistant to digestive enzymes in humans, which means it passes through the digestive tract without being broken down. It plays an important role in gastro-intestinal health and bowel function, especially in the prevention of conditions such as diverticulitis, irritable bowel syndrome (IBS) and Crohn's disease. It may also help in the prevention of colon cancer and diabetes, as well as controlling blood-sugar balance and lowering cholesterol.

Fibre found in vegetables, fruits, whole grains, nuts and seeds also helps to regulate testosterone levels by increasing the production of a protein called sex hormone binding globulin (SHBG). This protein binds to testosterone in the bloodstream, rendering it inactive, and can help to reduce the risk of prostate cancer. It improves the oestrogen:progesterone balance because excess testosterone is converted to oestrogen if it is not bound to SHBG (see 'Hormones', page 28).

There are two main types of fibre, categorized as insoluble and soluble, and each plays a different role in digestion.

Insoluble fibre

• Passes through the body virtually unchanged.

• Promotes the growth of certain beneficial bacteria.

• Fermentation makes the waste material soft and bulky, which in turn helps it to pass through the intestines more quickly.

• It has a high water-binding capacity which acts like a sponge in the gut, adding liquid and bulk to prevent and relieve constipation.

• In weight loss it can be beneficial as it promotes a feeling of fullness and therefore reduces appetite.

• Sources of insoluble fibre are wholegrain products such as wholemeal bread, wholegrain couscous and brown rice, fruit and vegetable skins, celery, nuts and seeds.

Soluble fibre

• This has the capacity to bind to bile acids which are rich in cholesterol. This in turn prevents the re-absorption of cholesterol, hormones and other detoxification products into the bloodstream, so aiding their excretion from the body.

• In the small intestine soluble fibre dissolves in water and forms a gel. This helps to slow down the digestion and absorption of carbohydrates, resulting in a more gradual release of glucose into the blood. This is important for people with diabetes as it helps to keep blood sugar balanced.

• It is metabolized by gut bacteria and then fermented to short-chain fatty acids (SCFAs) such as butyrate, which acts as fuel for our gut cells. Butyrate is thought to protect against colon cancer.

• Sources of soluble fibre are beans, pulses, most fruit and vegetables, oats, psyllium, flaxseeds, rye and barley.

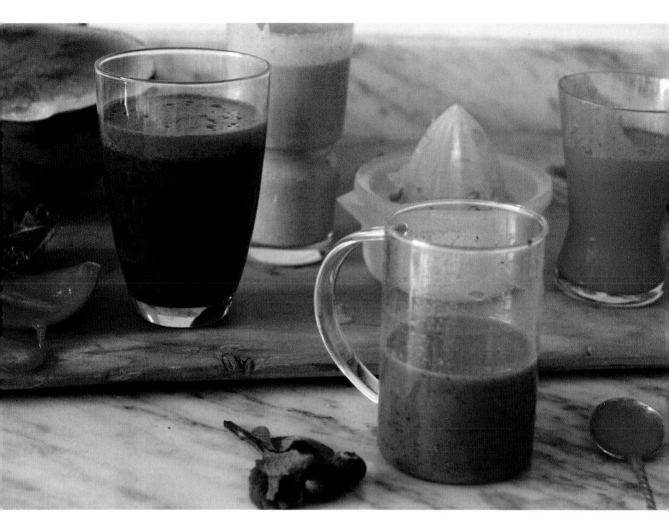

Vegetables and fruit – a rainbow a day

Vegetables and fruit are essential because they contain such an abundance of vitamins, minerals and phytonutrients (see page 52) which are incredibly healthy.

Although we recognize that both vegetables and fruit should be a component of our diet, the emphasis should always be on vegetables, as they contain less sugar than fruit. If you find that you are favouring sweet fruit over vegetables, try introducing a greater array of vegetables, especially green leafy varieties, which are the most nutrient-dense.

The current official government guidelines for vegetables and fruit recommend five a day, but there has been research to show that increasing this to between seven and ten portions reduces our risk of disease significantly, including cutting the risk of dying from cancer by 25 per cent. Therefore it is imperative that after a cancer diagnosis you should pack in as many vegetables and fruit as you can. Whenever possible, try to eat produce that is low in pesticide residues, as increasing our intake of these foods could mean we are consuming far more chemicals of the synthetic kind.

WHAT IS A PORTION SIZE OF FRUIT OR VEGETABLES?

Raw leafy vegetables such as spinach or lettuce	→	1 cup
Non-leafy cooked vegetables	→	½ cup
Salad	→	1 large cereal bowl
Cooked green beans/peas	→	½ cup
Fresh fruit e.g. apple	→	1 tennis-ball size
Fresh fruit e.g. plums	→	2 pieces
Fresh fruit e.g. grapes	→	½ cup
Dried fruit	→	¼ cup
Nuts	→	small handful

(adapted from wcrf-uk.org)

The recommended daily intake of fibre is 26–35g a day. If you increase your consumption, be sure to increase your intake of water too, otherwise it may actually cause constipation. Ongoing research by the WCRF that collates studies on cancer prevention and diet has shown categorically that vegetables and fruit reduce our risk of cancer, and this includes reducing the odds of a recurrence. However, many people struggle to eat a sufficient amount of these foods. To ensure an adequate supply, the number-one rule is to fill at least half your dinner plate with vegetables. For ideas, see our plate on page 42. You should also try to eat at least three varieties in one meal. Lunch could be a colourful salad and breakfast can include some veg and fruit too. Try mushrooms and tomatoes on wholemeal toast, or a poached egg on some asparagus. Fruit is, of course, a great accompaniment to porridge or muesli. If you are still struggling, add a green smoothie or a veg-and-fruit smoothie to your day as that is an easy way of packing in a good variety of produce. See our smoothie ideas on pages 68–9.

Phytonutrients

Phyto means 'plant' in Greek, and phytonutrients (or phytochemicals) are naturally occurring compounds found in abundance in vegetables and fruit – particularly in the brightly coloured pigments, giving rise to the expression 'Eat a rainbow a day' – as well as in other plant foods such whole grains, nuts, beans and tea.

A huge amount of research has been carried out into the health benefits of phytonutrient-rich foods, particularly in the field of cancer. A large review of 200 epidemiological studies showed that regular consumption of colourful fruits, herbs and vegetables was associated with lower rates of cancer of the lung, colon, breast, cervix, oesophagus, oral cavity, stomach, bladder, pancreas and ovary. So visualize that rainbow and make sure your daily vegetable and fruit choices imitate it.

Carotenoids are a group of phytochemicals found in a whole host of vibrantly coloured vegetables and fruits. One study demonstrated a significant relationship between a higher consumption of carotenoid-rich foods, such as leafy green vegetables and carrots, and a lower risk of breast cancer. Likewise, a higher intake of cruciferous vegetables, such as broccoli and asparagus, was seen to lower the risk of prostate cancer, while green tea, legumes, onions and soya lowered the risk of oesophageal, breast and prostate cancer. Consumption of onions has been associated with lower rates of lung cancer, particularly squamous cell, and dark chocolate has demonstrated a reduction in the risk of colon cancer. All of these foods are packed with phytonutrients.

Thousands of phytonutrients have been discovered, many of which are known as polyphenols (see the table on page 30) and their many anti-cancer roles include influencing the cancer process through their effect on our hormones – particularly the polyphenol compounds found in soy products, legumes, pulses and some cruciferous vegetables. Phytonutrients are not always easily absorbed in the gut and rely on being broken down by our microflora, which means absorption can be highly individual and dependent on a healthy gut (see page 82). Phytonutrients play a role in protecting plants from fungi, bacteria, bugs and other threats, and there is increasing concern that the use of fungicides and pesticides on our vegetables and fruit is reducing the levels of these extremely important natural compounds to the detriment of our health.

ESSENTIAL VITAMINS AND MINERALS

Vitamin/ Mineral	Top Food Sources
Vitamin A/ Beta-carotene	Liver, fish liver oils, eggs, meat, oily fish, dairy Yellow and dark green, leafy vegetables (carrots, red peppers, spinach) Fruit – mango, papaya, apricots
Vitamin B_1 (Thiamin)	Liver, pork, milk, cheese, eggs, wholegrain cereals, brown rice, beans, nuts, barley, lentils, vegetables and fruit, dried fruit
Vitamin B_2 (Riboflavin)	Milk, eggs, brown rice, mushrooms, green leafy vegetables, meat especially Liver and fish
Vitamin B_3 (Niacin)	Wholegrain cereals, eggs, milk, cheese, peanuts, avocados, meat especially liver and other organ meat, poultry and fish
Vitamin B_5 (Pantothenic acid)	Chicken, beef, oats, tomatoes, offal, yeast, molasses, eggs, milk, beans, brown rice and other whole grains
Vitamin B_6 (Pyridoxine)	Milk, eggs, whole grains, wheatgerm, vegetables especially cruciferous, meat, liver, yeast, beans, walnuts
Vitamin B_{12} (Cobalamin)	Foods of animal origin, meat especially liver, fish, dairy. Micro-organisms such as algae (spirulina/chlorella), yeast, seaweed
Folate	Green leafy vegetables, peas, chickpeas, yeast extract, brown rice, liver, bananas and oranges
Choline	Eggs, seafood, meat, liver, fish, cruciferous vegetables, spinach, asparagus, mushrooms, nuts
Vitamin C (Ascorbic acid)	Fruit and vegetables especially sprouted seeds and beans, broccoli and cabbage, potatoes, tomatoes, blackcurrants, oranges, red and black berries

Functions

Essential for maintenance of mucus membranes, skin and night vision

Stored in the body

Acts as an antioxidant

Necessary for the steady and continuous release of energy from carbohydrate and fat. For nerve function (may help neuropathy)

Energy from food, especially carbohydrates and fats. Essential for healthy skin, hair and eyes. Taken in supplement form makes urine bright yellow

Energy from food. Aids digestion and blood-sugar control. Skin, nerve and hormone health. A deficiency can cause a loss of appetite. Depleted by some chemotherapy drugs

Energy from food especially fats and carbohydrates. Production of stress hormones. Healthy skin. Neuropathy

Energy from food. Protein metabolism. Formation of haemoglobin. Hormone balance

For rapidly dividing cells such as those in the bone marrow forming red blood cells and making DNA. For healthy nerves. Difficult for vegetarians to obtain through diet. Absorption may be difficult in a compromised gut

Acts with B_{12} on rapidly dividing cells. Important for pregnant women. Readily destroyed by cooking – eat raw or steamed vegetables

Building DNA, nervous system, cell membrane structure. Useful when folate is deficient

Antioxidant. Aids detoxification of heavy metals, collagen formation – skin, gums, bones, arteries, joint health. Immunity

Vitamin/Mineral	Top Food Sources
Vitamin D	Sunshine, oily fish, eggs, mushrooms (left in the sun)
Vitamin E	Plant oils, nuts, seeds, wheatgerm, meat, poultry, dairy
Vitamin K	Spinach, cabbage, cauliflower, peas, cereals. Synthesized by certain gut microbiota
Zinc	Offal, eggs, meat, mushrooms, yeast, oysters
Copper	Eggs, wholewheat, beans, beetroot, liver, fish, spinach, asparagus, nuts
Selenium	Seafood, green leafy and root vegetables, chicken, egg yolk, whole grains, milk, mushrooms, garlic, nuts especially Brazil, pulses, meat, fish
Iodine	Seaweed, seafood, iodised salts, vegetables and cereals grown in iodine-rich soil
Magnesium	Soya, nuts, green leafy vegetables, whole grains, meat, fish, sunflower seeds, figs
Iron	Haem-iron – meat, offal, poultry, fish (blood). Non-haem – wheat, beans and lentils, vegetables especially green leafy, fruit and dairy
Manganese	Oats, wheatgerm, whole grains, nuts, tea, pineapple, plums, beans, dark green vegetables, beetroot

Functions

Helps regulate calcium (see page 62). Plays an important role in bone health, immune system. Cancer prevention

Healthy skin, eyes and immune system

Blood clotting. Healthy bones

Needed for wound healing, immune function, eye health, cell membrane structure, healthy skin and mucous membranes

Increases iron absorption for haemoglobin. Associated with a number of enzymes

Regulates thyroid function. Immune function. Antioxidant properties. Fertility. Energy system. Anti-cancer properties

Most soil depleted. Essential for thyroid hormones. Helpful for lumpy, fibrous breasts

Nerve transmission, energy production, building DNA, healthy heart and arteries. May reduce stress levels

For haemoglobin production (transports oxygen in the blood) and myoglobin in muscle. Deficiency causes anaemia

Antioxidant, enzyme activator, haemoglobin synthesis, urea formation, bone formation, reproduction, lactation

Hydration

Our body is comprised mainly of water and our hydration to electrolyte balance is key to the optimal functioning of our cells and in turn our body systems. There is a lot of different information on how many glasses of water we should drink daily, but it is very individual, depending on body weight, diet and exercise levels. As a rule, I would say drink enough that you need to pee every two to four hours and be guided by the colour of your urine. It should be light coloured; if it is dark, then it is too concentrated and you need more fluid. When we are dehydrated we can feel sleepy and lacking in energy; severe dehydration can bring about further symptoms including confusion and anxiety. Dehydration can also sometimes make it harder to yield blood for a blood test, so if extracting blood from your veins is problematic, drinking a glass of water can sometimes help. Dehydration will also increase inflammation within the body (see page 27).

Water is the best way of hydrating, but other fluids, including tea and coffee, can be counted. However, caffeinated drinks will have a diuretic effect, meaning a significant amount will be peed out. Herbal teas can be an ideal way to stay hydrated, and eating a diet high in vegetables, salad and fruit, which are around 90 per cent water, also adds to our intake, as do liquid foods such as soup. A sufficient intake of fluids will keep cells hydrated and working optimally, help remove toxins from the body and regulate bowel movements.

Getting into the habit of carrying water around with you is a good way of prompting yourself to drink more. Invest in a water bottle, preferably non-plastic, fill it and keep it with you during the day. It saves buying plastic bottles of water, which are not ideal due to chemicals from the plastic leaching out. Added to that, they are also an expensive way of keeping ourselves hydrated and an environmental disaster.

There is often concern about the quality of tap water and advising on filter systems is difficult because they can be so expensive. The one sure thing is that we need to drink water and the fact that we are not going to get cholera from our water supply puts things into perspective. Of course the ideal is to have water with as many impurities as possible filtered out. There are the cheaper jug systems available, or sports bottles with individual filters, but top of the range are the under-sink or whole-house systems. Remember to factor in the cost of regularly replacing the filters, which don't come cheap.

Salt

Although drinking too much water is rare, we do need to consider that our sodium levels will become diluted the more we drink. Eating a healthy diet with an increased intake of potassium-containing vegetables and a reduction in processed food, the main sources of salt, can lead to a considerably lower salt intake and potentially an imbalance of potassium to sodium.

The culprits for overconsumption of unhealthy salt are ready meals, breakfast cereals, tinned foods, sauces, pizzas, sandwiches, crisps, salted nuts, processed meats and bread. We do need salt in a healthy diet, but choose to add sea or Himalayan salt which has a healthy balance of other minerals. Do not use ordinary table salt, which is bleached and highly refined (see iodine, page 60).

The dietary guidelines for salt are no more than 6g (around 1 tsp) per day. On a food label, salt is often referred to as sodium; 1g of sodium is roughly the same as 2.5g of salt. It is the sodium that may lead to health problems such as high blood pressure.

The Top Anti-cancer Foods

I have talked a lot about a nutrient-dense diet with plenty of variety of coloured vegetables and fruits, but there are particular foods that research has shown to have some pretty impressive anti-cancer properties. However, remember that most of the evidence is based on results seen in a petri dish in a lab, or on mice, or in human epidemiology studies that rely on retrospective data. Also, studies looking at the therapeutic effects of food compounds often use large doses which would not be found in our general dietary intake. This is where supplements may provide the ideal therapeutic dose; however, I am a firm believer that if we regularly eat all these healing foods, many of which have therapeutic effects by working in synergy with each other, we are creating a diet that nature has cleverly created to keep us healthy. It is true to say, though, that in ill-health one may need to take large doses in supplement form to have a significant effect (see 'Nutraceutical Approaches', page 112).

It is also important to remember that the therapeutic constituents of many foods are reduced through the digestive process, meaning that the amount we absorb into our bodies is not as great as the amount actually present in the food before it is eaten. Therefore eat the following foods frequently as part of a balanced diet to keep up your intake of their beneficial properties.

Cruciferous vegetables (*Brassica* species)

These are all members of the cabbage family and include green, white and red cabbages, broccoli, cauliflower, Brussels sprouts, kale, spring greens, watercress, pak choi, mustard greens, turnip greens, rocket, kohlrabi, horseradish, wasabi, swedes and radishes. There has been some good evidence from research in humans to show that eating these vegetables produces favourable genetic changes within the body to protect against cancer.

Cabbage is the king of the crop, containing not only many vitamins and minerals but the greatest concentration of some very powerful anti-cancer phytochemicals. These include a group of substances known as glucosinolates which give rise to the pungent smell and bitter flavour of cabbage. Glucosinolates are broken down by the action of an enzyme called myrosinase which is released when these vegetables are chopped or chewed. This gives rise to active phytonutrients such as isothiocyanates, including sulforaphane and indoles including indole-3-carbinol and its product DIM (3,3'-diindolylmethane). These appear to have a plethora of anti-cancer roles, which include inducing apoptosis and inhibiting cell proliferation (see page 22), DNA repair, reducing angiogenesis (see page 29) and drug resistance, and inhibiting oestrogen metabolism, possibly by binding to oestrogen receptors and suppressing oestrogen-receptor expression (see page 29). In fact, indole-3-carbinol and DIM (3,3'-diindolylmethane) are thought to be particularly protective against breast cancer and act in a similar way to the drug Tamoxifen.

If you suffer from mastitis (inflamed breasts) or have any areas of inflammation, use a cabbage leaf topically (on the skin) to reduce the swelling. This is an old remedy that many a midwife will quote to women with mastitis due to breastfeeding and it also works for many acute inflammatory situations, especially swollen knees. Keep your cabbage (white cabbage works well) in the fridge. Peel off a leaf and scrunch it slightly to release the enzymes. Apply it directly to the inflamed area. The cold effect helps to reduce the heat and then as it warms on the skin the enzymes and anti-inflammatory compounds get to work to reduce the inflammation.

Eating raw cabbage or drinking the water after cooking your cabbage gently for 3 minutes has been found to help to heal stomach and duodenal ulcers. So, all in all, this is an extremely therapeutic food.

Broccoli has also been well researched and found to have high levels of these anti-cancer phytonutrients too. Fresh broccoli sprouts contain much higher levels of the phytonutrient glucoraphanin which breaks down to the sulforaphane on chewing.

The therapeutic properties of fermented cabbage or sauerkraut are vast. Have a go at making it yourself (see page 252). Not only does it provide us with beneficial *Lactobacillus* bacteria, but it can aid digestion, enhance the immune system and reduce inflammation in the gut.

Turmeric (Curcumin)

Curcumin is the most important active ingredient in turmeric. Apart from eating this in abundance there is plenty of research to suggest that turmeric supplementation may be a useful therapy to take alongside chemo- and radiotherapy and that taking it in high

doses is safe. It has been shown to increase the sensitivity of many types of cancer cells to these treatments, thus increasing the rate of cancer-cell death. But it has also been found to afford protection to normal cells, which in turn can reduce some of the damaging side-effects of these therapies. It is thought that this action is down to the antioxidant properties of curcumin (see 'Free Radicals', page 26), which is also anti-inflammatory and anti-thrombotic, and has been shown to induce apoptosis in certain cancer cells and to inhibit angiogenesis and metastasis (see page 29). Its anti-inflammatory action has been demonstrated to be particularly beneficial in the inhibition of colon cancer.

One of the main problems of curcumin is that it is not absorbed easily. Combining it with piperine, found in black pepper, has been found to improve absorption. In supplement form, choose a well-researched product from a reputable company and use organic *curcuma longa* if possible.

Fresh turmeric is much more readily available nowadays in the UK. Grate the root into many of the dishes you prepare. Just a little will not be too overpowering, but will turn both the food and your hands yellow. Always best to prepare it with gloves on unless you are happy with your hands and kitchen taking on a yellow hue. It can also be infused in hot water to make a tea, or in warm milk (almond, coconut, hemp) for a deliciously comforting nighttime drink. Add a little ground black pepper and a sprinkling of cinnamon.

Green tea

Green tea is made from the young shoots of *Camellia sinensis* and is far less processed than black tea, therefore retaining many more of its therapeutic properties. It is the polyphenols in the form of flavonols called catechins that are responsible for its powerful anti-cancer effects. The most important is epigallocatechin gallate (EGCG), providing about 50–80 per cent of the total polyphenols. Just like all polyphenols, these act as the plant's defence mechanism against bacteria and fungus, so buy an organic brand to ensure optimal amounts. Studies have shown that those who drink green tea may lower their risk of developing many types of cancer, especially hormonally related ones, as it appears to modulate oestrogen metabolism. It has also been shown to block the activity of VEGF, which is key to inducing angiogenesis (see page 29). Other benefits are that regular drinking of green tea appears to be helpful in preventing periodontal disease which is often experienced during cancer treatment.

There are various grades of tea, but Sencha and Matcha are two which are often heralded as the best. However, any good-quality green tea will be beneficial. Some studies use concentrated green tea extract, which would equate to an awful lot of cups of tea daily to gain the same results. Just exactly how much we need to drink has not been definitively established, but I would aim for around four cups a day if you have active disease. Green tea does contain caffeine, so be mindful of this if you are drinking it in the evening. The tea should be drunk with a meal, just as the Japanese do, or at least with a snack. If you drink it on an empty stomach it may be a bit strong and make you feel nauseous, especially first thing in the morning.

It is important to brew the tea properly in order to gain all the beneficial properties. Use freshly boiled water but not boiling water as this can make it bitter. Let it infuse for at least 10 minutes in a cup with a lid on it. Adding a slice of lemon can improve the flavour and is thought to preserve the antioxidant compounds for longer (see 'Free Radicals', page 26).

Blue/red/black berries

Included in this category are red or black grapes, cranberries and pomegranate seeds, along with raspberries, strawberries, blueberries, blackcurrants, redcurrants, blackberries and many more. The anti-cancer properties of these fruits are found again in their phytochemicals – namely anthocyanidins, proanthocyanidins and ellagic acid. These appear to block the induction of angiogenesis, stimulate the immune system, regulate apoptosis (see pages 22, 28 and 29), aid detoxification and have amazing antioxidant powers (see 'Free Radicals', page 26).

Red grapes contain the polyphenol resveratrol, which has been shown in animal studies to induce apoptosis in cancer stem cells (see page 22). The fact that resveratrol is found in the skin of the grapes is the reason red wine, which uses the whole grape, is touted as good for you – in moderation (see 'Alcohol', page 81).

Berries are also an extremely good choice of fruit because they are low in sugar and so do not impact on glucose levels as other very sweet fruits can. Strawberries are believed to be excellent binders of mercury in the gut, so eat them as a dessert after a meal of fish to eliminate any mercury residues before they are absorbed.

Mushrooms

There is extensive research on mushrooms which demonstrates their many anti-cancer benefits. Most of the investigation into these benefits has been conducted in Asia on the oriental types such as shiitake, maitake, reishi and *Coriolus versicolor*. Some of them are actually approved by the Japanese government for cancer treatments, as studies in that country have shown that mushroom extracts can shrink tumours, improve the effectiveness of chemotherapy and offset some of the side-effects of treatment, including enhancing white cell counts.

Common to all mushrooms are polysaccharides, which have immune stimulatory effects. It is believed the potent anti-cancer properties of mushrooms are mostly due to their ability to activate certain immune cells such as macrophages, natural killer cells and T-cells. They also appear to have immune-modulating effects, helping to dampen down inflammatory responses. A study in Australia found that eating the common button mushroom daily could reduce the risk of breast cancer in pre-menopausal women by 65 per cent.

Mushrooms such as shiitake and oyster are readily available in the supermarkets along with our more common varieties, so add mushrooms to many of your dishes. Have mushrooms on toast for breakfast, slice them raw in a salad for lunch and add them to a stir-fry for supper – just a few ideas for this wonderfully versatile medicinal food.

Garlic and onions

Both members of the Allium family, these sulphurous vegetables are renowned for their many health benefits. They are high in polyphenols, with onions being a particularly rich source, containing the flavonoid quercetin, known for its antioxidant and anti-inflammatory properties. Eating approximately half an onion a day appears to reduce the risk of colorectal, larangeal, lung and ovarian cancer. Garlic is thought to be protective against radiation, therefore it may be beneficial to eat plenty during radiotherapy treatment. Both onion and garlic have antimicrobial properties and may well help guard against bacterial infections, particularly those of the oral cavity.

Again, these are foods that release enzymes when they are crushed, chopped or chewed, which activates their therapeutic properties; you know when the enzyme has been activated because it is what causes the familiar pungent aroma of these vegetables. Remember that you get these benefits only by eating them fresh. With onions try not to peel off too many outside layers where the flavonoid content is highest. Red onions generally have a higher total of flavonoids than white.

To make the most of garlic's therapeutic effects, it should be chopped or crushed and allowed to rest for 5–10 minutes before cooking. This allows the compound alliin and the activated enzyme alliinase to come into contact and form allicin. Heating the garlic before allowing the allicin to form de-activates the enzyme and you will lose some of the health benefits and flavour, although cooking does unfortunately reduce these further. It is best to eat garlic raw, perhaps crushed in a salad dressing or popped into a smoothie.

The therapeutic properties of onions are also enhanced by letting them sit for at least 5 minutes after slicing or chopping before cooking.

Sea vegetables and iodine

There is a hypothesis that iodine deficiency may be the reason that there is a link between breast cancer and thyroid disorders. Iodine is necessary for thyroid function and an increasing number of people in the UK have been found to be deficient. Iodine deficiency is seen to cause fibrocystic breast tissue and breast lumps, which may lead on to cancer. Seaweed contains good levels of iodine and a daily intake of seaweed solution has been found to inhibit mammary cancer cells in rats, while in a test tube it induced apoptosis in human breast-cancer cells (see page 22). It was also seen to inhibit angiogenesis in tumours in rats (see page 29). Iodine is taken up by every cell in the body and has antioxidant and anti-inflammatory properties (see 'Free Radicals', page 26, and 'Inflammation', page 27).

Sea vegetables are another food consumed in abundance in Japan, where the incidence of breast cancer is low. It is difficult to obtain sufficient iodine through our Western diet. The levels in our plant foods are low because iodine is a rare element in soil, but it is found in concentrated amounts in oceans, hence its abundance in sea vegetables. Seaweed is gaining in popularity and accessibility in the UK. Brown-coloured seaweeds, such as kelp and wakame, are the richest in iodine but may contain up to 500 per cent of the recommended daily intake per serving, so you don't want to consume too much. A serving once a week can be adequate.

Seaweed can be an acquired taste, but there are plenty of varieties to choose from. You can add seaweed to stir-fries, salads or smoothies, or buy flakes to sprinkle on salads, soups and stews. You can also find seaweed mixed with salt for use in a grinder. It is possible to buy iodized salt, but it is highly refined. Himalayan pink salt is the best choice and does contain some iodine.

Fucoidan is a sulphated polysaccharide found in brown seaweed and kelp. It

has demonstrated numerous anti-cancer properties such as triggering apoptosis, improving immune cell activity and inhibiting metastasis (see pages 22, 28 and 29). It can be found in supplement form too.

Flaxseed

Flaxseed (or linseed) appears to have many remarkable therapeutic properties, mainly due to its anti-inflammatory omega-3 levels and its oestrogenic effects. There have been plenty of studies in animals but also some in humans where it was shown to reduce the proliferation of cancer cells in breast and prostate cancer patients.

The phytoestrogens in flaxseeds appear to have a hormone-modulating effect by latching on to oestrogen receptors on cells and blocking them from the harmful effects of the more powerful oestrogens within the body. It is thought that this can also enhance the effects of hormone therapies used after treatment in hormone-related cancers (see 'Hormones', page 28, and 'Soya and other phytoestrogens', page 80). They can also help to relieve the symptoms of menopause.

Those with hormone-sensitive cancers have often been told to avoid foods containing phytoestrogens as they may have detrimental hormone-stimulating effects. There is quite understandably much confusion over this issue; however, the research is far more conclusive about their protective elements than about any potential harm.

The omega-3 benefits of flaxseed oil were observed by the biochemist Joanna Budwig, whose protocol (see page 109) uses flaxseeds in a way that helps to incorporate the oils into our cells. It is also known for its soothing fibre content which is extremely beneficial for gut health (see page 82).

Use your flaxseeds freshly ground and sprinkle them into cereals, smoothies, yoghurt and fruit salads, or make a porridge by mixing them with boiling water – in any of these ways they make a great dish for aiding constipation. Also stir them ground into stews or bolognese just before serving for an extra creamy consistency and greater nutrient value. You can soak the whole seeds overnight, whereupon they will become gloopy. Flaxseed tea is also very healing on the gut – steep 1 tbsp of flaxseeds in a cup of boiling water for 10 minutes or overnight, strain off the seeds and drink the liquid.

Important Nutrients

A comprehensive list of all nutrients and their sources is found in the table on page 52. All are important in one way or another to keep the body healthy. The following are some that I feel it necessary to mention separately, either because many of us are deficient or because they are depleted by treatment.

Calcium and vitamin D

Those being treated with long-term steroid medication have an increased risk of osteoporosis or thinning bones. They are generally prescribed calcium and vitamin D supplements, but people are often concerned about sufficient dietary intake of calcium and bone health, especially in those who have decided to give up dairy (see 'Building healthy bones', page 86). However, if you are eating a healthy diet there are plenty of foods high in calcium and as a rule this is not a concern (see page 86 for non-dairy sources of calcium). Chemotherapy can also temporarily deplete calcium stores.

However, intake of Vitamin D needs to be considered too, as it improves the absorption of calcium and is very important for healthy bones. It also has a number of other roles to play in the body, including regulating cancer-cell division, restricting angiogenesis (see page 29) and increasing cancer-cell death. We obtain it mainly from exposing our bare skin to sunlight, where the action of the ultraviolet B (UVB) rays converts cholesterol to vitamin D3. It is actually a steroid hormone of which diet contributes only a small amount from oily fish and fish liver oils, eggs, and meat and dairy from pasture-fed cattle. Unfortunately, many of us who live in the northern hemisphere are deficient in vitamin D, and the darker our skin, the more likely this is.

Due to the increase in skin cancer the advice has been to wear sunscreen and a hat when out in the sun to prevent burning. This is important, but we must also sensibly expose as much of our bare skin as possible to sunlight during the summer months without sunscreen. You only need approximately 20 minutes of sunshine regularly on your face and bare arms to make enough vitamin D, which your body can then store. During the winter months we cannot make vitamin D from the sun as the rays are too weak, so the body uses up stored vitamin D. Women should remember that most facial moisturizers have a sun-protection factor and this will reduce the amount of vitamin D they can make.

Research has shown that a high calcium intake may be protective of colorectal cancer, both through diet and supplementation. However, only take large amounts of calcium if advised by a health professional and this should be in conjunction with vitamin D.

It is advisable to have a vitamin D test if you have had a cancer diagnosis. Your GP may be happy to do this. If you are deficient, then get advice on the levels of supplementation needed. Do not supplement with large amounts of vitamin D unless directed by a health professional. For further information on the links between vitamin D and bone health, and vitamin D and cancer, see the report by the Scientific Advisory Commission on Nutrition (SACN).

Vitamin A – retinoids and carotenoids

Vitamin A is found in some animal foods but it is particularly high in liver. It is also obtained in the form of beta-carotene from yellow and red vegetables (sweet potatoes, carrots, dried apricots, cantaloupe, papaya, red peppers, tomatoes) and green leafy vegetables. It is a fat-soluble vitamin and so needs fat in the diet to be absorbed.

Vitamin A and its derivatives – retinoids and carotenoids – are involved in the promotion of healthy cell growth Some carotenoids appear to block tumour progression, particularly lycopene in tomatoes which seems to reduce the risk of prostate cancer. It also helps in the healing of gut mucosal cells (see page 82) and supporting immune cells.

Coenzyme Q10

CoQ10 is a potent antioxidant and plays an important role in energy production in our mitochondria (see page 25), particularly in highly active tissue such as our heart muscle. Anthracycline chemotherapy drugs such as Doxorubicin and Daunorubicin are known to cause cardiotoxicity, which can lead to long-term heart problems. Research has shown

that supplementing with CoQ10 during this treatment appears to be safe and protects the important heart mitochondria from damage. Dosage levels have not been set, but general advice is 100mg a day.

CoQ10 is made in the body but can also be obtained from the diet. Organ meats and oily fish are the main sources, with some vegetables containing it too.

Selenium

Low levels of selenium have been linked to increased cancer risk, particularly those of the prostate, breast, skin and stomach. It plays a role in immune function, protects our cells by promoting the body's antioxidant defences and has anti-inflammatory properties (see pages 26–27 and 28).

Dietary intake of selenium has fallen significantly in the UK in the last few decades. As many people have low levels, we should ensure we have a sufficient intake of those foods richest in it. The best sources are Brazil nuts (although levels vary considerably from one nut to another), fish, meat, organ meat, eggs, nuts, seeds, seaweed and grains.

Tests for selenium deficiency are not readily available and supplementing with high amounts is detrimental unless you have a known deficiency. Do not supplement above 100mg a day without advice from a health professional. A couple of Brazil nuts each day will in general supply you with your daily needs, but make sure they are as fresh as possible and, to reduce oxidation, keep them in the fridge.

Zinc

Zinc is often depleted during chemotherapy treatments. It plays an important role in the healing of wounds, immune function and the activity of many enzymes. It is also involved in cell repair and division and has anti-inflammatory properties (see pages 22 and 27). A deficiency has been linked to many cancers, especially head and neck cancers. It is harder for vegetarians to get sufficient zinc in their diet as one of the main sources is meat, especially beef. Other sources are dairy, eggs, seeds and grains.

Supplementation should only be considered when guided by a health professional, as excess zinc can drive cancer growth.

If you are anaemic and have been prescribed iron supplements, do take them between meals: when taken with a meal the iron will interfere with zinc absorption. Be careful if taking supplements of zinc, because too much can actually impair the functioning of immune cells just as depletion can. It is always best to seek advice on supplementation from a health professional.

B vitamins

Again, these can be depleted by chemo-therapy drugs. See the table on page 52 for a comprehensive list of food sources for each B vitamin. Be aware that the drug Methotrexate is used in cancer treatment to interfere with the conversion of folic acid to its active form, therefore do not supplement without the advice of a health professional.

Choline is a nutrient linked to the B-complex family of vitamins and is necessary for healthy cell-membrane functioning and nerve communication; it also reduces inflammation (see page 27). Rich sources are seafood, eggs, poultry, meat and green leafy vegetables.

Culinary Herbs and Spices

Herbs and spices in your food not only add nutrient value and enhance flavour, but they can also aid digestion and detoxification, and may have anti-inflammatory and antibacterial effects. They can be useful for overcoming the metallic taste induced by chemotherapy.

The following is a list of some of the herbs and spices you should be including in your diet on a regular basis. There are of course many more, so experiment with other flavours too. Fresh is always best, but build up a supply of dried ones too for convenience – just remember to use them! Organic dried herbs and spices are readily available in supermarkets.

Store fresh cut herbs in a plastic bag or glass of water in the fridge. Once chopped, many herbs will freeze well in a container for several months. This makes a very convenient source of ready-prepared herbs. Always use double the amount of fresh herbs to dried herbs as they are less pungent, and add them towards the end of cooking to preserve the aromatic oils and delicate flavour.

HERBS

Basil

The volatile oils of basil can relax the smooth muscle of the digestive tract and dilate small blood vessels, making it a good digestive and anti-spasmodic aid. Try chewing on a leaf to counteract chemo tastebuds.

Basil is a particularly great accompaniment to tomatoes, but can work well with many other dishes and herbs. It mixes well with garlic, thyme and oregano.

Dill

Dill is a carminative (prevention or relief of flatulence) for any digestive disturbance; it has also shown antimicrobial and anti-cancer effects. It is useful for promoting detoxification reactions in the liver to help rid the body of toxic chemicals. It is delicious with fish.

Lemon Verbena

This herb, with its wonderful lemon fragrance, has many medicinal properties. It is an easily grown deciduous plant, producing many leaves which can be used fresh or dried for tea infusions.

Lemon verbena is extremely calming and can help to relieve indigestion, flatulence, nausea and diarrhoea, whilst also stimulating appetite. It is anti-inflammatory and has antiviral properties too. Due to its slightly sedative nature, it may also help to relieve insomnia when drunk as a tea before bed. Try it with chamomile for an even greater sedative effect.

Mint

This herb is rich in compounds that have been shown to inhibit the growth and formation of cancer. It is an excellent carminative and aids digestion, and is well known for its effective relief of indigestion and symptoms of irritable bowel syndrome.

Use it to make a wonderful fresh mint tea by steeping the leaves in hot water and leaving to infuse for several minutes. Make up a cafetiere of mint tea and keep it in the fridge as a cooling, refreshing drink.

Oregano

This herb also has amazing antioxidant properties (see 'Free Radicals', page 26), ranking higher than other herbs, fruits and vegetables in this respect – even including blueberries! It is also particularly known for its antimicrobial activities, due to its volatile oils thymol and carvacrol. Both have been shown to inhibit the growth of bacteria, including *Staphylococcus aureus*.

Oregano is closely related to marjoram and both are members of the mint family. In some parts of Europe oregano is known as wild marjoram, but marjoram is a little milder and sweeter. Both herbs are easy to grow in the garden or in a pot and their fresh leaves are wonderfully aromatic, bringing a subtle and delicate flavour to dishes.

Parsley

Parsley has long been used for medicinal purposes and is regarded as an excellent nerve stimulant and detoxifier. Its volatile oil components have been shown to have antiseptic and anti-cancer properties. It is rich in chlorophyll and carotenes and is a very good source of vitamin C, folic acid and iron, as well as many other minerals.

Parsley is a member of the same family as carrots and celery, with the most popular types being the curly variety and the Italian flat-leaf. The latter has more fragrance and a less bitter taste than curly parsley.

Rosemary

Rich in flavonoids and volatile oils, rosemary may help to reduce inflammatory conditions (see page 27), stimulate the immune system, increase circulation and improve digestion. In ancient times it was believed to stimulate the memory, and in fact it has been shown to increase blood flow to the brain.

Rosemary is a member of the mint family and has a wonderfully pungent taste and smell. It is an evergreen shrub, with pine-like needles, and is easy to grow. To prepare rosemary, run your fingers down the stalk to remove the leaves and chop them with a sharp knife. Chewing on a rosemary needle can be helpful in overcoming the metallic taste often experienced after chemotherapy. Just chew it to release the oils, then you can spit it out if you prefer.

Tarragon

Rich in antioxidants (see 'Free Radicals', page 26), tarragon has also been shown to have potent anti-fungal and antimicrobial properties. Its sweet anise flavour goes well with fish, chicken and many vegetables.

Thyme

Used by the ancient Greeks and drunk in a tea in the Middle Ages, thyme is rich in antioxidants (see 'Free Radicals', page 26) and has been shown to possess anti-spasmodic, antibacterial and carminative actions. Research also indicates that it may help brain function. It is delicious when used with garlic and lemon to flavour roast chicken.

SPICES

Cardamom

This versatile spice can be used in both savoury and sweet dishes. It is usually sold and used in pods, but the seeds can be extracted and ground. It is very calming on the gut and can aid digestion. It is also good for refreshing the mouth and may help to counteract the metallic taste often produced by chemotherapy drugs.

Chilli

Capsaicin is a carotenoid and is the active component of the chilli. It appears to have abundant anti-cancer properties, although there is concern in some studies that its heat may damage healthy cells too and so cause cancer, so perhaps go easy on the very hot ones. In the main, however, studies have found that the benefits outweigh the negatives and chillis probably should be used liberally in our food.

Capsaicin has been found to prevent liver damage and cream preparations containing it may help if you are suffering from the nerve pain often induced by cancer treatment. In one study with prostate cancer cells, capsaicin was also found to promote apoptosis (see page 22). Another found it able to interfere with the mitochondrial activity in cancer cells but not in healthy cells (see page 25).

The hotter the chilli, the more capsaicin it contains, but be careful if you have a sore or ulcerated mouth.

Cinnamon

Medicinally, research has shown that cinnamon has the potential to be a circulatory stimulant, a digestive aid, an anti-convulsant, a diuretic, and that it has antibiotic and anti-ulcerative properties.

A small study published in 2003 in the journal *Diabetes Care* looked at sixty men and women with type 2 diabetes. It found that just 1g (approx. ¼ tsp) of *Cassia* cinnamon lowered blood glucose over a period of time. More research needs to be done in this area, but adding it to your food as a flavouring can be a great substitute for sugar: it adds a subtle sweetness, yet it may have the additional benefit of controlling blood glucose.

Cinnamon comes from the bark of trees. There are two types: *Ceylon*, grown in South East Asia, South America and the West Indies; and *Cassia*, grown in Central America. You can use cinnamon sticks to flavour food or buy the spice ground. In ancient history cinnamon was once so highly treasured that it was more precious than gold. It has useful flavouring properties, as it can be used to enhance both sweet and savoury dishes.

Cloves

Cloves are rich in eugenol, which has been shown to reduce the effects of environmental toxins in the body. It is anti-inflammatory (see page 27) and protective against cancers of the gut. Cloves were traditionally used by dentists to help relieve toothache – they act as a mild anaesthetic and antibacterial agent. They may also aid healing of mucositis (inflammation and ulceration) of the mouth when chewed.

Coriander

Coriander seeds help to aid digestion, calm the digestive tract and may help to balance blood sugar. They also have anti-inflammatory (see page 27) and antibacterial properties and could even reduce feelings of anxiety.

Coriander leaves are a good source of iron and magnesium, as well as vitamins C and K.

Cumin

Cumin is known for its digestive properties, particularly its stimulatory effect on pancreatic enzymes, so drinking cumin tea with a meal will aid digestion. It may also have a cancer-protective effect due to its antioxidant (see 'Free Radicals', page 26) and detoxification abilities.

Cumin is used widely throughout the world, probably due to its wonderfully complex flavour which works beautifully with so many foods. Use it in rice, with vegetables and rubbed on meat. To make a tea, lightly boil 2 tsp cumin seeds in 2 cups water, cover, then allow to steep for 10 minutes.

Fenugreek

Fenugreek is used for digestive problems and upset stomachs and has anti-inflammatory properties (see page 27). It has been used in the past to relieve menopausal symptoms due to its oestrogenic effects. It also appears to enhance blood-glucose control.

Fenugreek seeds are roasted, then ground and used in spice mixes and for flavouring curries. The leaves are also used in Indian cooking, either dried or fresh in salads.

Ginger

Ginger is an excellent spice for calming down typical IBS symptoms, such as spasm and wind. It is probably best known for its anti-nausea properties and has been trialled alongside anti-emetic drugs, where it was found to increase the anti-nausea effects, although it may be just as effective when used alone. From my observations it is fair to say that some people find it very useful, whilst for others it appears to have no effect. The best way to use it to reduce nausea is by making ginger tea. Cut two thin slices of ginger root and infuse in hot water in a covered cup or cafetiere; sip throughout the day.

Daily consumption of 3g of ginger in a capsule has been found to reduce fasting blood sugar and insulin resistance, and to increase insulin sensitivity.

Ginger is also highly anti-inflammatory (see page 27) and has been used with some success in those with rheumatoid arthritis. Use it grated to pep up some of your dishes, but remember it can pack quite a punch.

Saffron

Saffron comes from the stigma of the crocus. It is a very labour-intensive procedure to produce just a small amount and the cost reflects this. However, a little goes a long way and its vast health benefits make it worth its weight in gold!

The carotene found in saffron's orange pigment produces its antioxidant and anti-cancer properties (see 'Free Radicals', page 26). When tested on human cells in a lab, it was found to inhibit cancer cells and trigger apoptosis (see page 22), whilst stimulating healthy cells, including those of the immune system. It also appears to protect healthy cells from the damaging effects of carcinogens and aids their detoxification.

Turmeric – see page 58

Juices and Smoothies

Juicing is an excellent way of increasing our intake of fruit and vegetables. It breaks down the food, making it highly absorbable and therefore extremely nutritious, which is particularly useful in cases where gut function may be compromised such as during treatment or after surgery.

Fresh juices contain an abundance of enzymes responsible for the digestion and absorption of food, thus ensuring optimal metabolism. Cooking destroys these enzymes. Juicing and blending raw green vegetables and living greens such as sprouted seeds provides a source of chlorophyll, which has antioxidant (see 'Free Radicals', page 26) and anti-cancer properties.

Smoothies use the whole fruit or vegetable and therefore contain fibre, which supports liver detoxification by binding to excess oestrogen, cholesterol and toxins and eliminating them from the body. Fibre also helps to maintain bowel function. Smoothies are more filling than juices and make a good breakfast option.

For advice on juicers and smoothie makers, see page 137.

Juicing and smoothie tips

• Green vegetable juices should be favoured over fruit juices because they are more healing, regenerating and detoxifying, with far more minerals and oxygen. Fruit juices have a much higher sugar content and should be diluted with water to avoid inducing a blood-glucose spike.

• Juices and smoothies start to oxidize as soon as they are made, so it is best to drink them immediately. If this is not possible, store in an airtight container in the fridge for a maximum of 24 hours. Drink immediately on taking out of the fridge.

• Wash all ingredients well before juicing or blending. Use organic where possible, but make sure they are very fresh.

• Cucumber and celery make a good base for green juices as they are watery and can help to dilute other strong-tasting vegetables.

• Wheatgrass juice is extracted from young shoots of grass grown from wheatgrain and is extremely nutritious. A maximum dose is 50ml twice daily. It is best taken on an empty stomach on its own and should be absolutely fresh for full benefit. It is possible to buy dried wheatgrass and, although not quite as beneficial as fresh, it is worth taking if fresh is unavailable. Fresh can be bought online. Freshly made juice can be frozen in ice-cube trays.

• Sprouted seeds contain levels of nutrients that are up to fifty times higher than in the plants or vegetables, and juicing or blending them is a great way of incorporating them in your diet. Use sunflower and snow-pea shoots, alfalfa, fenugreek, broccoli, onion, radish sprouts, etc.

• During chemo- or radiotherapy, limit your intake of green juice to one glass a day, otherwise you could affect your body's response to medication by altering the rate of liver detoxification.

INGREDIENT IDEAS FOR JUICES AND SMOOTHIES

Almond milk	Lemon/lime juice
Aloe vera	Mango
Apples	Melon
Avocado	Nuts/nut butters
Bananas	Okra
Basil	Onion
Beetroot	Papaya
Berries	Parsley
Broccoli	Pears
Cabbage	Pineapple
Carrots	Seaweed
Celery	Seed oils (unrefined)
Coriander leaves (fresh)	Slippery elm
Courgette	Spinach
Cucumber	Sprouts
Fennel	Tomatoes
Garlic	Watercress
Ginger	Wheatgrass
Grapes	Yoghurt
Kale	

Dietary Debates

Organic food – is it worth it?

I find it sad that eating a predominantly organic diet is so often dismissed as merely a middle-class fad. I also find it sad that much of the research on organic food puts the emphasis on taste and nutrient levels rather than discussing the merits of lower levels of herbicides, insecticides and fungicides. Most people who choose organic do so as much for the health benefits of consuming fewer pesticide residues as for the significant improvement in taste, although this is a distinct bonus.

To date, research into organic versus conventional diets has been limited, and there is a dearth of large-scale studies into health implications. However, some significant findings have emerged.

Research has suggested that higher levels of phytonutrients (see page 51) – which have known anti-cancer properties – are present in organic products, while at the same time concentrations of cadmium (a toxin) are lower. There is evidence that organic meat and dairy products from grass-fed animals also have significantly higher levels of anti-inflammatory omega-3 fatty acids, whereas non-organic products from grain-fed animals are higher in omega-6, which may be pro-inflammatory (see pages 45–6).

There have been suggestions that organic produce may carry a small risk of bacterial infection – but washing it or cooking it well should reduce the risk. Non-organic produce, however, carries a much higher risk of contamination from bacteria resistant to antibiotics – a major health concern today, and one which organic farmers avoid because they do not routinely vaccinate their livestock with antibiotics. Studies of children have revealed much lower levels of pesticide residues in those eating organic foodstuffs compared to those following a conventional diet. Other research has indicated that pesticide levels may be 30 per cent lower in organic produce, while non-organic foodstuffs – especially citrus fruit, pineapples, grapes and wheat – are increasingly likely to contain high levels of pesticide residues; some have even been found to exceed safe limits.

Cutting the cost of organic food

So we can see organic may well be the healthier option, but how to afford it? There is no doubt that, in general, organic produce is more expensive than its conventionally grown equivalent. However, there are ways in which you can keep the cost down:

• Consider a weekly organic box. Some box schemes are significantly cheaper than buying the equivalent produce from a supermarket, and they are often a good way of increasing your intake and variety of vegetables (see page 49). You may find a small local farm who will deliver; alternatively, the larger retailers usually offer anything from fruit and vegetables to meat, dairy and store-cupboard items. Don't automatically assume that organic is more expensive. It's always worth having a look: you may be surprised to find some items are a similar price, or you may find bargains amongst the reduced items. But beware of buying produce that is past its best just because it is organic: given the choice between a tired-looking organic cabbage and a fresh-looking non-organic one, I would go for the non-organic because its freshness will mean it has greater nutrient value.

• Decide where it's worth spending extra on organic produce. The Pesticide Action Network website gives a list of the best and worst foods for pesticide residue. This will enable you to be more discriminating about foods it's important to buy as organic and those which aren't such a concern and can be bought as less expensive non-organic.

• The Environmental Working Group (EWG) is a US-based site with a wealth of information on best and worst organic buys, from food to cleaning products and cosmetics.

• Eat a mainly plant-based diet to cut costs, as meat is certainly the most expensive of organic foods. Organic beans and pulses are cheaper.

• Buy cheaper cuts of organic meat such as stewing steak and use a slower cooking method.

• Eat wild, sustainably caught fish. Organic farmed fish can be expensive.

• Find a local farmers' market or a farm tha sells products direct. Get to know the producers and you may find the food is of high provenance but not necessarily organic. It costs a lot and takes years to get registered, but there are farmers who are choosing more sustainable and natural farming methods but just lack the accreditation.

• Animals that are predominantly grass fed have a healthier fat profile whether organic or not (see page 44). Non-organic New Zealand lamb may be a good choice as it is naturally reared on open pastures – not so good on food miles, though!

• Try growing your own organic produce. This may seem idealistic to some – and as someone who struggled to manage an allotment organically I am not a zealot in this department – but a few pots or growbags of vegetables and herbs can usually be grown on a patio or balcony. A kitchen windowsill with herbs and a pot or two of salad leaves can work well.

• Forage for wild food. There are courses on foraging that can teach you where to look for everything from wild mushrooms to herbs and berries.

• If you have space, keep your own chickens and bees.

WORDS OF WISDOM FROM AN ORGANIC FARMER

Guy Watson, Riverford Organics, Devon

A cabbage grown slowly on a Devon hillside, which has fought off pest attack, rooted deeply and extensively in a healthy soil to find its nutrients, and arrived at a modest weight in the fullness of time will be a very different vegetable from the same variety grown in the same season on the Fens in a soil awash with soluble nitrogen, repeatedly sprayed with insecticides and fungicides and harvested in half the time at twice the weight. The two cabbages look and taste so different that it would be absurd to think they would not be different nutritionally as well. Science may not yet have demonstrated the difference, but that is the fault of science and its application, not of my cabbages.

Modern medicine and nutritional science has done a fine job of explaining the impact of diet on scurvy and rickets – in each case one easily identified nutrient and one relatively acute ailment. But it has virtually nothing to contribute towards understanding the relationship between the complex, whole diets we eat and most chronic ailments. To design an experiment to measure the relationship between, say, green vegetables and cancer in a way that will meet scientific criteria and pass peer review would be prohibitively expensive and might take decades to become conclusive. To go further and investigate the relationship between the particular way those vegetables are grown and chronic disease is unlikely to happen in my lifetime. Apart from all the considerable technical problems of experimental design and time, there is no one with a substantial commercial interest to fund such a study.

My frustration with scientists, and medics in particular, is the implication that the absence of evidence *for* a relationship between eating, say, cabbage (organic or not) and cancer is evidence for the *lack* of a relationship. All we can say is that, to date, *science doesn't know* – something science should be far more willing to say. In the absence of firm scientific knowledge, we must make up our own minds. Peripheral indicative studies might give some guidance, as might tradition and folklore, but their interpretation is subjective; in the end we are left largely with our own intuition. Intuition is open to influence and stands dangerously close to prejudice, but there can be little doubt that animals avoid toxic plants and self-medicate (our cows do anyway); why should we not be capable of the same? Faced with a supermarket shelf of processed foods or a vending machine, this may be a challenge; an addiction to, and the constant availability of, sugar, caffeine, salt and fat might lead us astray at times but, given a little help and availability, most of us know what is good for us.

My intuition and common sense tell me the less our food is messed around with, the fewer additives and the less processing, the closer it is to the diet our bodies evolved to cope with, the better our chances of a long and healthy life. That 'messing around' applies as much to farming as it does to food processing, which is why we converted Riverford to organic farming thirty years ago.

Dairy – good or bad?

Due to a lot of conflicting advice in the media, the question of whether to consume dairy is a confusing one, especially if you have a hormonally driven cancer. Dairy contains natural hormones and growth factors (IGF-1; see page 28) and modern intensive farming methods mean there is the possibility of added ones too. Population studies of Asian women have shown that those who consume less dairy have a lower risk of hormone-related cancers. Also, studies investigating hormones in dairy products and high IGF levels have equally concluded that dairy may be related to a greater incidence of breast and prostate cancer. However, this research is by no means conclusive, as other studies have found no such correlation.

My advice is that consuming moderate amounts of dairy from high-provenance, grass-fed organic animals is probably fine. This eliminates worries about added hormones and high levels of antibiotics and provides you with the beneficial fats omega-3 and conjugated linoleic acid (see pages 45 and 46). So if you especially like dairy milk in your tea, a bit of butter and cheese, and some health-promoting bio-yoghurt, then it is probably fine. I find that cheese is the hardest thing for many people to give up; however, you can find high-quality, unpasteurized, unprocessed natural cheese from some small producers. Dairy in its raw form from a reputable producer is best in many respects because it still contains beneficial bacteria which are good for our gut (see pages 82–4) – although it can of course also contain non-beneficial and distinctly harmful bacteria. Food-borne illness is always a concern, so you certainly should be very careful if your immune system is at all compromised.

If you would prefer not to consume dairy because you have a hormone-related cancer or are simply not keen on it, then there are plenty of alternatives to choose from. Ensure you are eating a balanced diet rich in fish, nuts, pulses and vegetables so that you are sure of getting sufficient calcium. There are plenty of milk alternatives on the market, such as almond (see page 264 on making your own), coconut, hemp, hazelnut or oat milks, along with coconut milk bio-yoghurts, and all of them supply us with plenty of nutrients. I would not particularly recommend rice or soya milk due to the potential presence of toxins.

The other problem with dairy is that it can be difficult to digest. Many people are intolerant of lactose (milk sugar), often as a result of treatment during which damage to the gut reduces the amount of enzymes produced and the sugars do not get broken down. If you find that drinking milk causes bloating, you may well be lactose-intolerant, but most people experiencing this problem can tolerate around 300ml daily.

Some people have an allergy to cow's milk due to the proteins casein, whey or albumin and this may manifest as bloating, diarrhoea, constipation, vomiting or rash as the body mounts an immune response. Others may have difficulty breaking down the proteins in cow's milk and may find goat's or sheep's milk easier to digest. Butter, which is mainly fat, does not generally cause any of the detrimental effects of dairy, but ghee is even healthier.

Sugar – how bad is it?

Sugars are simple carbohydrate molecules which all end in '-ose': fructose, glucose, maltose, lactose, galactose, dextrose, high-fructose corn syrup. Sugar is an 'empty calorie' food and is therefore not needed by the body and should be avoided in all its processed forms. It is also known that many cancer cells need an abundance of glucose to thrive (see Warburg effect, page 25). However, if cutting out carbohydrates, and hence sugars, were the complete answer, then dealing with cancer would be simple and of course this is not the case. But there is enough evidence to show it is an important factor in the fight against cancer and is certainly a driver of inflammation.

When we think of sugar we tend to think of the processed white powdered table variety or the assumed healthier choice, Demerara. Both of these are sucrose, made up of equal parts glucose to fructose. Sucrose can be metabolized efficiently by the body but sends our blood sugar soaring and is not good.

Fructose is increasingly used as a sucrose substitute as it does not affect blood-sugar levels in the same way, but it is still damaging to our bodies when consumed in large quantities and in the absence of sufficient glucose. While glucose suppresses parts of the brain that make us feel hungry, fructose does not and we are therefore far more likely to consume more. The fructose in natural, whole fruit is not bad because there it is combined with glucose, which aids its metabolism; it is also in a small enough amount that the body can handle it efficiently. Without glucose, fructose is rapidly absorbed by the gut and produces a significant inflammatory response before travelling to the liver to be metabolized into fat. A high intake can lead to non-alcoholic fatty liver disease which increases the risk of type 2 diabetes.

White flour and its products, and other starchy carbohydrates such as potatoes, break down upon digestion to glucose very quickly, causing an immediate and greater effect on blood sugar than even table sugar (see 'Blood-sugar control', below).

Sugar is extremely addictive. It hits the reward centre in our brain just like other addictive drugs and this releases large amounts of dopamine, which makes us feel good and leaves us craving more and more and more. I am a firm believer that a treat every now and then may be a good thing, but if you find it difficult to curb your sweet tooth you really need to learn to resist by having healthy alternatives in place for when you have a sugar craving. It is said that if you wait ten minutes a craving will dissipate, whereas true hunger won't. But it is only by abstinence that you can train your brain and tastebuds to let go of the cravings. The good thing is that when you stop eating so much sugar it very quickly tastes too sickly whenever you do eat it, and when you learn about some of the potential consequences of eating a diet filled with refined sugars and starches it can put you off so much that you really don't fancy it any more. Breaking old habits and undoing learned behaviour is the key.

The glycaemic index (GI) and blood-sugar control

When we eat or drink carbohydrates, glucose is released into the bloodstream and insulin takes it to our cells for energy. Any glucose not used by cells for energy is stored in the liver and as fat cells. This is why insulin is known as the fat-storage hormone.

The glycaemic index (GI) provides a ranking system which measures how the food you eat reacts in your body and the effect it has on blood glucose. Foods with a high GI value generally cause sharp increases in glucose and insulin. These include refined carbohydrates and sugars, which, when digested, release glucose almost immediately in very high amounts. When glucose spikes quickly the body panics and releases large amounts of insulin to deal with it. This rapid response is because high amounts of glucose are toxic to our cells, especially our brain cells.

Continually high levels of sugar can lead to glucose intolerance and diabetes, and high levels of insulin lead to increased amounts of insulin-like growth factor (IGF-1; see page 28) which may be implicated in the promotion of tumour growth. Most cancer cells require a large amount of glucose for energy (see 'Cellular respiration', page 25), therefore limiting intake makes sense.

In addition to the health consequences mentioned above, a rapid spike in glucose also means that our blood sugar crashes pretty quickly too. Low blood sugar can make us feel tired and irritable, and it can also lead us to crave more sugar. It is in this moment of weakness that we are likely to reach for unhealthy, sugar-loaded food.

A low-glycaemic diet includes foods that are more slowly converted into the body's preferred fuel of glucose, thus helping to stabilize blood-glucose levels. These include complex, unrefined carbohydrates, which contain plenty of fibre (see page 48), slowing digestive processes and the release of glucose. This means that the levels of insulin released and the uptake of glucose in our cells happens in a more controlled manner. Eating our carbohydrates alongside proteins and fats also helps to slow down the release of glucose because protein and fat take longer to digest. So if you do fancy a sugary treat, the best thing is to eat it as part of a meal or snack that includes foods from these groups.

You may also come across the term 'glycaemic load' (GL). This is a slightly more complex way of determining the effects of a food on blood glucose by taking into consideration the actual amount of carbohydrate in the food. You need to aim for low GL, but to be honest, once you grasp that, in general, the less processed a food is, the less effect it has on blood glucose, you can't go too far wrong. So when you are eating whole foods containing plenty of fibre alongside a balance of protein and fats, you can guarantee you will get a slower release of the glucose into your bloodstream than with processed foods.

Physical activity can help to control blood sugar by making your cells more sensitive to insulin. It also causes your muscle cells to take up more glucose, thus reducing the amount circulating around the body and available to any cancer cells. Regular exercise can have long-term beneficial effects on the balance of blood sugar. (See 'Exercise', page 93.)

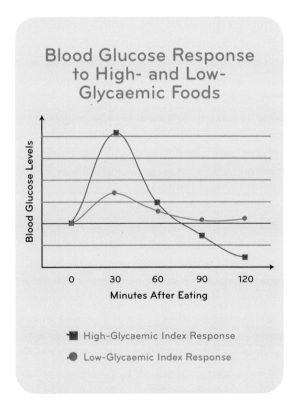

Blood Glucose Response to High- and Low-Glycaemic Foods

Blood Glucose Levels

Minutes After Eating

0   30   60   90   120

■ High-Glycaemic Index Response
● Low-Glycaemic Index Response

Foods to eat, foods to avoid

Low-glycaemic foods include whole, unrefined grains such as wholemeal bread, wholewheat pasta, brown rice and wholegrain cereals. These are the preferable starchy carbohydrates as they contain higher levels of fibre and nutrients.

Milk and fruit contain the natural sugars lactose and fructose respectively. These will not raise glucose levels in the same way as a spoonful of sugar, as there are other constituents such as fat and fibre which slow down digestion and glucose release. However, they should be eaten in moderation when following a low-GI diet. Green leafy vegetables and berry fruits are the best choices as they contain less sugar. Root vegetables such as carrots and parsnips are healthy but contain higher sugar levels.

The worst high-GI culprits are the highly refined carbohydrates such as white bread and pasta, refined breakfast cereals, biscuits, cakes, fizzy drinks and sugary juices, along with some foods we tend to think of as healthy, such as energy drinks, fruit juice, rice cakes, cornflakes and baked potatoes. However, as explained above, we can lower the glycaemic effects by combining these foods with fats and protein: for example, make a potato lower GI by adding some cheese or butter, or have some nut butter on your rice cake. Eat your dried fruit with some nuts and seeds, or add ground nuts or seeds to a smoothie for a lower glycaemic effect.

Anyone following a very low-carbohydrate diet (see Ketogenic Diet, page 106) and monitoring their blood-glucose levels will know that the body actually keeps it at a fairly consistent level of between 3.5 and 5.5mmol/l. This is because our cells do need some glucose and the body will release stored glucose in small amounts into the bloodstream. But by cutting back our carbohydrate intake and eating them in only their low-glycaemic form we maintain a flatter glycaemic response after consuming food. This healthier way of eating avoids the detrimental effects of spikes in blood glucose and insulin.

How much sugar is hiding in your food?

Sugars are everywhere in our processed foods, and if you are eating these foods you would be hard pressed to avoid consuming far too much. Don't be fooled by supposed health-food products labelled 'low fat' or 'free from': these need to be made palatable and what can do that better than sugar?

If you are buying processed food, read the label. One of the most important considerations after trans-fats is 'total carbohydrates', under which will be listed 'of which sugars' and 'fibre'. Always aim for foods with the highest fibre content, as this is not digested and will not affect blood sugar. The sugars listed may include natural sugars in milk or fruit, which aren't so bad. If you take the sugar and fibre amounts away from the total carbs you get an indication of the starches, which are actually sugars too. A good example is to look at the labels on cereal packets. Refined cereals have less fibre and higher sugar and carbohydrate levels, whereas a wholegrain variety has more fibre and less sugar and carbohydrate, making this the healthier option. Remember: higher sugars and starches in a refined form will cause a spike in blood sugar and insulin levels which is inflammatory and potentially cancer-enhancing.

THE LOW-DOWN ON SWEETENERS

The question of sweeteners is another minefield in the world of nutrition and can be very confusing. These are my thoughts after dissecting all the information and evidence.

Firstly, I am not a fan of sweeteners. They can be very sweet and I would always advocate that we try to train our tastebuds and brain to get used to less sweetness in our diet. Whatever form of sweetness it is, the more you have the more you crave.

However, where some sweetness is needed in our food, I would recommend that you use the most natural form of sweetener. One way of doing this is by adding fruit to breakfast cereals or dried fruit to home baking. When making recipes that require sugar, you can often cut the amount by at least half and still have great-tasting food. Remember that once you acclimatize your taste to less sugar you'll find regular sugar usage to be too sickly. In this book you will find some tasty recipes for baking without added refined sugars or sweeteners. Our recipes use healthier, nutrient-dense choices such as blackstrap molasses or date paste, coconut palm sugar and pure maple syrup.

Blackstrap molasses is a by-product of sugar-cane production that retains all the nutrient value of the plant, including many minerals such as iron, calcium, magnesium, manganese and potassium. It also contains significant amounts of vitamin B_6. This nutrient-dense food can be used in baking or is great as a sweetener for porridge. It has a very rich, treacly taste and may not be everyone's cup of tea.

Coconut sugar is made from the sap of the coconut palm and has a lower glycaemic index (see page 73) than honey or maple syrup but is low in fructose too, making it a healthier option. It also retains many nutrients, meaning that unlike ordinary sugar it is not just empty calories but has a taste and texture similar to brown sugar.

Maple syrup is relatively unprocessed and still retains plenty of mineral content. It contains less fructose than honey, which makes it a slightly healthier choice. Ensure you buy a good-quality, naturally processed brand. It may be an expensive option, but in my opinion it is worth spending that bit extra. A little can go a long way – and remember we shouldn't be overdoing it on the sugar front even with these healthier options.

Honey has a higher fructose to glucose content than sucrose but cannot be thought of as being any healthier unless you buy it in its raw form, in which case it has other benefits. Raw honey is not always easy to obtain and it is expensive, but because it is not heated, processed or pasteurized it retains all its natural vitamins, minerals and enzymes. This puts raw honey into the more nutrient-dense category, so seek it out from your local health food store or farmers' market. If you meet a local beekeeper, befriend him!

Incidentally, if you suffer from hay fever and you eat raw honey from your home area, you may find it relieves your symptoms by priming your immune system. But you do need to start eating it well before the season begins.

There are some sugar substitutes that are marketed as natural, healthy sweeteners, such as stevia, xylitol and agave syrup. Stevia is often promoted as the healthiest, but the most common brand is highly processed and not recommended. Natural green stevia powder and liquid is considered to be the best option. It does not affect blood-sugar levels, has no calories and is 300 times sweeter than sugar. Xylitol is a sugar alcohol that does not affect blood-sugar levels and has no calories. Agave syrup has a high fructose content and contains calories. It was thought to be a healthy alternative as it does not affect blood-sugar levels; however, it does raise blood-fructose levels which is now seen as problematic (see page 74).

These sweeteners can be useful to diabetics, but some research has suggested that the sweetness on the tongue triggers the pancreas and gut to release hormones such as insulin even when no sugar will reach the bloodstream. The mechanisms are not totally understood, but non-caloric sweeteners may have more knock-on effects than previously considered and could be detrimental to our health.

Other research has suggested that artificial sweeteners such as saccharin, sucralose and aspartame drive glucose intolerance in mice and humans by altering the intestinal bacteria. These have also been linked to certain cancers and a host of other disorders, although the studies have been refuted by many in the food and health industry. Known as non-calorific artificial sweeteners (NAS), they are often found in diet sodas, cereals and sugar-free desserts. As with all non-caloric sweeteners, they avoid digestion in the small intestine and therefore arrive intact in the colon. Here they appear to exert negative effects on our gut bacteria which in turn increase blood-sugar levels. Therefore it would seem that these sweeteners may be increasing type 2 diabetes and obesity – the very disease they are trying to protect against. More research needs to be done, especially on natural non-caloric sweeteners such as stevia and xylitol, as these may well have the same effect. In view of this, I would strike a note of caution on consuming too many non-caloric sweeteners.

Be aware that among the worst culprits for NAS are soft drinks and, contrary to popular belief, not just the diet ones. Drinks manufacturers are increasingly using NAS in sugar-laden drinks because they are cheaper than natural sugar. This means you are getting a double whammy of sugar and chemicals. It just goes to show how important it is to read the ingredients list. Pepsi have, however, recently bowed to pressure and are removing aspartame from their Diet Pepsi.

What is so wrong with gluten?

Gluten is a protein found in grains such as wheat, barley and rye and is the culprit in the autoimmune condition coeliac disease. It is diagnosed by testing for antibodies and taking a tiny biopsy from the gastro-intestinal tract during an endoscopy. Many gastroenterologists believe that a large number of people have undiagnosed coeliac disease. The symptoms are chronic diarrhoea, anaemia, weight loss, malnutrition and osteoporosis. Even those who test negative for the disease itself may still be extremely sensitive to gluten and these days many people without a diagnosis decide to follow a gluten-free diet, some because of an obvious gluten intolerance and others because they feel it is a healthier alternative to the usual wheat-laden foods. In relation to a cancer diagnosis, the less the body, especially the liver, is stressed the better. By reducing the amount of gluten in your diet you may well be supporting your immune system and lowering inflammatory processes in the body.

If you have coeliac disease then there must be total exclusion of gluten from your diet, and anyone who has symptoms that could suggest gluten sensitivity should see their GP to eliminate anything more serious. The problem is that many people are self-diagnosing and by eliminating gluten products they may leave themselves at risk of vitamin and fibre deficiency.

Gluten is present in many products, not just the obvious ones such as bread, cereals and pasta. It frequently appears as a binder, thickener or flavour enhancer, which makes it very difficult to eliminate from the diet completely. Gluten also makes our food chewy and tasty. There is a burgeoning 'gluten-free' industry, but to make these products as palatable as possible extra fat and sugar may be added, which renders them less healthy.

You may suspect gluten sensitivity but in fact have wheat intolerance, which is a different disorder although there is often a crossover in symptoms. Sometimes just reducing the amount of wheat you eat can make a difference to the way you feel, and diet-wise this is easier to manage. People often find that they can help to reduce the side-effects of treatment such as joint pain, neuropathy and brain fog by the elimination of wheat or gluten from their diet, but do see your GP for any necessary tests before you start to cut them out, as the antibody tests may not give an accurate picture if they are done once you have already reduced your intake.

Modern wheat has been bred for its high gluten content, but there are alternatives, some of which are listed below. These include some ancient grains, which are gaining in popularity as people recognize their health benefits, and some from other parts of the world where wheat is not predominant. Grains that are gluten-free are amaranth, quinoa, corn, buckwheat, millet, sorghum and rice – though rice can contain worrying levels of arsenic. All are very good sources of fibre. Alternatives to grain flours are coconut, rice, quinoa flour and ground almonds, all of which can be used in baking (see below).

Spelt versus modern wheat

Although it is a type of wheat, spelt contains less gluten than ordinary wheat and is a good alternative flour to keep in your kitchen cupboard. It is a primitive form of the grain and fell from favour when mass farming techniques were introduced in the mid-twentieth century. Modern wheat replaced it because it gave higher yields, was easier to thresh and possessed higher levels of gluten, giving it a greater rising ability in bread making.

Consumer desire for fluffier, lighter bread promoted the use of this high-gluten product still further, and this is what may lie behind the growing numbers of people with wheat intolerance or, worse still, gluten sensitivity and coeliac disease.

Spelt, with its strong husk, is naturally protected from insects, pollutants and disease. Wheat is less resistant to disease, and it therefore requires greater levels of pesticides and fungicides, with the result that it and its products are high in pesticide residues.

The chemical bonds holding the gluten protein together in spelt are more fragile than those found in modern wheat, making it more easily digestible. This means that, although spelt does contain gluten, it is generally better tolerated in wheat-sensitive individuals.

Spelt is a great form of fibre and has a high nutrient value. The flour can be used for tasty homemade bread and, because it has a more fragile form of gluten, it requires less kneading and proving time, so is quicker to make.

Barley

Another grain that fell out of fashion, barley is gaining in popularity again and is a useful addition to soups and stews. It can also be used as a replacement for risotto rice, although it will take longer to cook. You can buy wholegrain barley, which has the highest fibre and nutrient content; pearl barley, which is polished and less nutrient-rich; or pot barley, which falls between the two in terms of processing. Barley does contain gluten.

Buckwheat

This has no connection to wheat, but is a seed related to rhubarb and sorrel. It is gluten-free. Buckwheat grains can be made into porridge or added to soups to give texture, but rinse it thoroughly before using to remove any bitterness. Buckwheat flour is readily available and can be mixed with wholemeal flour for baking and making pancakes.

Amaranth

This is one of the earliest known plant foods and is gluten-free. It requires quite a bit of water when cooking: 6 cups water to 1 cup amaranth. Gently boil the amaranth for 15–20 minutes, rinse and then fluff it with a fork. Amaranth can be added to soups, salads and stir-fries, and amaranth flour can be used in baking.

Quinoa

Pronounced 'keen-wah', quinoa is actually a seed, not a grain. It is gluten-free and contains all the essential amino acids, making it a complete protein and a useful food for vegetarians. Quinoa needs to be rinsed well before cooking to remove the saponins, which produce a slightly bitter taste. It is excellent in casseroles, soups, stews, stir-fries and salads. The seeds are prepared in a similar way to rice and cook in about 15 minutes.

Millet

This is also a seed and is a staple food in Asia and Africa. It has a mild, sweet, nut-like flavour and is gluten-free. It is high in fibre and B vitamins and can be made into a creamy porridge or a fluffy whole grain like quinoa. When cooking millet, you will need 1 part millet to 2–3 parts water, depending on the consistency required. Once the water has come to a boil, lower the heat and let the millet simmer for 25 minutes with the lid on. Raw millet can be used in baking to add fibre or to thicken soups.

Kamut® (Khorasan wheat)

This is an excellent alternative to modern wheat because it has a higher nutrient profile. It contains 40 per cent more protein and it is also rich in magnesium, selenium and zinc. It has a natural sweetness and a nutty, buttery taste. When cooking Kamut®, it is best to soak the grain overnight. Use 3 parts water to 1 part Kamut®. Once the water has come to the boil, reduce the heat and allow the grain to simmer for 30–40 minutes, depending on how tender you like it to be. It is available as flour for baking too.

Chia

Native to Central and South America, chia seeds have gained a reputation as an ideal fuel for athletes because they are high in calories, a complete protein, rich in omega-3 fatty acids, and a good source of calcium, magnesium, manganese and phosphorus. They have a similar nutritional profile to flaxseeds, but do not have an outer shell and so can be digested without the need to grind them. Chia seeds also provide plenty of fibre and are therefore best introduced in small amounts (1–2 tbsp a day) to minimize gas and abdominal discomfort.

Chia seeds expand in size and become glutinous once exposed to moisture, making them a useful replacement binder for breadcrumbs and egg. If you are allergic to eggs you can use them as a substitute in baking – soak 1 tbsp chia seeds in 3 tbsp water, leave them for approximately 15 minutes until the water has been absorbed and the mixture is gel-like, then use in place of the egg in a recipe.

The most impressive aspect of chia seeds is that a 28g serving contains approximately 5g of important omega-3 fatty acids, which is more than double the amount in a serving of salmon. They therefore make a very beneficial addition to the diet of anyone who doesn't like oily fish.

Soya and other phytoestrogens

Soya is a cheap, high-protein food, often used as a filler and preservative in other foodstuffs, and it is literally everywhere. Take a look at almost every manufactured food product, including bread, and you will find it lurking; and, unless you buy organic, it is more than likely to be genetically modified (GM). GM soya has been found to have high residues of the herbicide glyphosate, which has been classified by the WHO as 'probably carcinogenic to humans'. What's more, an allergic reaction to soya is now very common because we are subjected to so much of it.

Soya is the subject of much debate in nutrition workshops, particularly amongst those who have a hormone-driven cancer. This is because soya has a high concentration of active phytoestrogens known as isoflavones which can mimic the activity of our natural oestrogens and modulate other steroid hormones; they therefore have the potential to stimulate hormone-related cancer cells.

Soya was initially thought to be protective of breast and prostate cancer due to the fact that people of Asian origin who had consumed it regularly throughout their lives had a low incidence of these diseases. If they moved to a Western country with a Western diet, they very quickly had the same incidence rate as others born there. Clearly there is some protective element in their diets, but it could be the amount of fish or seaweed they eat, not just the soya. Also, variations between individuals' gut microflora lead to further inconsistencies in studies.

Much of the thinking now, particularly for breast cancer, is that plant oestrogens have a very weak oestrogenic effect and when they bind to oestrogen receptors on cells they block those receptors, preventing the body's natural oestrogens from having a stronger stimulatory effect and therefore actually providing protection. Consuming some soya, then, would seem to be beneficial. In men, soya intake may decrease testosterone and other androgens, therefore possibly providing some protection against prostate cancer, but again this is not conclusive. For those taking Tamoxifen or Anastrozole therapy, phytoestrogens do not appear to interfere with activity and in animal models have been shown to enhance the effects, but I would still advise a moderate intake of no more than one serving a day.

Most studies conclude that if people start eating soya at a young age it may have a protective effect and if eaten in moderation it is safe. However, it has some other adverse effects, such as inhibiting the uptake of some minerals in the body due to its phytate content and possibly also affecting thyroid function. In many forms it is a highly processed food that does not resemble the type of soya that is part of the Asian diet. If you do eat soya, choose the fermented, less processed products such as tempeh, miso and natto (both of which are good for bones) or good-quality organic tofu. If you like to use soya milk, I would recommend this highly processed product only in moderation. It would be far better to use other non-dairy milk substitutes – see page 72.

Phytoestrogens occur naturally in a wide variety of plants, nuts and seeds, primarily in the form of lignans. Flaxseeds are a source of these, but again our gut bacteria need to convert them into active oestrogens which are not well absorbed by the gut and so they may have only a very weak oestrogenic effect (see 'Flaxseeds', page 61). They have been shown to inhibit aromatase, which synthesizes oestrogen in the body, and along with this they are healthy in many other respects too.

Individuals who have an oestrogen-dependent cancer or are at risk due to a familial history should not take any form of concentrated phytoestrogens – such as supplements – unless directed to do so by a health professional.

Alcohol

When alcohol and healthy eating are mentioned together people often justify alcohol consumption by quoting the health benefits of red wine. It is true that red wine contains the polyphenol resveratrol which is found in red grape skins and it is also true that this appears to have beneficial health properties, particularly for the heart. However, encouraging the drinking of alcohol is not a good idea. Plus you can get the resveratrol from simply eating the red grapes.

So what are the guidelines on alcohol consumption after a cancer diagnosis? Ideally, abstaining is best, especially during treatment when the liver has more than enough detoxifying to contend with. However, for many people a drink in the evening relaxes them and this in itself can be a health benefit. So if you like a drink, only have one, don't have it every night and don't binge-drink. Binge-drinking can significantly lower your immune system, albeit temporarily. Alcohol has also been shown to increase circulating IGF-1, which is implicated in cancer-cell proliferation (see page 28).

Recent research has found that just three alcoholic drinks a day can cause liver cancer. There is also strong evidence that alcohol is linked to breast, bowel, mouth and throat, and oesophageal cancer.

Essential Wellbeing

Gut health

'All disease begins in the gut' – Hippocrates

As a nutritional therapist, I believe that gut health is key to overall wellbeing and this is certainly backed up by research. Our gut is like a hose that runs through the body, stretching from the oral cavity to the anus, and its lining is the interface between the outside world and our internal environment. When it is working well it does a fantastic job, but all too often damage to our gut lining or to the micro-organisms within it means it can let us down. Unfortunately, many things can cause damage to our gut or at least cause it to work less efficiently. Stress, what we consume, illness, aging and antibiotics can all have a direct effect; add to that treatments such as chemotherapy, radiotherapy and other medications, and our gut will struggle to stay healthy. Therefore before any treatment is started it is a good idea to ensure that your gut is as healthy as possible.

Having a clear understanding of the workings of our gut and the cells that line it can motivate us to give it some tender, loving care.

Leaky gut

The term 'leaky gut' is used to describe the gut when it has become highly permeable. The cells in the gut are held together tightly and they are very selective in what they allow to be filtered through into the bloodstream. When this barrier is damaged or stressed through medication, poor diet, stress or surgery, the cells become loose, allowing undesirable or large molecules to leak between the cells and cause problems. These rogue molecules can then trigger an immune response and cause allergic reactions or food intolerances. Foods which help to heal the gut, maintain gut integrity and keep it healthy should be consumed at all times (see the table on page 98).

Food intolerances

A damaged gut may result in food intolerances manifesting during treatment. One of the most common is lactose intolerance. Lactose is milk sugar and it requires the enzyme lactase to break it down. Symptoms of lactose intolerance are bloating and stomach pain after consuming dairy. Generally around 300ml of milk a day can be tolerated, and live yoghurts, traditionally made cheeses and butter (particularly clarified butter) have low levels of lactose and so may not cause symptoms.

A compromised gut may also struggle with breaking down gluten. Reducing the amount you consume may be helpful and the easiest way to do this is by consuming fewer wheat products (see page 78).

If you suspect food intolerances or allergies, these should be identified to avoid additional stress to the body. Symptoms may include bloating, a skin reaction, diarrhoea, stomach pain or a runny nose and sneezing. The symptoms of a food intolerance tend to manifest over time and may come on many hours after eating the offending food, whereas a food allergy causes a rapid response by the immune system.

Food allergies are potentially serious and the problem food should be eliminated from the diet. Food intolerances may be more difficult to pinpoint and the only way to be absolutely sure is to eliminate suspected foods in a systematic way and reintroduce them individually in order to monitor any response. A food and symptom diary can be a helpful way of identifying trigger foods (see pages 270–71). Beware of eliminating whole food groups from your diet without seeking advice from a health professional.

Gut microbiota

I have previously mentioned the importance of a healthy terrain in the body and I would certainly include the gut microbiota in this. These are the bacteria that live in our gut, which contribute to about 2kg of our body weight and which total at least 20 per cent more than the living cells in the rest of our body – you could say that we are an ambulatory system for bacteria! Having always been of great importance in nutritional therapy, the health of our gut microbiota is now considered very much a part of mainstream medicine. In fact, we ignore it at our peril, because these microbiota are so important for healthy digestion, metabolism, our immune system and nutritional status. They also have a vital role to play in reducing inflammation (see page 27). Those beneficial little microbes synthesize B vitamins and help our gut absorb calcium and vitamin K, both vital for healthy bones. They also help to break down excess cholesterol, hormones and toxins, allowing them to bind with fibres and enabling them to be excreted.

Recent research has identified a link between gut microbiota and depression. We already know that our gut communicates with our brain and vice-versa, but it has now been seen that the brain influences gut and immune functions that shape the make-up of our microbiota, which in turn make compounds, including chemicals known as neurotransmitters, which act on the brain.

Non-beneficial microbes can work against our health. They can cause digestive upset and increase an enzyme in the gut called beta-glucuronidase which breaks apart bound oestrogens and allows them to be re-absorbed into the circulatory system. So right from diagnosis, through treatment and out the other side, the gut microbiota should be nurtured and fuelled to keep them healthy and prevent any imbalance occurring.

Among the worst culprits in upsetting the delicate balance of our gut microbiota are oral antibiotics. These can eliminate many of our healthy bacteria, so it is essential that after a course of antibiotics we give our gut a helping hand in re-colonizing with the good bacteria it needs. Non-organic animal products such as meat and dairy may also contain antibiotics which upset the balance.

Eating plenty of prebiotic foods encourages the survival of beneficial microbiota. These are foods which contain certain soluble fibres, such as fructo-oligosaccharides, that our microbiota love to break down and use as fuel to thrive. The highest concentrations of prebiotic fibre are found in Jerusalem artichokes, leeks, onions, beans, peas, lentils and oats.

Probiotic foods are those containing the beneficial bacteria we want to encourage in the gut and these are found in fermented foods such as bio-yoghurt, sauerkraut, kimchi and miso. It is also worth taking a probiotic supplement after a course of antibiotics. The best ones have a broad spectrum of bacteria and can be bought in a health store or pharmacy, or may be prescribed by your GP.

If you have had investigative tests such as a colonoscopy you will have cleared the colon in preparation for this procedure. If you have any sort of bacterial overgrowth in the gut you may find symptoms are relieved initially, but it is vital that you repopulate your gut with the right bacteria in the days and weeks following the procedure, which will have left it open to colonization by bacteria you really don't want to encourage. Be aware also that a high-sugar and processed-food diet is just what non-beneficial microbiota love to munch on, so don't give them the chance: make sure you stick to the low-sugar, high-fibre foods our friendly microbiota love and in turn they will reward you well. Again, a probiotic supplement may be a good idea at this time.

We are also in danger of damaging our internal environment by using products containing antibacterial agents such as soaps, toothpastes, cleaning products and kitchen utensils, plus being exposed to agricultural chemicals like fungicides and herbicides.

Love your liver

Do so because it works extremely hard to keep you healthy. The liver has many functions within the body and is consequently one of the most overworked organs, but it has the amazing capacity to regenerate, even after 75 per cent of it has been removed. It is responsible for manufacturing bile, regulating blood sugar, making and breaking down hormones and cholesterol, processing all foods, nutrients, alcohol and drugs, and neutralizing environmental toxins. Ensuring a healthy gut (see above) is crucial to supporting the liver, as the fewer the toxins, hormones and cholesterol absorbed through the gut, the easier the job of the liver.

We are subjected to an increasing number of toxic compounds in our everyday life, from the air we breathe to what we ingest. An individual's ability to detoxify is a key factor in overall health, and the food we eat has a greater influence on our liver than many people would believe. We are all aware that alcohol stresses our liver, but how aware are we that high-sugar foods damage it significantly too?

We are also probably unaware how much influence certain compounds in our food can have on our liver enzymes, either slowing down or speeding up the detoxification process.

Naringenin, found in high levels in grapefruit juice, is a good example. It can interfere with the blood levels of certain pharmaceutical drugs by inhibiting the clearance of the drug by the liver. I would therefore recommend that you never take any form of medication along with grapefruit juice. On the other hand, green leafy vegetables, dark berries and green tea have been found to be particularly supportive of optimal detoxification.

The importance of caring for your liver during cancer treatment cannot be overstated. Liver function is checked throughout treatment and if raised enzymes indicate that the liver isn't coping, then treatment is stopped. Luckily, supporting your liver through a nutrient-dense diet can be very beneficial. Nutrients are crucial to its functioning and the detoxification process requires the help of certain vitamins and minerals, such as B vitamins, zinc, magnesium, iron, selenium and many antioxidants.

An adequate supply of protein is important too, as many of the detoxification pathways are protein-based and require a ready supply of essential amino acids. We cannot store protein and therefore a consistent intake is needed in our daily diet.

Avoid large amounts of fructose derived from processed foods, as recent research has revealed the toxic effects this can have on the liver. Isolated fructose, found in products such as sweetened and concentrated drinks, energy drinks, sweeteners and many other processed foods, has a particular effect on metabolism which may lead to damaging free fatty acids being deposited in the liver. This does not appear to occur, however, when vegetables and fruit are eaten in their natural form in plentiful amounts; in fact, it is these very foods, when eaten in variety, that help maintain a balanced detoxification system.

CHEMICAL OVERLOAD

Numbers of cancer cases are increasing year on year and it would be short-sighted to ignore the fact that the ever-growing array of chemicals in our environment is probably having an influence. In fact, there is plenty of evidence that chemicals such as parabens used in cosmetics and toiletries, bisphenol A found in plastic bottles, food-can lining and till receipts, and phthalates in nail varnish and liquid soaps (to name just a few) have an influence on hormonally related cancers such as breast cancer and prostate cancer. These chemicals are xenoestrogens, which can mimic our body's natural oestrogens and are referred to as endocrine disruptors. It is argued that the amounts in such products are so low that they are not a cause for concern, but what is not understood is the exact way they work within the body; what level of exposure is needed to have an effect; whether exposure when we are young is worse; and the effects of being subjected to a cocktail of different xenoestrogens. New chemicals are trialled for safety as individual entities and interactions with other regularly used chemicals are not researched.

The range of ways in which we are exposed to xenoestrogens is wide – pollution, food and drink packaging, pharmaceuticals, pesticides, detergents, cosmetics, furnishings, food additives, electrical equipment . . . Frightening, isn't it? And there are whole rafts of other chemicals and environmental factors that have been shown to be carcinogenic too.

Worrying over things about which we can do nothing just induces unnecessary stress. What we need is to have faith in our body's ability to restore balance, but we must support it where possible. Be discerning about the food you eat, the cosmetics, deodorants, bath, shower, hair and cleaning products you buy. Avoid drinking water from plastic bottles and do not re-use the bottles. If you have new furniture or carpet, ventilate the room as much as possible initially to reduce the levels of toxic fire-retardant, also known to be an endocrine disruptor. Some people believe you should also avoid using electronic devices too much. The Environmental Working Group (ewg.org), an American online resource, has plenty of useful information to support a healthier lifestyle by reducing exposure to carcinogens.

Building healthy bones

You are very likely to be prescribed steroids during your treatment and if you have to use them for a long time your medical team will talk to you about the increased risk of osteoporosis. Some chemotherapy may also contribute to calcium loss, therefore looking after your bones is very important. Many people worry that if they cut out or cut down on dairy then they will struggle to provide their body with enough calcium, but there are many other non-dairy sources of this important mineral.

BEST NON-DAIRY SOURCES OF CALCIUM
In descending order:

Sardines/mackerel (canned), with bones

Greens (lightly cooked)

Kale (lightly cooked)

Rhubarb (lightly cooked)

Spinach (lightly cooked)

Almonds

Pink salmon (canned), with bones

Oysters

Beet greens, leaves and stems
  (lightly cooked)

Amaranth

Quinoa

Brazil nuts

Scallops

Sesame seeds

Tofu

Shrimps

Blackstrap molasses

Okra pods

Brussels sprouts

Broccoli (lightly cooked)

Asparagus (fresh, lightly cooked)

Butter beans (cooked)

Green beans (cooked)

Cabbage (fresh, lightly cooked)

Pak choi

Carrots (cooked)

Parsnips (cooked)

Onions (cooked)

Tomatoes (canned, solids and liquid)

Red kidney beans (cooked)

Lentils (cooked)

Chickpeas (cooked)

Wheatgerm

Oats

Oranges

Hazelnuts

Cauliflower

Celery

Turnip

Olives

Parsley

Peas (cooked)

Grapefruit

Kiwi

Figs, dried (uncooked)

Pears (raw)

Raisins

Sunflower seeds

Eggs

Milk alternatives with added calcium

- Nutrients good for bone rebuilding are calcium (see opposite), vitamin D (see page 62), vitamin K (leafy green vegetables, natto, miso), magnesium (nuts, seeds, leafy green vegetables, fish, beans and pulses, whole grains), boron (chickpeas, nuts, vegetables), copper (nuts, shellfish, offal), manganese (tea, nuts, grains, vegetables), zinc (meat, shellfish, dairy, whole grains), and silicon (fruit, vegetables, whole grains).

- Vitamin D aids the absorption of calcium. Safely expose your skin to sufficient sunlight, responsible for making vitamin D, during the summer months (read about vitamin D on page 62). Remember the sun's rays can penetrate cloud cover – which is just as well if you live in the UK!

- Avoid excessive salt (more than 1 tsp daily) in your diet, as this leaches calcium from your bones.

- Eat an alkaline-based diet which focuses on vegetables, fruits, nuts and legumes. An acidic environment means that calcium may be re-absorbed from bone to increase alkalinity.

- Avoid all soft drinks containing phosphates, as these also leach calcium from your bones.

- Avoid refined sugars and starches. Also avoid artificial sweeteners as these create an acid environment. If you need to sweeten foods then blackstrap molasses is a good choice as it contains many minerals, including plenty of calcium.

- Canned fish such as sardines and salmon *with bones* are a high source of calcium: the calcium is in the bones and the canning process softens them, making them more easily digested.

- Green leafy vegetables are high in calcium but it is not so readily absorbed as that from animal sources. Cooking the vegetables helps calcium absorption.

Acid/alkaline balance

The pH scale measures the level of acidity or alkalinity in a substance or solution. The desired pH for the human body is 7.4, which is slightly alkaline and optimal for body functions. Our stomach pH is much more acidic – 3.5 or below – so that it can break down foods, and our urine should be between 6.5 and 7.25, though this will vary according to our hydration levels, foods consumed, pollution, toxicity and even stress levels.

The body works hard to maintain optimal pH levels, but we should give it a helping hand by eating a diet that has an alkalizing effect. Generally, foods that are high in minerals such as potassium, sodium, magnesium, calcium, zinc, copper and iron are alkalizing, so a diet rich in vegetables and fruits is the best way to achieve the correct balance.

Junk foods high in sugars and unhealthy trans-fats can cause the blood to move towards a slightly lower, more acidic pH. Although blood pH is tightly controlled between 7.35 and 7.4, small fluctuations towards acidity can have profound negative consequences for the body by affecting enzyme activity, protein structure, cellular processes and hormone function, and impairing insulin sensitivity and glucose tolerance. A more acid environment in our body tissues also damages mitochondrial function (see page 25), destabilizes our genes and may encourage tumour growth. Protein foods, dairy, grains and caffeinated drinks tend to be acidic too, but this effect is negated when combined with alkaline vegetables and fruit.

Pack plenty of foods from the following list into your diet to ensure a healthy terrain and a hostile environment for cancer cells.

FOODS TO SUPPORT ALKALINITY

Vegetables

Asparagus
Broccoli
Brussels sprouts
Cabbage
Carrot
Cauliflower
Celery
Cucumber
Dulce
Garlic
Green beans
Kale
Lettuce
Mushrooms
Onions
Parsley
Parsnips
Peas
Peppers
Potato
Pumpkin
Radishes
Sea vegetable
Spinach
Spirulina
Sprouts (from seeds)
Sweet potatoes
Tomatoes
Watercress

Fruits

Apples
Apricots
Avocados
Bananas
Dates
Figs
Grapes
Mango
Peaches
Pears
Prunes
Raisins
Raspberries
Rhubarb
Strawberries
Tangerines
Tropical fruits
Watermelon

Acidic fruits with an alkalizing effect

Berries
Cantaloupe
Cherries
Cranberries
Currants
Grapefruit
Honey melon
Lemons
Limes
Nectarines
Oranges
Pineapples
Plums

Grains

Amaranth
Brown rice
Buckwheat
Kamut®
Millet
Quinoa
Spelt

Beans and legumes

Butter beans
Cannellini beans
Chickpeas
Kidney beans
Lentils
Mung beans
Pinto beans
Soy beans

Nuts and seeds

Almonds
Brazil nuts
Chestnuts
Coconut
Flaxseeds
Hazelnuts
Macadamia nuts
Pumpkin seeds
Sesame seeds
Sunflower seeds

Condiments and spices

Apple cider vinegar
Cinnamon
Curry
Ginger
Miso
Turmeric

Good Mood Foods

The gut is often referred to as the 'second brain'. It is linked to the brain via the vagus nerve, and the gut and brain communicate continuously through the enteric nervous system, hormones and the immune system. The chemicals responsible for this communication – known as neurotransmitters – are made in our gut, so if the gut is damaged or irritated in any way this can have an immediate impact on our mood and our ability to deal with stress. This could explain why our emotions and anxieties are so often felt in the gut; we even say we have a 'gut feeling' about something.

Our neurotransmitters serotonin, dopamine, adrenaline, noradrenaline and gamma-aminobutyric acid (GABA) are synthesized in a complex process through the action of enzymes which are dependent on a plentiful supply of specific minerals and vitamins, particularly magnesium, zinc and vitamin B$_6$. Nutrient deficiencies will impair the production and function of these neurotransmitters, all of which have very specific and important functions within the body. For instance, serotonin stabilizes our mood and promotes sleep; dopamine enhances our drive and motivation; GABA helps us to relax; and acetylcholine aids memory. They are also depleted by an excess of refined, processed foods, alcohol, caffeine and other stimulants.

Eating carbohydrates, which break down into glucose, will supply our cells – particularly our brain cells – with energy. No doubt we are all aware of how sapped of energy, irritable and foggy-brained we feel when our blood sugar is low. Consuming slow-release, unrefined carbohydrates helps to regulate blood-sugar swings and keep our mood on a more even keel. Refined carbohydrates, on the other hand, give us a quick fix of energy which just as quickly plummets, leading to fluctuating blood-sugar levels which are liable to cause mood swings. People consuming a low-carb, high-fat Ketogenic Diet (page 106) often find that it has a stabilizing effect on mood and energy when the brain switches to being fuelled by ketones.

Protein is an important nutrient for good mood, as tryptophan, an essential amino acid (see page 90), makes serotonin in the body. Serotonin is our most important 'feel-good' neurotransmitter and maintaining a supply of it in the body is the basis of many antidepressant drugs. Although tryptophan converts to serotonin, it needs to be eaten in abundance relative to other amino acids in order to be utilized otherwise the body directs it down another pathway. Eating complex carbs alongside a high-protein source of tryptophan enhances its absorption. The main sources of tryptophan are meat (especially turkey), fish, eggs, dairy and whole grains, but eating many of the vegetarian options from the list below will supply you with both tryptophan and carbohydrate.

There are a few foods, such as avocado, bananas, plums, pineapples, kiwis, plantain, tomatoes and walnuts, which naturally contain serotonin, but unfortunately this is unlikely to reach the brain.

5-HTP is a derivative of tryptophan and can be bought in supplement form. Research has found it to be as beneficial as SSRIs (selective serotonin reuptake inhibitors), drugs used to treat depression, but larger studies are needed to determine dosage levels, so it is best to take this supplement under the guidance of a nutritional therapist. It should never be taken alongside antidepressants.

Healthy essential fats such as omega-3 can help brain function and people with depression are often found to have a deficiency. Trans-fats found in processed foods can block the uptake of these good omega fats. (See pages 45–6.)

TOP VEGETARIAN SOURCES OF TRYPTOPHAN

Food	Portion size	Amount of tryptophan/portion
Kidney beans	170g	180mg
Rolled oats	85g	175mg
Lentils	200g	160mg
Chickpeas	200g	140mg
Pumpkin seeds	30g	120mg
Sunflower seeds	30g	100mg
Baked potato with skin	1 large	75mg
Tahini (sesame seed paste)	1 tbsp	56mg
Brazil nuts	25g	50mg
Almonds	25g	40mg
Walnuts	25g	40mg

B vitamins are the most important vitamins for lifting mood. A deficiency can lead to tiredness and feeling depressed or irritable. Vitamin B_6 particularly supports the production and function of serotonin. Good sources of B vitamins are meat, fish, dairy and whole grains.

Niacin is a B vitamin which can be made in the body from tryptophan. As we want our body to convert tryptophan to serotonin rather than getting side-tracked by a need for niacin, a good intake is essential. Liver, poultry, fish, whole grains, eggs, dairy, peanuts and avocados are good sources of niacin.

Folate is another B vitamin that influences mood. It can easily become depleted, particularly as we age. To ensure a good intake, eat foods such as liver and other offal, green leafy vegetables, nuts, eggs, bananas, oranges and pulses.

A deficiency in iron can result in anaemia, where we have low levels of haemoglobin which carries oxygen in the blood. This can make us feel very tired and lethargic and is one of the first things to test for if you are feeling this way. Red meat, poultry, fish, eggs, beans, spinach and some dried fruit will provide iron. Eat these foods along with vitamin C-rich fruits and vegetables to enhance your absorption of iron. Zinc, another mineral obtained from similar food sources, plays an important role in the regulation of neurotransmitters and there is some evidence to show that a deficiency may predispose a person to eating disorders.

So we can see that a diet lacking in nutrients leaves a person susceptible to low mood. Eating an array of nutrient-dense foods will also help to protect the brain from damaging free radicals (see page 26), assist in incorporating essential fatty acids into the brain and help to convert tryptophan to serotonin.

Don't forget that exercise increases the release of endorphins, which work to enhance our mood and also act as natural pain killers. (See page 93.)

Foods that trick the brain

Caffeine, chocolate, alcohol, nicotine, foods high in sugar, and chemical additives all have a stimulatory effect on the brain. If consumed in excess, they can stimulate it to the extent that it becomes less sensitive to the body's own neurotransmitters and less able to produce healthy patterns of activity. When the brain is flooded with artificial stimulants, the receptors on our brain cells respond by closing down until the excess is metabolized away. A vicious circle can ensue, because the brain then needs more stimuli to have an effect, resulting in cravings.

Consuming a diet as close to nature as possible ensures a natural balance of any stimulants and ensures that there are no nasty additives.

Cooking Methods

Slow and gentle cooking methods are the best for most food. Cooking meat at the high temperatures used in grilling, frying and barbecuing causes the formation of carcinogenic compounds such as heterocyclic amines (HCAs) and polycyclic aromatic hydrocarbons (PAHs). These have been linked to some cancers, possibly due to the damaging effects they might have on our DNA. We probably need to eat an awful lot of these compounds for them to have a significant detrimental effect on our health, but it is still worth bearing in mind and in general sticking to slower methods of cooking protein-rich foods such as meat and fish. Great alternatives are stews, casseroles and slow pot roasts. Incidentally, if you marinade meat and fish in spices or rub garlic into the flesh before cooking on a high heat the production of the carcinogenic compounds is reduced.

Smoked foods should be eaten in moderation, as the smoking process causes carcinogens to form.

Carbohydrate-rich foods containing sugars and starches also produce carcinogenic compounds when baked or fried at high temperatures. These are known as acrylamides and are found in many processed, pre-cooked goods such as biscuits, crackers and crispbreads, French fries, crisps, bread and even some baby products. Oven chips fare particularly badly mainly because they are treated with a sugar solution, partly cooked and then cooked again at home. Cigarette smoke and roasted coffee also contain significant amounts of acrylamides. Studies have shown that high levels of acrylamides in the blood increase the risk of developing cancer, but research in humans is limited.

As with meat, it is best to avoid grilling or frying carbohydrate at a high temperature. Brown toast only lightly, and avoid burnt foods. Bake at lower temperatures where possible – see our recipe for crackers, page 159.

When sautéing vegetables such as onions, just cook them gently and never heat the cooking oil to smoking point. Steaming vegetables is the best way to conserve water-soluble vitamins such as vitamin C. It is cheap to buy a simple steamer to fit on top of a regular saucepan, but electric steamers are available too. Whether boiling or steaming, the key is not to over-cook your vegetables, as some important plant chemicals and nutrients may be lost; for instance, the important anti-cancer compound sulforaphane found in cruciferous vegetables such as kale, cabbage and broccoli is destroyed when over-cooked.

The use of a microwave is somewhat controversial. I would advocate never using it for actually cooking food, only for the convenience of reheating. When heating food, stir it and let it sit for a couple of minutes before you eat it to allow the heat to distribute and ensure there are no cold spots where bacteria could lurk. Microwave ovens use radiation, zapping the food with high-frequency waves of heat, which causes changes to the molecular structure of the food. It has been suggested that this may make it harder for the body to digest and absorb the nutrients, although this has not been proved.

Eat Mindfully

Mindfulness is a word that pops up a lot nowadays (see page 125) and it can certainly be applied to eating. When we eat mindfully – in other words with an increased awareness – we gain a deeper connection with our food, our senses are heightened and our food is better digested. Research has shown that mindful eating can help with weight management and digestive problems.

Enhancing digestion allows us to gain more nutrients from our food. The digestive process begins in the mouth, so chewing your food slowly and thoroughly starts to break it down before you swallow. Enzymes in the mouth also work on the food to break it down further. This is particularly important if your gut is working less than perfectly, as it reduces some of the digestive burden. Chewing also increases the surface area of insoluble fibres in the food, enabling them to bind to toxins in the gut and so eliminate them more efficiently.

We tend to eat more quickly when we are stressed, so make sure you eat in a calm manner, seated at a table and not whilst on the move or working at your desk. Take time out for meals, maybe making it a social event as this can often lead to more relaxed eating.

When we are on the go or stressed our body diverts the blood supply needed to digest our food to our muscles or brain. Also eating quickly and less mindfully does not allow time for the brain to receive signals telling us when we have had enough, therefore potentially leading us to eat more than we need.

Exercise

There is plenty of research to show that regular exercise of at least three hours a week can be beneficial for those with a cancer diagnosis. Exercise is seen to lower hormone levels, balance blood sugar, reduce inflammation, support the immune system, keep the bowel regular, enhance circulation and increase oxygen levels. This will all be helping your healthy cells and hampering the cancer cells.

Whilst it is sometimes difficult to exercise when you are feeling fatigued and anxious, getting out for a walk can give your energy levels a boost and make you feel significantly brighter. If you are really struggling, even a little armchair exercise is better than nothing at all. Some of the gentler exercises such as yoga, tai chi or qigong can be good for clearing the mind.

If you feel up to it, regular periods of more intense physical activity in short bursts can be beneficial. Incorporate some skipping, dancing or jogging on the spot, if you can, and build it into your week or day on a regular basis. Those with greater fitness levels during treatment seem to experience fewer side-effects.

EXERCISE AFTER CANCER: THE EVIDENCE

Carolyn Garritt, Personal Trainer

There is a broad and rapidly growing body of evidence about the benefits of physical activity to people with cancer. In the UK, Macmillan Cancer Support produced the Move More campaign – a series of projects and interventions that provides very specific yet wide-ranging information on exercise and its relevance to cancer recurrence rates and to helping people manage the consequences of cancer treatment.

Their report 'Physical activity the underrated wonder drug' is a very useful synthesis of the evidence that supported the campaign and some of the interventions that arose from it. Macmillan also provide an evidence guide for those commissioning services and a motivating and creative information pack available free to anyone wishing to begin exercising.

One of the clinicians who is a key driving force in the Move More campaign is Professor Robert Thomas, a consultant oncologist at Addenbrooke's Hospital and clinical teacher at Cambridge University. He has written widely on the links between lifestyle and cancer outcomes, and is currently conducting the world's largest prospective lifestyle study in men with prostate cancer.

Professor Thomas designed the UK's first formal training course for fitness professionals who work with people recovering from cancer and this is now a nationally accredited qualification (Level 4 Exercise in Cancer Rehabilitation). It allows personal trainers and fitness instructors to study to a level where they understand the effects of cancer and its treatments on the body so that they can adapt exercise programmes accordingly.

4 Coping with Common Side-effects of Cancer and Its Treatment

MANY, BUT NOT ALL, PEOPLE with cancer experience one or more of the following side-effects in varying degrees of severity, as a result of either the cancer itself or from treatments and medication. A body well nourished by food, exercise and mindset stands more chance of combating some of these side-effects and creating an environment which optimizes the benefits of treatment.

Eliminate Stress – Easier Said Than Done!

If you or a loved one has just had a cancer diagnosis it can seem pretty insensitive if someone advises you to deal with any stress issues. However, it is something that needs to be faced and strategies thought through, because stress does have significant consequences through the body releasing inflammatory chemicals. Read the section on mindfulness (page 125) as this can be an excellent approach to addressing anxiety and stress.

Cancer-related Fatigue

Cancer can be absolutely draining, physically, mentally and emotionally. This is most likely due to inflammatory processes, metabolic changes in cancer cells and altered energy production. Add to that the toxicity of treatment, along with anxiety, poor sleep,

possibly a reduced intake of food (see pages 96 and 101) and reduced nutrient absorption, and it is no wonder that some people describe the fatigue as overwhelming and affecting every part of their life.

During chemotherapy you may find that a pattern emerges of when the treatment most depletes your energy reserves. This is usually during the first few days, after which it gradually improves until the next round. With radiation the fatigue tends to build up as treatment goes on.

If the fatigue seems excessive and you are not coping, discuss it with your medical team. There may be another underlying cause such as a thyroid imbalance, anaemia or depression.

Ways to reduce cancer-related fatigue:

• Improve nutrient intake and blood-sugar control (see pages 52 and 73).

• Stay as active as possible. Think about what form of exercise would suit you best and plan a schedule. Short, regular walks can often be a good boost and are easy to organize.

• Try to get about seven or eight hours of good-quality sleep at night. Ensure your bedroom is dark to boost your melatonin levels – this will help to regulate your circadian rhythm.

• You may want to schedule some naps throughout the day: keep them short, rather than sleeping for too long and disrupting your sleep pattern.

- Attend a stress-management class.

- Organize help with meals or other chores. If you know the times you are likely to feel extra fatigue during treatment, you can plan ahead and arrange help.

Weight Loss and Cachexia

Weight loss is a common issue for those with cancer. It is mainly due to cachexia, which is the breakdown of skeletal muscle mass. The primary cause is abnormal metabolism brought on by an increase in inflammatory chemicals released by both the tumour and the body's reaction to it (see 'Inflammation', page 27). The result is loss of appetite (see page 96), often due to feeling full early on in a meal, and fatigue. Weight loss usually follows. Simply eating more food to try to regain weight is not the answer, as it is the underlying factors that need to be addressed.

Concern over a patient losing too much weight often leads to an oncology team advising on increased amounts of high-energy, sugary, fatty foods. The reason is that glucose-rich, high-glycaemic foods give a quick release of energy without calories being used up in the digestive process (see page 73). However, excessive sugar and unhealthy fats are not the answer; instead, there are plenty of very healthy high-energy foods that can give you the extra calories you need.

Build-up drinks (see page 156) can be a helpful way to increase calorie intake, as they are easy to sip and digest and often a liquid meal is easier to tolerate than solids. You can pack in lots of the extra macronutrients – fats, protein and carbs – and tailor your drink to your particular needs and taste. The addition of whey, hemp or pea protein powder provides the branched-chain amino acids leucine, isoleucine and valine which can help to ameliorate cachexia symptoms and improve body composition and quality of life. If using protein powder, try to buy a good-quality, non-denatured, additive-free product, which you will find in a good health food shop or online.

Concentrate on increasing dietary protein by eating fish (especially oily fish), meat, chicken, eggs and dairy, along with vegetarian sources such as beans, pulses, nuts and rice for beneficial amino acids. Add in plenty of extra healthy fats such as coconut or olive oil, dairy (butter and cream), nut and seed butters, and oils.

Use our Super Stock (page 256) as a hot drink or as a base for a high-protein fat-and-vegetable soup; it is packed with proteins which help to maintain muscle mass and reduce inflammation. The gelatine in the broth promotes healthy digestion, so all in all it is wonderfully healing and comforting.

Ensure your soups are as energy-dense as possible by choosing high-energy root vegetables such as pumpkin, squash, sweet potato, swede, turnip, celeriac, carrots and parsnips. Adding anti-inflammatory herbs and spices can help dampen down inflammatory responses and oxidative stress, and also improve taste (see 'Culinary Herbs and Spices', pages 64–8). If you can't face a meal served to you on a plate, you can always liquidize it, as giving your digestive system a helping hand means you use up fewer calories in breaking down the food. Interestingly, though, soup has been shown to keep you fuller for longer than solid food so, because you want to increase your intake of food, have it little and often throughout the day.

Fish oils contain the anti-inflammatory omega-3 fatty acid eicosapentaenoic acid (EPA) and have been shown to prevent the loss of muscle mass, especially if taken early on before cachexia really takes a hold. The cannabinoids in medicinal cannabis are known to have appetite-stimulating effects and may be helpful to those suffering from cachexia, but trials have failed to prove this (see page 119).

To help build muscle, do not exercise on an empty stomach and make sure you are well hydrated. Eat a protein-rich meal or have a build-up smoothie within a couple of hours of exercising to repair and support the exercised muscle.

Poor Appetite

After a cancer diagnosis it is not surprising that many people lose their appetite through increased anxiety and stress. Whilst I am of course advocating a healthy diet, it's also true that sometimes simply eating what you feel like does you good. When my son Sebastian was feeling extra poorly all he ever really wanted was an awful, plastic-looking microwavable pizza full of carcinogens, additives and trans-fats. I really felt that I couldn't always deny him, so I found ways of incorporating good stuff to offset the nasties!

To increase appetite and calories:

• Find ways of reducing anxiety and stress. Increase your exercise levels if you are able, although it does not have to be strenuous. A walk, especially in the countryside, can increase endorphin levels, making us feel more relaxed and perhaps stimulate our appetite too.

• Establish an eating schedule and plan ahead for days when you have hospital visits to ensure you have a ready supply of nutrient-dense, appetizing food and don't have to rely on hospital cafeterias and vending machines.

• Eat little and often. This may help you to consume more food and also means you are not faced with large, off-putting portions.

• If you are not managing to consume enough calories and are losing weight because of it, make sure that the foods you do eat are higher in energy by adding in extra healthy fats and ensuring you have sufficient protein throughout the day (see 'Weight Loss and Cachexia' above). Fish is often a good choice when feeling poorly (see 'Protein', pages 42–3).

• Try to have nutrient-dense food when you are hungry to avoid deficiencies when you aren't eating very much.

• Whilst sufficient hydration is important, try not to fill up with too many fluids that have little nutritional or calorific value, such as tea and coffee. Although water is important, do not drink a glass before or during a meal as this will fill you up more.

• Try nutrient-dense soups and smoothies which can be easily digested and are not too daunting to eat (see 'Weight Loss and Cachexia', page 95, and the recipe section).

Weight Gain

There is plenty of evidence to link excess weight with an increased risk of cancer and if you are carrying some extra pounds it will probably be mentioned by your oncology team, particularly for breast and prostate cancers. Unfortunately, some cancer treatments increase the likelihood of putting on weight, which can seem very unfair.

Following a healthy eating plan during treatment, keeping blood sugar balanced and remaining as active as possible can significantly help in warding off too much weight gain and keeping body composition healthy. During treatment is not the time for any drastic diets unless you are following a protocol under the guidance of a health professional (see page 106).

Digestive Issues

During chemotherapy or radiation treatment DNA damage occurs to both healthy and cancerous cells, but it is the rapidly dividing cells such as those in our mouth, gut and hair follicles that are most affected. Treatments are administered to slow down cell replication, so in the gut, where the turnover of the cells is one to two days, cell renewal is soon depleted.

The cells particularly affected are the mucosal cells that line the whole of the gut: the term used for any damage and inflammation of this mucous membrane is 'mucositis'. Although there will undoubtedly be damage to these cells during treatment, not everyone will suffer significantly from the consequences. In general, symptoms can range from difficulty in swallowing to indigestion and heartburn, nausea, constipation, diarrhoea and malabsorption of nutrients. However, much can be done to ameliorate some of these by eating a diet that includes an abundance of healing foods. Preparing the gut prior to the start of treatment can be most beneficial (see page 82 and the table on page 98).

Cancer treatments such as chemotherapy or radiotherapy and steroids can alter our gut microflora because when the mucosal lining gets damaged the micro-organisms lose their attachment sites and are very easily sloughed off and eliminated from the body.

Be cautious in taking probiotic supplements if your immune system is compromised, which can often happen through treatment when white cells become depleted. Probiotics, which you might take for gut health, although sold as the good guys, are nevertheless bacteria and there is a small risk that they could set up an infection within the body if the bacteria pass through the gut membrane into the bloodstream. If you are neutropenic (see 'Neutropenia', page 101), do not take probiotics.

Chemotherapy and radiation therapy increase inflammation within the body (see page 27). Ensuring a high intake of anti-inflammatory foods can help to dampen this down. Foods that contain a balance of healthy fats have a direct effect on the production of anti-inflammatory chemicals in the body, whilst those containing polyphenols can help block key inflammatory enzymes (see the table overleaf).

Dry Mouth and Swallowing Difficulties

Chemotherapy, radiation, surgery or other medication can cause damage to the salivary glands and this makes it difficult to swallow and can affect your ability to speak too.

• Choose soft, moist foods such as soups, eggs, avocados, yoghurts. Add gravy, sauces or oils to food to ease swallowing.

• Sip water regularly.

• Make a nutritious smoothie.

• Liquidize meals or use nutritious build-up drinks (see page 156) as meal replacements.

• Avoid salty and spicy food.

• Chewing gum can sometimes stimulate saliva production.

Mouth Sores

Sores in the mouth and an inflamed, sensitive gut are common with some chemotherapy drugs or radiation near to the mouth or digestive tract. Again soft, non-scratchy foods can ease the pain of eating. Drinking through a straw can help too. Be careful of acidic or spicy foods which might irritate the mucosal lining.

Herbal mouthwashes, turmeric mouthwash, aloe vera juice, yoghurt and many anti-inflammatory foods can be very healing (see the table on page 98).

Taste Changes

It is very common to have a strange taste in your mouth during chemotherapy. It is usually described as either a metallic or a bitter taste and can often put people off even their favourite foods. Which foods are affected and which help to overcome the taste varies from person to person, but spicier foods often do the trick. My son Sebastian at the age of seven would happily chomp through a very spicy curry, which he wouldn't have touched before. However, for others this might make matters worse. Remember to avoid very spicy food if you are suffering from a sore mouth (see page 97).

Chewing or sucking on some mouth-cleansing herbs or spices such as lemon verbena, mint, rosemary, basil, cardamom pods or cloves can help the situation, but be

TOP FOODS FOR HEALING THE GUT

Ingredient	Action
Cabbage/kale	Very healing. Excellent for stomach ulcers, stomach discomfort, pain, bloating and hyperacidity. Can be added to juices in small amounts.
Shiitake mushrooms (fresh)	Boost immunity by increasing white blood cells. Excellent source of enzymes. Have shown anti-cancer activity. Use in cooking or add 4–5 to a smoothie. Put your mushrooms in the sun for an hour and they will make vitamin D.
Pineapple	Contains the enzyme bromelain which is anti-inflammatory and appears to have other anti-cancer properties. This may be too acidic for some people, but the enzymes can help to heal a sore mouth. Also aids digestion.
Papaya	An excellent source of papain, an enzyme that can aid protein digestion. Use the seeds too by soaking them in water for 24 hours in the fridge, then strain and drink the water as a refreshing tonic.
Jerusalem artichokes	A good source of inulin, a prebiotic food for fuelling beneficial microbiota.
Garlic/onions/leeks	Prebiotic foods. Anti-tumour activity. Anti-inflammatory. Garlic possesses considerable antimicrobial properties.
Beans and lentils	Prebiotic food. Excellent source of fibre for relief of constipation.

careful if they are very strong as that can make matters worse. Grow some of the herbs on your windowsill for a ready supply of very healthy chewing gum – what's more, they are very anti-inflammatory (see the table on page 98). Adding plenty of herbs to cooking to increase the flavour can help overcome an unpleasant taste.

Keep a list of foods that you can tolerate and those you can't and stick to the ones you can eat. Luckily the taste alteration generally passes as soon as treatment finishes.

Nausea

Nausea is much better controlled nowadays with anti-emetic drugs. Tips for alleviating the symptoms are:

• Sip ginger tea (a slice of root ginger infused in hot water).

• Drink a mint and lemon verbena infusion. Use fresh or dried leaves and steep in hot water for at least 10 minutes.

• Drink sparkling mineral water. Add a little ginger cordial.

Ingredient	Action
Apples	Eating apples regularly (2 per day) has been found to balance our gut microbiota. Pectin is a gelling agent which can improve gut transit time and nutrient absorption.
Oats/barley	Excellent prebiotic foods and sources of fibre.
Flaxseed/pumpkin/ hemp seeds	Flaxseeds/linseeds can help to relieve both constipation and diarrhoea and make a very healing tea (see page 62). Eaten after soaking they have the ability to buffer excess acid and protect the gut. Seeds are good sources of fibre and have anti-inflammatory effects. Hemp seeds have an excellent balance of omega fats.
Walnuts	Contain a balance of omega fats with anti-inflammatory effects.
Live yoghurt	Contains probiotics and if eaten before a meal can help to protect the gut by coating the lining.
Fennel	The bulb, leaves and seeds may help to relieve gas, indigestion, vomiting and nausea.
Ladies' fingers (okra)	Mucilaginous – i.e. contains a gloopy substance which helps to lubricate the gut and may assist swallowing. Reduces the action of acid on the stomach and can help nausea. Add about 4 to a smoothie.
Dark green leafy vegetables	A good source of vitamin A, which helps to heal the gut (do not supplement with high levels of vitamin A without professional advice). Also high in magnesium and potassium.
Oily fish	Omega-3 has anti-inflammatory properties which will help gut function.

Ingredient	Action
Mint leaves (fresh)	Help digestion, nausea, bloating and wind.
Slippery elm	Mucilaginous – lines the stomach, protecting it from high acidity, and may help relieve nausea, vomiting and heartburn. Add 1 teaspoon powder per glass of juice/smoothie or take 1 teaspoon mixed with water before a meal. Can be bought in any health food shop.
Bone stock	Helps to repair the lining of the gut and reduces inflammation.
Aloe vera	Very healing. Add 2 tablespoons aloe vera juice to juices or smoothies and drink before breakfast. Can be bought in a health-food shop.
Lemon or lime juice	Although acidic in its pre-digested state, this has a highly alkalizing post-digestive effect. Add freshly squeezed to juice and smoothies.
Fresh ginger	May relieve nausea and vomiting. However, may be too acidic for some, so could aggravate acid reflux. Anti-inflammatory.
Whey powder	Contains specific amino acids which can aid in healing the gut. Add to smoothies and use only when necessary.
Turmeric	Dissolve in water and use as a mouthwash up to six times a day for radiotherapy-induced oral mucositis (see above). Anti-inflammatory. Can also make a soothing drink when added to warm dairy or non-dairy milk (see page 58).
Herbal teas – liquorice/camomile/lemon verbena	Many herbal teas have anti-inflammatory properties along with being calming and healing on the gut. Use freshly dried herbs if possible. • Liquorice helps to protect the mucous membrane of the gut, is anti-inflammatory and has a mild laxative effect. It also improves circulation and increases blood pressure. Have only one cup a day if you have high blood pressure. • Camomile is calming and has antibacterial properties. • Lemon verbena helps to settle the stomach and calm nausea.
Berries	Red, blue and purple berries (blueberries/cherries/strawberries/pomegranates) contain anthocyanins, which have important anti-inflammatory effects. Be careful with seeded berries if you suffer from diverticulitis.

- Avoiding strong-tasting or fatty foods may help.

- If strong cooking smells make you feel sick, plan cold meals or food you have cooked in advance and frozen so it only requires defrosting and heating up.

- Eat little and often.

- Make a frozen juice lolly or small ice cubes to suck on.

- Try nibbling on our dry seeded crackers (see page 159).

Heartburn

This appears to be a very common complaint when people are under treatment. Any damage to the gut can weaken the valve that stops food and stomach acid backing up. This results in the burning sensation in the oesophagus that we know as heartburn. Again, eat small, frequent meals and afterwards do not lie down for about an hour until your food is digested. It can be useful to keep a food symptom diary to determine which foods aggravate the situation. Saturated fat, coffee, citrus juices and fruits can irritate the oesophagus and exacerbate the problem.

Constipation and Diarrhoea

Quite often the digestive issues experienced during treatment are similar to those of irritable bowel syndrome (IBS), especially in the case of alternating constipation and diarrhoea. Both complaints can be remedied by foods that have the capacity to absorb water and become gel-like. (These foods have many other health benefits too.)

Psyllium husk, an indigestible, soluble fibre found in most health food stores, can be taken for both diarrhoea and constipation. In cases of diarrhoea it will absorb excess fluid in the colon and bulk up the stool. For constipation, take the psyllium husk with plenty of water and it will swell up into a gel and increase movement within the gut. Flaxseeds (linseeds) can work in a similar way. Use ground flaxseeds for diarrhoea; to relieve constipation, soak the flaxseeds overnight and eat as a porridge. Chia seeds soaked overnight are also good for keeping the bowel regular. Try our Porridge and Chia Breakfast Bowl (page 146).

If you are constipated, ensure you are drinking plenty of fluids, especially water and herbal teas. Also keep active as much as possible, as this helps to keep the gut moving.

Diarrhoea may be helped by eating live yoghurt and fermented foods, or by taking probiotics to balance the gut microbiota, especially if it is caused by antibiotics.

Insomnia

Many people with cancer suffer from insomnia. It may be that you have difficulty falling asleep at night; or that you wake in the middle of the night and cannot get back to sleep; or you just don't achieve a restful sleep. Try some of the following to see if they help:

- Adopt a regular bedtime routine, preferably early to sleep and early to rise.

- Do not fall asleep watching television – try to clear the mind before sleeping.

- Don't use a computer, tablet or phone for two hours before going to bed, as this stimulates the brain when you want to calm it.

- If you wake in the middle of the night it may be due to low blood sugar. Try a snack just before bedtime, such as a banana and some warm oat milk mixed with turmeric and cinnamon.

- Other foods rich in melatonin are oranges, pineapples and barley.

- Try a herbal sleep remedy. A medical herbalist will recommend a mixture of herbs that can help. Camomile tea can also be very calming as a bedtime drink.

- Avoid alcohol at bedtime.

- Sprinkle your pillow with lavender oil, or have a lavender bag next to you, as it is a tried-and-tested traditional way of aiding relaxation.

Neutropenia

Neutrophils are types of white blood cell that are our primary defence against bacteria and fungi. Neutropenia is an abnormally low level of neutrophils and is common in those being treated by chemotherapy and radiotherapy, both of which affect the bone marrow, and in those with blood cancers. During this time be extra careful about hygiene and cleanliness to reduce the risk of infection. Try to avoid going into crowded places such as on public transport, and ask your friends and family not to visit or get too close if they have anything contagious. If you have to visit your GP's surgery, don't sit in a packed waiting room. Tell the staff you will wait outside and they should call you when the doctor is ready.

Certain foods should be avoided, such as raw eggs and undercooked meat, soft cheeses, shellfish, live yoghurts and unpasteurized milk. All vegetables and fruit should be very well washed, particularly bags of salad leaves. Adding some vinegar to the water used to wash fruit and vegetables can help to eliminate some bacteria.

Menopausal Symptoms

Some treatments cause early menopause: this is known as treatment-induced menopause. It can be caused by removal of the ovaries, chemotherapy, radiotherapy to the pelvic region and hormonal therapy. Apart from the removal of the ovaries, other therapies can lead to either temporary or permanent menopause. Hormone therapy may not induce permanent menopause but may cause menopause-like symptoms.

Symptoms may include:

- Hot flushes/night sweats

- Fatigue

- Muscle aches and joint pain

- Mucous membrane dryness

- Depression

- Anxiety

- Memory loss

- Insomnia/sleep disturbance

- Weight gain

- Water retention

The nutritional approaches already covered in this book may help to alleviate symptoms:

- Support the gut and liver, and control blood sugar (see pages 98, 52, 91 and 73–5).

- Eat a variety of fresh, colourful vegetables and fruit along with other anti-inflammatory foods.

- Eat a phytoestrogen-rich diet (see pages 80–81).

- Include plenty of fibre in your diet (see pages 48, 78–9).

- Include foods to aid bone health (see page 86).

- Include foods to help mood (see page 89).

Some herbs may be helpful, but you should consult a qualified herbalist for advice. Vitamin E oil used topically can help alleviate vaginal dryness, as can omega-7 found in sea buckthorn supplements.

Chemo Brain

Short-term memory loss and difficulties in concentration and coordination can be a consequence of the cancer itself and of anxiety, in which case they should be short-lived. However, they may arise from treatment, and in this case may linger on. In particular, 5-fluorouracil (5-FU) has been shown to have an effect on the cells in the central nervous system that produce myelin, a fatty substance that insulates our nerve fibres; without adequate myelin normal nerve signalling is disrupted, causing messages from the brain to slow down.

Unfortunately there is a dearth of research in this area, although there has been awareness of it for some time. Late-effects clinics for childhood cancer survivors are especially aware of this potential problem and in fact allowances can be made for them in exams taken at the time or in the future.

Although there is no research to prove it, it would seem that anything we can do to protect our healthy brain cells during treatment must be of benefit and may reduce cognitive impairment. The brain needs lots of good fats to stay healthy, so pack these into your diet along with plenty of plant foods, especially broccoli and turmeric which are amazingly protective of healthy cells. A high-fat, low-carb diet such as the Ketogenic Diet (see page 106) may well afford brain protection during treatment.

Other ways of coping with chemo brain are:

- Make sure you get enough rest and sleep.
- Take regular exercise.
- Use a planner to remind you of appointments, etc.
- Keep to a daily routine.
- Stay hydrated.

Peripheral Neuropathy

Peripheral neuropathy is a result of nerve damage and can cause mild to painful tingling or numbness in the body, especially the hands and feet. You may also experience twitching muscles, loss of reflexes, cramping and spasms, along with a loss of sensation. It can develop at any stage of cancer, even some time after treatment has finished.

The nerves do have the ability to heal, but it can take several months. Peripheral neuropathy can be difficult to treat but a nutrient-dense diet and possible supplementation may help to relieve it. Taking a B vitamin complex or using capsaicin cream can be helpful.

Eating Well After Bowel Surgery

People's experience of gastro-intestinal disturbance after surgery or with a stoma – a surgical opening from the intestine to the outside which bypasses the rectum – is extremely individual. After such surgery, some people will have no problems at all; or foods that one person tolerates may disagree with another. However, initially extra care is generally needed to avoid complications.

After two or three weeks you may well be back to eating a normal and varied diet, but it is advisable to re-introduce foods one at a time and to keep a food diary to document any resulting symptoms. This way you will immediately know which, if any, are problematic. Remember, however, that any foods that cause problems during the early days after surgery may be fine further down the line.

Stomas

General guidelines are:

• Chew your food well so that enzymes in the mouth start the digestion process.

• Drink plenty of fluids: 1.5–2 litres a day.

• Eat as much fibre as you can tolerate to lessen the risk of constipation.

• Eat regular meals.

• Initially, add salt to your diet to replace the increased sodium lost after surgery.

• To reduce flatulence and odour, avoid foods such as onions, garlic, cabbage, Brussels sprouts, cauliflower, cucumber, radishes, beans, nuts, soy, carbonated drinks, alcohol, excess fruit, dairy and wheat. Also avoid talking too much during a meal or chewing gum, as both increase the amount of air in the gut.

• To neutralize odour, include parsley, fennel tea, cranberry juice, tomato juice, yoghurt.

• Avoid sugar substitutes such as stevia or xylitol which may cause bloating and diarrhoea.

• If you experience loose or watery stools, ensure you drink plenty of fluids. Coconut water can be useful for replenishing electrolytes.

• Do not use bulking agents unless instructed.

Dumping Syndrome

This condition can affect people who have undergone an operation to bypass or remove part of the stomach. It manifests either as severe discomfort in the digestive tract or immense fatigue after eating, and is caused by the stomach emptying its contents into the intestines at a faster rate than normal. If you eat a big meal – especially one high in carbohydrates – a large amount of fluid is absorbed quickly and in response to the sugar concentration the intestine may contract vigorously, leading to an almost immediate loose bowel movement. This happens to a limited extent to all of us when we eat, but if you are recovering from this sort of surgery the effects can be drastic and difficult to deal with.

For some people dumping occurs very quickly after eating; for others it is delayed. Eating small but frequent meals, avoiding sugars, starches and excessively acidic foods and drinking only between meals rather than along with them can help. Those with early dumping should aim to have meals high in protein and fat and low in starches and sugars. For those with late dumping, increase the complex carbohydrates for a slow release of sugars. Symptoms tend to resolve over time, or you simply learn to avoid those foods that aggravate the condition.

Low-fibre/Low-residue Diet

You may have been advised to follow this diet if you have had any digestive tract surgery, an ileostomy or colostomy. It basically includes only those foods that leave a minimal amount of undigested material in the digestive tract. This can often be a source of frustration for anyone trying to follow a healthy diet centred around whole, unprocessed foods with plenty of fibre, but it is generally a short-term solution to prevent any blockages and allow healing to take place. Once things settle down you may be able to be less restrictive and gradually test out more fibre-rich foods.

The table below gives a list of foods to include or avoid in a low-fibre or low-residue diet. Consult your hospital dietitian for a more comprehensive or personalized list.

When you are following a low-fibre/low-residue diet, try to do the following:

- Eat little and often.

- Chew your food slowly and thoroughly.

- If eating a varied diet is very difficult, ask your treatment team about multivitamin and mineral supplements.

- Re-introduce foods slowly and use a food diary to monitor symptoms.

- Make your own clear and strained vegetable and fruit juices to maximize nutrient intake (see page 68).

- Boil up meat bones to make a restorative stock to aid healing (see page 256).

LOW-FIBRE/LOW-RESIDUE DIET

Foods to eat	Foods to avoid
Cooked vegetables – peeled, de-seeded and de-stalked Raw lettuce Strained vegetable juices Sieved tomato sauces/passata/purée Finely chopped leaves of herbs or dried herbs Spices – in moderation and as tolerated Smooth nut butters	Raw vegetables and any with seeds, stalks, skin and stringy fibres – whole tomatoes, cucumber, peas, sweetcorn, mushrooms, celery, cabbage, kale, fennel, leeks, okra, peppers, pumpkin, spinach, sprouts, yam, cassava, chopped herbs (unless very fine and without stalks) Beans, pulses, nuts and seeds
Fruits – puréed fruit, banana, tinned fruits without seeds or skin, honeydew melon, watermelon (without seeds) Fruit juices Coconut milk Herbal teas Weak tea and coffee	Fruits with seeds, stalks and skin Dried fruit Whole/desiccated coconut Smoothies Caffeine drinks – strong tea and coffee, Red Bull and cola
Eat in moderation – white bread, rice, pasta and noodles, cornflakes and rice crispies	Wholegrain products – breads, pasta, rice, couscous, noodles, pearl barley, quinoa, oatmeal, wheatgerm, bulgur wheat, digestive biscuits, Ryvita, oatcakes Cereals – Weetabix, Shredded Wheat, muesli, porridge, All-Bran
Meat and fish – all types Homemade bone broth Eggs/tofu Dairy – all milk products	Gristly, fatty meat, fish bones and skin Dairy products containing nuts, seeds or cereal

5 'Outside the Box' Approaches to Cancer

THIS CHAPTER LOOKS AT complementary or alternative approaches to cancer treatment, many of which lack solid scientific research – see the earlier discussion of evidence-based medicine on pages 20–21. I am sure we are all aware that non-conventional strategies exist, and a quick search of the internet brings up a veritable host of them, usually leading to utter confusion for those seeking reliable advice. Some are options that may work effectively alongside standard treatments, or they may have benefits as standalone treatments; but one thing that unites them all is that there is not a large enough body of evidence of their efficacy in humans for them to be recommended by many doctors working in mainstream medicine.

Described below are some investigational therapies, some emerging research and some treatments that I have experienced cancer patients finding beneficial and safe. Included are diets, nutraceuticals, herbs, and off-label pharmaceuticals but there are plenty of others that may be beneficial too.

In describing some of these treatments, my aim is to present the facts in order to clarify them and, hopefully, avoid confusing you further. It is important to remember that to date no treatment, conventional or otherwise, has been found to be a definitive cure for cancer. I am not endorsing or making claims about any of the therapies mentioned here, but by setting out the evidence – or lack of evidence, as is mostly the case – I hope to enable people to make informed choices and to feel confident about asking questions and seeking answers. In the resources section there are useful websites where you can obtain reliable information on a range of therapies – see page 279.

Dietary Approaches

The Ketogenic Diet

Growing interest in the Warburg hypothesis, that cancer is a metabolic disease (see page 25) has led to thoughts on how we can utilize the metabolic difference between cancer cells and normal cells to our advantage in cancer treatment. Limiting the amount of glucose available to the cancer cells appears to be a sensible approach and ketogenic therapy, particularly in the area of brain cancer, is showing some promise.

The Ketogenic Diet is a low-carbohydrate, adequate-protein and high-fat diet which has been used successfully and safely for many decades to treat childhood epilepsy. By eating a diet high in fat with very little in the way of carbohydrates, a physiological shift takes place whereby fats are converted to chemicals called ketones and these are used by normal cells as a replacement fuel for glucose. Circulating levels of glucose and insulin are maintained at the lower end of the normal range and, as cancer cells struggle to adapt to ketones and have insufficient glucose, it is hoped that they will fail to thrive and will effectively starve to death.

The Ketogenic Diet does include restricted amounts of carbohydrate in the form of vegetables and some fruit, particularly green leafy vegetables and berries. Some argue that the cancer cells will lap up any glucose produced from these and deprive our healthy cells. However, our healthy cells, including brain cells, appear to function very well on ketones without any major side-effects. In fact, most people, once they are 'keto-adapted', report increased energy and concentration levels. There is also concern that cancer patients may lose weight. If insufficient fat is consumed then this may well be the case, but of course for some this is desirable. Where a

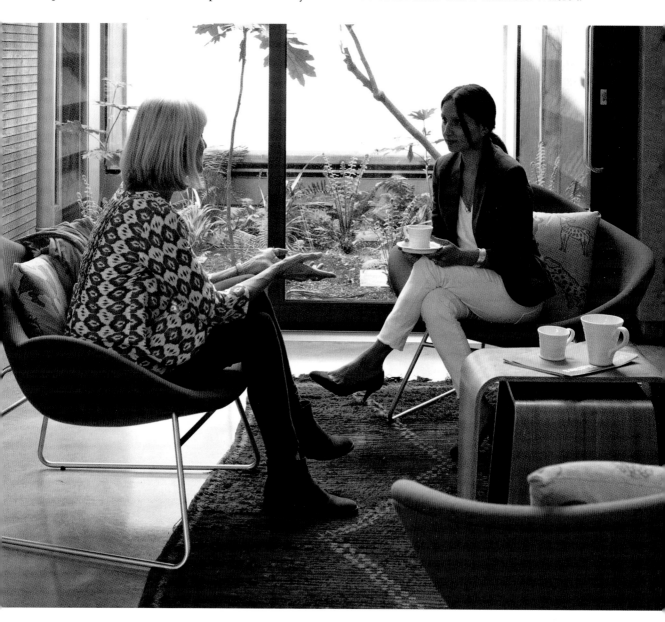

person needs to maintain or increase weight, sufficient or extra fats in the diet is important. A Ketogenic Diet can actually help to protect against cachexia (see page 95).

Most of the research has been in mice; however, small-scale studies have deemed the diet to be safe in humans with cancer. It also appears to enhance the effects of treatment whilst protecting normal cells. There are many plausible biochemical mechanisms to explain why low carbohydrate intake and, possibly more importantly, low insulin levels weaken cancer cells and halt progression. Once the cancer cells are weakened through glucose restriction it makes them more vulnerable and less resistant to chemotherapy and radiotherapy. Hyperbaric oxygen therapy (see page 122) has also been shown to be effective in promoting cancer-cell death when used in conjunction with the Ketogenic Diet, but this is not as yet scientifically proven.

From an evolutionary standpoint, we could say that consuming an abundant supply of carbohydrates only began with the introduction of agriculture, particularly grains, around 12,000 BC. In the evolution of man this is a fairly recent phenomenon and it is probably safe to say that before this first agricultural revolution it's more than likely that man was fuelling his body mostly with ketones as opposed to glucose, relying mainly on animal protein, nuts, seeds and berries, alongside periods of famine. Many would argue that as humans we were most certainly not designed, nor have we evolved, to consume the amount of starchy carbohydrate in a typical modern Western diet.

Most cancers are avid consumers of glucose, but there are just a few that aren't so glucose-dependent – such as 80 per cent of prostate cancers, some colon and lung cancers, and high-functioning cancers such as thyroid.

I would advise anyone with a cancer diagnosis to consider following a low glycaemic load diet (see page 74). To follow a true Ketogenic Diet it is best undertaken in conjunction with your medical team alongside expert supervision (see panel overleaf).

Calorie restriction and intermittent fasting

There has been growing interest in the effects on cancer-cell growth when calories are restricted. Similar to ketogenic therapy (see above), fasting triggers the body to convert fat to ketones for use as fuel. Proponents of the Ketogenic Diet often advise an initial period of fasting to jump-start the body into a ketotic state.

Animal studies have shown that restricting calorie intake is an effective cancer-preventative strategy. In an analysis of all relevant animal studies it was concluded that calorie restriction may be superior to intermittent fasting for cancer prevention; however, small studies of intermittent fasting in humans have shown positive results too, possibly due to the fact that this is an easier diet to follow.

Intermittent fasting has also been studied for its weight-loss effects. Rather than total fasting, calories are restricted to around a quarter of the usual intake for two days of the week. The '2-day diet' was put together by researchers at the University of Manchester who were studying breast cancer and treatment-induced weight gain (see 'Weight Management', page 129). Both calorie restriction and intermittent fasting have been found to improve blood levels of inflammatory markers and insulin-like growth factor (see pages 27 and 28) alongside weight loss. However, fasting for longer periods should never be undertaken without the advice of a health professional.

Short-term fasting during chemotherapy

Ongoing research is investigating the benefits of fasting for 24 hours before chemo is administered. This puts the body into a mild ketotic state (see 'Ketogenic Diet', page 106), which means fat is burned for energy in the form of ketones. Benefits may include the protection of normal cells during treatment, the sensitizing of cancer cells to the chemo drugs, and a reduction in side-effects such as fatigue and gut problems.

Research suggests that if cancer cells have limited access to glucose they cannot repair the oxidative stress caused by chemotherapy or radiotherapy. This leaves them more vulnerable to the treatment. So far only small studies have been carried out in humans.

Gerson Therapy

Working in the 1920s, Dr Max Gerson maintained that the best way to treat disease was to correct metabolic disturbances, thereby maintaining harmony throughout the body. In his own words: 'the onset of metabolic disturbance constitutes the beginning of disease . . . the task is to bring the body back to that normal physiology . . . the next task is to keep the physiology of the metabolism in that natural equilibrium'.

One important aspect of his therapy was the promotion of an oxygen-rich environment within the cell to increase oxidative metabolism – the process by which oxygen makes energy from carbohydrates. Gerson had been convinced that an abundance of oxygen within the tissues could slow the rate of tumour growth after encountering the work of Otto Warburg (see 'Cellular respiration and the Warburg effect', page 25).

Gerson Therapy is a gruelling regime and would be difficult to manage without support, as it involves juicing huge amounts of fruits and vegetables several times a day. The Gerson Institute runs courses but many people simply take aspects of the therapy, such as juicing and increasing their consumption of vegetables and fruit as part of a more manageable healthy diet.

Budwig Protocol

Dr Joanna Budwig was a German biochemist who studied the role of fatty acids in protecting the body from cancers and other diseases. Her work on cancer was sparked by Otto Warburg's hypothesis that damaged cells which fail to respire properly and use excessive glucose in the absence of oxygen become cancerous (see 'Cellular respiration and the Warburg effect', page 25).

Dr Budwig understood the importance of good fats in the diet and was in fact one of the first to be critical of trans-fats in food production back in the 1950s (see page 43). She researched and devised a protocol using a blend of electron-rich flaxseed oil with sulphur-rich protein, such as quark or cottage cheese, which enabled the oil and sulphur to enter cells and oxygenate them. She also advised plenty of vitamin D from sunshine, along with ample exercise and other selected foods and nutrients. There is plenty of anecdotal evidence of the beneficial effects of following the Budwig Protocol and, as it has no side-effects, it may be worth trying.

I actually love the creamy combination of flaxseed oil and cottage cheese and we have included its use in one of our recipes (see page 177). But for more information on the complete protocol, see our additional resources, page 279.

THE KETOGENIC DIET

Sue Wood, Dietitian, Matthew's Friends Clinics, supported by Matthew's Friends Charity and Astro Brain Tumour Fund

Matthew's Friends Charity was set up in 2004 to provide support, education and information to patients, families and professionals involved with ketogenic therapy, a specialist treatment option for drug-resistant epilepsy. With growing interest in the use of the therapy in oncology we started supporting our first brain-tumour patient in 2011, liaising with his neuro-oncology team so that they were aware of the principles of the therapy, the preliminary research and the need for monitoring. Since then we have supported around 40 individuals with a range of brain tumours, with the associated medical and biochemical monitoring component being delivered by their local neuro-oncology teams and GPs.

This shared experience is teaching us that for those with low-grade glioma [a malignant tumour that starts in the brain or spine], ketogenic therapy has the potential to deliver real benefits in seizure control and fatigue management where these are impairing day-to-day life. Most report that this sense of taking control, with visible results, is really important to them. Beyond this, we know little about the impact [of the diet] on low-grade glioma, as no research has been conducted in this sector and the time taken for these tumours to progress varies markedly from one individual to the other.

For those with high-grade gliomas, many of which may not have significant seizure symptoms, the benefits may be less tangible, although fatigue is a common symptom and can readily improve. [The diet] is often undertaken alongside radiotherapy and chemotherapy, so major dietary changes can add a further layer of complexity to an already highly stressful time and it is not suitable for all. However, the need to take control in a situation that feels beyond control is a powerful driver to those seeking support for this approach.

Is there any evidence?

The use of a ketogenic diet as an additional component in the management of two paediatric cases of high-grade glioma was first reported in 1995, where they noticed a significant reduction in glucose uptake at the tumour sites. Both were reported to be enjoying a good quality of life four and five years after diagnosis. In 2007, the use of a calorie-restricted ketogenic diet (around 600kcals/day, leading to a 20% loss in body weight) was reported in a 65-year-old woman. Standard therapy was maintained and progression was tracked using PET scans. After two months' treatment, no discernible brain-cancer tissue was detected. However, 10 weeks after suspension of the strict dietary therapy, MRI evidence of recurrence was found.

A small study of 53 patients with glioblastoma multiforme, of which six were on a ketogenic diet alongside standard therapy, was published in 2014. The authors reported that the ketogenic diet was safe and well tolerated and appeared to significantly reduce circulating blood-glucose levels even when high-dose steroids were used alongside. They concluded that this may improve the response to standard treatment and prognosis and recommended that further research be carried out to confirm this.

What do animal studies tell us?

In 2010, studies on a mouse model of glioblastoma multiforme reported that an unrestricted ketogenic diet (a) specifically retarded tumour growth; (b) prevented increases in reactive oxygen species associated with tumour growth; and (c) shifted overall gene expression in cancer tissue to that seen in the normal brain. In 2012 the same research group reported that a ketogenic diet significantly enhanced the effect of radiation in the same model. This team [and others] are currently undertaking a human trial to see if ketogenic therapy can increase survival and enhance the effects of standard radiation and chemotherapy treatments used to treat glioblastoma multiforme. However, there is still much to be learned about the therapeutic mechanisms of action and how to monitor the impact on the tumour, enabling adjustment of the regime or additional components to maximize its effect.

Please see www.matthewsfriends.org and www.astrofund.org.uk for further information.

Nutraceutical Approaches

Taking supplements is always a thorny issue, but the majority of people I talk to who have had a cancer diagnosis take them in one form or another. Of course it goes without saying that a varied, nutrient-dense diet must come first and just swallowing a handful of nutrient supplements should not be seen as a substitute for this. Foods work in synergy to benefit the body, and I hope we illustrate their very important functions in this book, but there is certainly a place for supplementation after a cancer diagnosis.

Advice can often be to take a significant amount of supplements, but it is important to be cautious and supplement wisely. Vitamin, mineral, herb and food supplements have a very safe track record and most of the research cited against them is simply that there is no evidence to prove that they have a beneficial effect. This is often because the dosage used in trials has been too low.

That said, I would advise anyone considering supplementing with anything other than the basic nutrients (see the table opposite) to seek professional advice. Consult a well-qualified nutritional therapist/doctor, or a dietitian who works in the field of oncology and who can advise you on an individual basis, depending on your diet and lifestyle, the type of cancer and your treatment protocol.

Research on supplementing with isolated vitamins and minerals in cancer has, in some cases, found them to be beneficial only when the person has a deficiency. In fact, some studies have shown that when a person has sufficient levels of certain nutrients, then supplementation may actually be harmful. This was clearly illustrated in trials into selenium and prostate cancer. Selenium appeared to be beneficial when given as a supplement to those who were deficient, but was detrimental when high doses were administered to those with no deficiency.

Another example of why caution should always be taken is provided by studies investigating the effects of beta-carotene supplementation in the general population and those in high-risk groups. Some but not all studies found that in heavy smokers beta-carotene increased the risk of lung cancer. It is not known why there appears to be a negative interaction between smoke carcinogens and beta-carotene, but it may be the form of beta-carotene used or, again, the fact that isolated compounds do not work in the same way as the synergy of mixed carotenes. Cases like this highlight the need for professional advice.

Many supplements have been shown to have beneficial effects, but they need to be prescribed in line with an individualized treatment plan. The following is a basic supplement protocol that I would recommend; however, do advise your medical team of any supplements you are taking.

There is increasing interest in whole-food supplements which get away from the isolation of certain therapeutic compounds and utilize the potentially beneficial synergistic effects of using the food as near to its natural state as possible. The research on the polyphenol supplement Pomi-T, with which oncologist Dr Robert Thomas has been involved, has produced some very exciting results. In the panel overleaf he explains about the supplement and its research.

BASIC SUPPLEMENTS AND THEIR BENEFITS

Supplement type	Reasons
Multivitamin and mineral	If nutrient intake is low or your gut is compromised. Use a good-quality brand containing a cross-section of vitamins and minerals, particularly iodine, selenium, B vitamins and vitamin D. A daily multivitamin and mineral tops up your levels, provides a good balance of nutrients and may be more easily absorbed than a single vitamin or mineral. Unless your iron stores are low, I recommend choosing a brand that does not contain iron.
Probiotics	The importance of healthy microbiota cannot be overemphasized. If your diet is lacking in vegetables and fruit, or if you have been on antibiotics, then a course of broad-spectrum probiotics can be useful. Do not take during times of low immunity.
Omega oil	If your diet is lacking in oily fish and healthy oils you may need to top up your omega-3 intake. Fish oils provide the best source, but flaxseed oil is beneficial too. Add in hemp or pumpkin oil for a balance of omega-3.
Phytonutrients	Recent research has found benefits in taking an array of phytonutrients such as turmeric, green tea, pomegranate and broccoli. Choose a whole-food capsule (see panel below).
Vitamin D	As many of us living in the UK are vitamin D deficient, taking a supplement is a good way of ensuring an adequate supply, especially during the winter months. Drops taken sublingually (under the tongue) can be the best way of ensuring absorption. Before embarking on this, it is best to have vitamin D levels tested to ensure accurate supplementation.

CAN CONCENTRATING FOODS INTO SUPPLEMENTS ENHANCE THEIR ANTI-CANCER EFFECT?

Dr Robert Thomas, Consultant Oncologist, Addenbrooke's and Bedford Hospitals

If certain whole foods have clinical anti-cancer effects, then it is reasonable to hypothesise that concentrating them into a pill may be a good way to supplement individuals with a poor diet or further enhance the benefits in those whose diets are already adequate. People living with and beyond cancer are certainly attracted to the potential health benefits of food supplements as over 60% report regular intake. Unfortunately most studies of mineral and vitamin supplements have shown no anti-cancer benefit and some even an increased risk so this is not generally recommended unless correcting a known or measured deficiency.

More recently academic attention has turned towards the evaluation of concentrated whole foods in supplement form, particularly foods rich in polyphenols such as herbs, spices, green vegetables, teas and colourful fruits which have the most robust laboratory data highlighting their anti-cancer properties.

So far, the largest trial analysing whole food extracts was the National Cancer Research Network Pomi-T study. This study combined four different foods rich in phytochemicals, particularly polyphenols (pomegranate, green tea, broccoli and turmeric). This non-commercial academic study was designed in conjunction with the UK government-funded National Cancer Research Network and involved a panel of scientists, doctors, nutritionists and dietitians. After an extensive review of the international literature, these ingredients were chosen, by the panel, because they provide a wide spectrum of synergistically acting nutrients, whilst at the same time

Antioxidant (phytonutrient) supplementation during treatment

One of the most frequent nutrition questions asked by those going through cancer treatment is about antioxidant supplementation. This is a confusing area to which there is no conclusive answer. A recent study looking at antioxidant usage in North American cancer centres found that, in general, guidelines were more restrictive than some research findings suggest is necessary. The complexity of the effect of antioxidants in the body and the conflicting research findings no doubt leads to healthcare providers being fairly conservative and working on the important principle of 'first do no harm'.

avoiding over-consumption of one particular phytochemical. Although this supplement was designed with all cancers in mind, the first major evaluation of its effect involved 200 men with localised prostate cancer managed with active surveillance or watchful waiting experiencing a PSA relapse following initial radical interventions.

The results were announced to the world during an oral presentation at the American Society of Clinical Oncology Conference, Chicago, which is the largest and most prestigious cancer conference. Men taking the supplement were reported to have a statistically significant, 63%, reduction in the median PSA progression rate compared to placebo. A further analysis of MRI images, presented in Copenhagen in 2015, showed the cancers' size and growth patterns seen on these images correlated with PSA changes, excluding the possibility that this was just a PSA rather than tumour effect. The supplement, named by the UK manufacturers as Pomi-T after the trial, was well tolerated apart from some mild loosening of the bowels in a minority and an improvement in the bowels in others. Another further analysis presented at the National Cancer Research Network conference in Liverpool, 2014, showed that, at six months, significantly more men opted to remain on surveillance rather than proceeding to expensive radiotherapy, surgery or hormones, which can cause considerable distress to the men and cost to the country.

In order for this supplement to be evaluated in this government-backed trial the manufacturers had to adhere to a strict quality-assurance programme testing for contaminants and authenticity which they have maintained for the current commercially available product (www.pomi-T.com).Following the success of the evaluation of Pomi-T, major studies are now being planned for other cancer types. In the meantime, studies are under way exploring its potential to treat hot flushes and arthritis following numerous anecdotal reports of it helping these common symptoms.

It is thought by some that antioxidants may reduce the efficacy of chemotherapy by protecting the cancer cells; however, research has shown that in many cases antioxidant supplementation may in fact protect the healthy cells and enhance the effects of chemotherapy on cancer cells whilst ameliorating side-effects.

I gave my son high doses of the antioxidant vitamin C daily throughout much of his treatment and then panicked one day when the newspaper headlines shrieked 'Vitamin C causes cancer'. I felt sick with worry, but on summing up the evidence realized no conclusion could be drawn from it and so decided that, as he had been doing so well,

I would continue. A couple of years later I came across a paper specifically on childhood leukaemia and the use of antioxidant supplementation during treatment. I could hardly bear to read it, thinking I may have done harm. However, the paper concluded that those children taking antioxidants suffered fewer infections and side-effects. My relief was palpable!

When the research is unpicked, it certainly shows that there is an evidence base for the use of antioxidant supplements in some – and maybe all – cancer cases, but some of the other effects of antioxidants on cells mean that their use is not straightforward. The antioxidant glutathione has been found to protect cancer cells and should not be supplemented. Again, individual advice is recommended.

Enzymes

Pancreatic enzymes are now a fundamental addition to many anti-cancer nutritional protocols as they are seen to play a vital role in reducing tumour mass. The hypothesis goes back to Professor John Beard, who first proposed in 1906 that the cancer cell shared tissue and behavioural characteristics with the pregnancy trophoblast, one of the most primitive of the embryonic cells that form the placenta. The evidence for a shared fundamental genetic identity between cancers of all types and trophoblasts has grown over the last century. In the 1940s it was found that cancer cells produce the pregnancy hormone human chorionic gonadotrophin, also produced by the trophoblast, and this has been confirmed in recent studies.

Around the eighth week of pregnancy the foetal trophoblast cells stop dividing and are destroyed. Beard confirmed that enzymes released from the foetal pancreas digest the outer coat of the trophoblast, exposing it to digestion by cells of the immune system. Following his findings, scientists began experimenting with pancreatic enzymes to break down the outer coat of a tumour to expose it to immune cells.

Gerson Therapy (see page 108) includes the use of digestive enzymes, but the best known of the enzyme therapies is that of the late Dr Nicholas Gonzalez in New York. He analysed the successful work of Beard with cancer patients and from the late 1980s used it to develop his own protocol, still used in his clinic. In addition to supplementing with digestive enzymes, Gonzalez also advised a large intake of nutritional supplements, an individualized diet and juicing plan, and detoxification through coffee enemas. It is an expensive therapy to undertake.

A clinical trial led to the conclusion that Gonzalez's protocol brought no additional benefit. He himself recommended that this therapy should not be used in conjunction with chemotherapy and radiotherapy.

Mistletoe extract

Mistletoe is used extensively in Germany, generally in conjunction with chemotherapy and radiotherapy. This is where much of the research has been undertaken and positive outcomes have been seen, with an improvement in quality of life and increased survival rates. A trial in the US on colon-cancer patients also showed decreased toxicity from chemotherapy and improved anti-cancer benefits.

Mistletoe extract has been found to enhance immunity against cancer cells and inhibit tumour growth. Iscador, the brand name, is licensed in the UK and is available on the NHS through some practitioners, mainly at the integrated and homeopathic hospitals in London, Bristol and Glasgow. It is given by injection, usually two or three times a week.

Apricot kernels (B$_{17}$)

Many foods contain the compound amygdalin, also known as B$_{17}$, but apricot kernels have the highest concentration. Amygdalin has been shown to kill cancer cells in a laboratory setting, but published research on Laetrile, derived from amygdalin, found very little evidence of benefit in cancer patients. Despite this, some alternative doctors use Laetrile injections and tablets and claim there is significant benefit. There is also plenty of anecdotal evidence from people with cancer who describe beneficial effects from eating the kernels. There is certainly no evidence that B$_{17}$ alone cures cancer.

As amygdalin contains benzaldehyde and cyanide, both of which are toxic, care should be taken when consuming apricot kernels, especially if you have any liver problems. It is thought that amygdalin itself is harmless because the toxic elements are bound to another molecule and are harmful only when freed. Any anti-cancer properties are thought to be due to cancer cells containing significantly more of the enzyme beta-glucosidase – which unlocks the bound benzaldehyde and cyanide within the cell – and none of the enzyme rhodanese, which in healthy cells would normally mop these toxins up. It is claimed this may lead to cancer cells being destroyed whilst healthy cells are preserved.

Amygdalin, or B$_{17}$, is a nitriloside and is what gives some foods their bitter taste. Unfortunately we have eliminated many bitter foods from our diet as our taste for sweetness has increased and this means we are no longer eating amygdalin in the quantities our ancestors did. Tribes that have been found to have no cancer amongst their population are noted for their diet high in amygdalin – a fact that may be of immense importance.

Adjusting our diets to include a higher proportion of plant-based foods will increase our intake. Foods containing high levels are wild blackberries, cassava, barley, buckwheat, alfalfa, bamboo and mung bean sprouts, and most nuts, seeds and beans – in fact, many of the ingredients used in our recipes.

Essiac tea

Herbs in general can be extremely helpful in supporting cancer patients (see page 64) and I highly recommend seeking the advice of a medical herbalist; they have lengthy training. To me it makes sense to use whole plants and their synergistic therapeutic properties rather than isolated compounds which can cause more side-effects (see page 112).

Essiac tea is a combination of herbs originally used by a nurse in Canada who sought out plant remedies from indigenous tribes and put together a concoction to help a friend who had breast cancer.

The herbs included are:

• **Burdock root** This provides a wide spectrum of therapeutic benefits, including blood-cleansing and immune-boosting functions. It has mild anti-blood-clotting properties. The herb also protects the liver and aids digestion and appetite by stimulating the production of bile. It is therefore known to be a mild laxative and diuretic, helping to clear toxins from the body.

• **Slippery elm** Taken in powder form and available in health food shops, this has anti-inflammatory qualities, helping to soothe the mucous membrane that lines the digestive tract. This makes it especially useful during chemotherapy. Slippery elm is also effective in soothing gastritis, enteritis, haemorrhoids and gastric and duodenal ulcers, as well as sore throats. It is easily absorbed and its nutritious qualities make it a valuable food during convalescence. It has gentle astringent properties as well, and helps to ease diarrhoea. In powder form it is an excellent source of soluble fibre, which may help to reduce cholesterol levels, as well as bulk up the stool when constipated.

• **Turkey rhubarb** This has bitter, astringent properties and is known as an effective digestive stimulant and liver tonic. At varying doses it can be used to treat both constipation and diarrhoea and therefore has a regulatory effect on digestion. It stimulates the appetite and promotes the flow of bile from the liver, thus optimizing the action of digestive enzymes, reducing liver congestion and preventing the formation of gallstones.

• **Sheep sorrel** This has a whole range of therapeutic properties and is a vital component of Essiac tea.

I have known many people who have used this herbal concoction to support them through treatment. It has anti-inflammatory properties and supports the gut and the liver, so can be very beneficial.

The Clouds Trust is a charity that can provide more information, and can supply the dried herbs ready for brewing into tea along with a recipe.

Detoxification

There is often fierce debate about the need to detoxify regularly. During treatment it is important not to undergo any radical detoxification as the drugs need to do the job they are designed to do. Eating the right foods in abundance will be doing an adequate job. However, a couple of weeks after finishing chemotherapy you can give your liver a helping hand – though I would never recommend aggressive detoxification without the advice of a health professional, as it can make you feel extremely unwell and may be detrimental.

Coffee enemas

Enemas have a long history and were part of medical practice in the West until relatively recently. Coffee enemas are probably the most infamous aspect of Gerson Therapy (see page 108) as, having observed that liver function was often impaired in cancer patients, Gerson recommended them as a means of removing accumulated toxins.

When a coffee enema is used, caffeine is absorbed through the haemorrhoidal veins, which are part of the rectal plexus of veins. From here the caffeine passes into the portal system, which carries the blood supply to the liver and the gall bladder. The caffeine acts as an irritant to both these organs, and as the gall bladder is irritated it begins to spasm. This leads to a flushing of bile down through the bile duct into the small intestine. Bile is partially an excretory product, helping remove substances that the liver has detoxified. As bile enters the small intestine, the hormone secretin stimulates secretion of bile by the liver cells, causing it to flow into the gall bladder. Coffee also contains substances that promote the activity of the liver's detoxification enzymes.

Coffee enemas are used alongside other therapies, notably enzyme therapy, and can be effective for pain relief. Only use alongside conventional treatments after consulting your medical team or a health professional.

Cannabis

The question of cannabis oil has cropped up on a few occasions in my workshops. This is an absolute minefield because of course cannabis is an illegal drug in the UK and most other countries.

Cannabis had been used as a medicine for many years until 1973, when its use for this purpose became illegal. Since then there has been considerable debate about whether or not it should be legalized for medicinal use. There is an abundance of interesting old and emerging research on the use of the plant in many areas of health, including its anti-cancer properties. Cannabis oil – which is made from industrial hemp and contains only cannabidiol (CBD) and none of the psychoactive tetrahydro-cannabinol THC – is now legal in the EU, but it is incredibly expensive and out of reach of most people's budgets.

Research has shown that cannabidiols have potent anti-inflammatory and anti-cancer effects. A pharmaceutical product called Sativex is being trialled with some cancers alongside chemotherapy. An earlier trial investigating the efficacy of Sativex on cancer pain was inconclusive, but has been found to be safe. To date it is prescribed only for multiple sclerosis patients.

Many argue that cannabis does not need to be made into a pharmaceutical product but just needs to be legalized for medicinal purposes in its natural form, which would mean the synergistic effects of the whole plant were retained. A significant amount of research on the benefits of cannabis and further research on medicinal cannabis is being carried out in the US in relation to cancer and many other health problems.

The hallucinogen psilocybin found in magic mushrooms is also being researched with cancer patients to see if it can help reduce anxiety and depression in end-of-life situations.

Homeopathy

One of the best-known complementary therapies, homeopathy is based on the principle of treating 'like with like'. In other words, a substance that, when used in a large quantity, causes symptoms similar to those of a particular ailment, can also, when used in minute doses, cure that ailment. It is considered a safe treatment, but there is no scientific evidence to support its use.

Homeopathy causes some very heated debates, not least in our household. I have always been interested in it, but can understand the scepticism. My son Sebastian is a biochemist and a complete sceptic, even though I feel a homeopathic remedy may have had a hand in turning his health around after his diagnosis and the start of his treatment.

Sebastian was, of course, extremely poorly, and when he left hospital after his initial treatment he was really struggling to regain any energy. I took him to see a homeopathic medical doctor who sought the approval of Sebastian's oncologist and proceeded to treat him. I am grateful to his oncologist, because she took the positive stance that, although she knew nothing about homeopathy, she trusted it would do no harm and felt it important we tried anything we believed in. Sebastian was duly given just one dose of a remedy before bedtime and, from going to bed a lethargic, pale child, he awoke the next morning having, as they say, turned a corner and seemingly back to his old energetic self. He was unaware of taking the remedy, as he was swallowing many tablets, so any placebo effect was negligible. Of course, maybe it was a coincidental improvement and purely down to the chemotherapy. We can't prove it was the remedy and we can't prove it wasn't, but I do feel we are in danger of dismissing potentially beneficial and fundamentally safe therapies to our detriment because we cannot prove them scientifically. After all, there are many mysteries in life!

The Royal London Hospital for Integrated Medicine is an NHS hospital that integrates the best of conventional and complementary treatments. It has a complementary cancer-care clinic offering therapies such as homeopathy, acupuncture and dietetics. There are also NHS homeopathic hospitals in Bristol and Glasgow, Liverpool and Tunbridge Wells.

Acupuncture

An acupuncturist uses fine needles which are inserted through the skin to stimulate special points on the body that activate the

THE ARGUMENT FOR DETOXIFICATION

Liz Butler, MSc, BSc, Dip ION, Nutritional Therapist, Body Soul Nutrition

The concept of detoxification has a bad reputation in some circles due to its association with faddy diets endorsed by celebrities and the often questionable products that form part of the lucrative detox industry. Scientists and health experts have at times spoken out against detoxification, making the case that our body is designed to perform its own internal cleansing and needs no help in this. And yet, despite these arguments coming from those with academic qualifications and scientific training, I disagree with their thinking. It's true that we possess sophisticated systems of purification and elimination evolved over thousands of years to protect us against toxins, but we're living in unprecedented times when it comes to toxicity and our chemical burden has grown extremely rapidly in just a short space of time. Our bodies have not had time to adapt to this onslaught and they are struggling to cope, as demonstrated by figures charting the rapid rise of many chronic diseases. Coupled with this, our modern Western diet is nutrient depleted and without adequate nutrition our detoxification systems, just like any other body system, are compromised.

Another anti-detox argument often cited is that no evidence exists to suggest it's possible to enhance the body's detoxification processes. This is simply not true. While it is the case that very few studies have investigated detox in a clinical setting (apart from in relation to addiction), there are many studies showing that a wide range of nutrients and plant extracts, for example rosemary, cinnamon and turmeric, have the ability to upregulate the body's detoxification enzymes. This was something recognized by scientists Margaret Sears and Stephen

nervous system. This is claimed to improve the functioning of the body and relieve pain by stimulating the release of the body's natural painkillers. It has an adequate body of evidence and may be prescribed on the NHS.

Hyperthermia

Hyperthermia involves high heat treatment of cancer cells, either at a localized site or to a region of the body or, in cases of metastatic cancer, to the whole body. Cancer cells are more sensitive to heat than normal cells, which may mean they can be damaged or killed with minimal injury to healthy cells. Heat treatment may also enhance the effects of chemotherapy and radiotherapy and assist with pain reduction.

More research is needed to establish better techniques and to evaluate the therapy, especially in conjunction with other treatments.

Genius in their recent research paper 'Environmental Determinants of Chronic Disease and Medical Approaches: Recognition, Avoidance, Supportive Therapy, and Detoxification'. One of their recommendations for a clinical approach to detoxification was the use of 'a combination of optimal diet and supplemental nutrients'.

When it comes to cancer, a disease well recognized to have associations with environmental toxins, I believe detoxification has an important role to play in supporting the healing process. A recent study showed that one of the key mechanisms of herbs and spices known to have a role in cancer prevention was their ability to upregulate the detoxification enzymes found in the liver and other parts of the body. However, detoxification should not be taken lightly. Over the years that I have used it to support those with cancer it has become clear that internal cleansing done in the wrong way or at the wrong time can do more harm than good.

When I, or others in the field of natural health and functional medicine, talk about detoxification we are essentially describing ways to support and enhance the body's systems of elimination and the biotransformation that takes place in the liver when toxic chemicals are altered to make them safe for removal. In my own practice this involves a several-stage process focusing on the final routes of elimination first (bowel and kidneys) before moving on to the liver, and then the blood and lymphatic systems. Foods, nutrients and herbal supplements can all be utilised at these different stages along with particular techniques such as saunas and colon hydrotherapy.

As mentioned, caution is required with detoxification as there are contraindications. A gentle but thorough approach under the supervision of a health professional would always be advised.

Hyperbaric Oxygen Therapy (HBOT)

HBOT involves saturating the body with pure oxygen by breathing it in at higher than atmospheric pressure in an enclosed chamber. This process causes oxygen to be absorbed by the body fluids, cells and tissues, even those with blocked or reduced blood flow.

In tumours, disordered capillary networks mean the blood supply often cannot reach all the cells to supply them with oxygen, so the cells adapt to functioning adequately in a hypoxic (oxygen-reduced) state. Lack of oxygen leads to the cells producing hypoxia-inducible factor (HIF-1; see page 29), which induces angiogenesis (see page 29) and increases genetic instability and cell proliferation. A high oxygen level in the body can switch oncogenes (genes with the potential to cause cancer) off.

The efficacy of radiation therapy is relative to oxygen levels within the tumour. If the tumour is saturated with oxygen prior to radiation, it causes more free-radical damage and may enhance the therapy. If the tumour is in a hypoxic state the cancer cells are leaky, which makes it more difficult for chemotherapy drugs to penetrate and damage them. It is this increased vulnerability and sensitivity of oxygenated cancer cells which may lead to treatments working more effectively.

HBOT was first used back in the 1950s to increase the effectiveness of radiotherapy and there is evidence to show that it can be effective in treating delayed radiation injuries. It has also been shown to be particularly beneficial in reducing the side-effects of radiation to the pelvic area, including rectal bleeding. The increased flow of oxygen stimulates and restores function to damaged cells and organs, including those of the liver and brain, making this a potentially useful post-treatment therapy for many cancer patients.

However, in the 1970s experiments with HBOT failed to show the expected benefits when it was given concurrently with radiation, as in addition to sensitizing the tumour cells it also increased the sensitivity of the normal tissues, causing significant toxicity. Unfortunately, this technically challenging treatment then went out of favour.

HBOT has been investigated recently alongside the Ketogenic Diet (see page 106) and the combination appears to have enhanced benefits during treatment and in tumour shrinkage. HBOT has also been shown to be beneficial for those suffering from lymphoedema. However, more studies are needed to ascertain its best use.

Intravenous ozone therapy is another treatment used to saturate the body's cells with oxygen. As it increases the number of free radicals in the cells and may also increase the toxicity of radiation treatment, it should always be discussed with your medical team before it is used alongside standard treatment.

Intravenous (IV) Vitamin C

Vitamin C is well known as an antioxidant and is often recommended in supplement form. However, high levels of vitamin C in the blood can be achieved only by injecting intravenously and if this is done it appears to have several anti-cancer mechanisms.

Cancer cells have an increased number of glucose transporters on their cell membranes and these also transport vitamin C into the cell. Within the cancer cell the vitamin C is transformed into hydrogen peroxide which is toxic to cancer cells and kills them, but it is not toxic to healthy cells and leaves them undamaged.

IV vitamin C has been investigated in humans alongside standard therapies and has been found to reduce side-effects of treatment such as fatigue and nausea, but unfortunately it has not gained a place in routine practice.

Low-dose Naltrexone (LDN)

Naltrexone is a pharmaceutical product which was originally approved at a high dose to help heroin addicts, as it blocks opiate receptors in the brain. Some doctors then found that at a low dose it can have a beneficial effect by regulating the immune system. Since then it has been used by a few clinicians in the treatment of diseases linked to immune dysfunction, including cancer.

The drug works by stimulating the body into producing more opiates. Immune cells have opiate-receptor sites and preliminary research has shown that the opiates latch on to the immune cells and modulate their behaviour. Studies on LDN are small and much of the evidence is anecdotal, but side-effects appear to be minimal and, as it seems to have anti-inflammatory effects by balancing and regulating immune function, its potential for treating autoimmune disease and cancer may be huge.

There is growing interest in well-tolerated, cheaper drugs that were designed for one condition but are now being seen as potentially useful in the management of cancer. Trials in this area are continuing – see the panel overleaf.

Lymphatic Stimulation

The lymph system bathes every cell in our body and is responsible for removing metabolic waste from cells. It does not have a pump like the cardiovascular system, and the only way for it to move is by our muscle contractions when we move. This is another example of the importance of exercise, especially because tumour cells that break away from the primary tumour tend to accumulate in areas of sluggish circulation. Aiding our circulatory and lymphatic system will help with the oxygenation of cells and detoxification processes.

Walking, jumping and jogging are all great ways to get your lymph moving, but one of the best exercises is rebounding. This is basically jumping on a trampoline and the reason it is particularly good is because every muscle in your body is expanding and contracting due to the G force – an extremely efficient way of pushing your lymph around the body. Rebounding, like any resistance exercise, can also reduce the risk of osteoporosis.

Dry skin brushing is also good for lymphatic drainage and circulation. It is easy to buy a skin brush and you can use it each day before you shower. You need to brush towards the heart from your toes, fingers and head. There are plenty of videos on the internet that demonstrate how to do this.

Massage

Massage can also help with lymphatic drainage, but in addition people report that after a massage they feel more relaxed, sleep better and their immunity improves. Choose a qualified massage therapist who is experienced in the field of oncology and if there are any concerns check with your medical team.

NEW USES FOR OLD DRUGS

Jerome Burne, health journalist

A clinic in London has collaborated with a small drug company who have gathered a stack of research material on a large number of old (and consequently cheap) drugs which appear to have a positive impact on cancer. The convincing evidence is from cell research, animal studies and small clinical trials on humans and these drugs are now being trialled at the clinic.

In general, whether the treatment was an old drug or a vitamin, the official 'scientific' approach would have said: 'No proper evidence, can't use it.' Old drug or vitamin stays on the shelf with all the rest. It can't get a trial, not because it is known to be ineffective or dangerous, but because they cost tens of millions of pounds and no one is going to spend that on a compound that is dirt cheap because it has no patent. That's not science, that is hard commercial logic.

To get round this fake-science blockade the doctors at the clinic – two of whom are oncology professors – are prescribing the drugs off-label (a standard and perfectly acceptable practice) with the intention of carefully monitoring the patients and writing up the results for a journal.

This is the sort of imaginative following up of a promising idea that proper science is all about. The clinic gives a cocktail of four drugs, all old, so besides being cheap there is good information on side-effects and dosage.

Total cost of the drugs for a year? Between £200 and £400, which is unheard of in the cancer world. If the results are positive this alternative approach to EBM will have produced a treatment that is effective, cheaper and safer.

Sometimes aromatherapy oils are used in massage, which can enhance wellbeing and healing – but again they should be used only by an experienced therapist. Many Maggie's Centres offer this complementary therapy.

A special type of massage known as manual lymphatic drainage (MLD) may be recommended if you have lymphoedema. A specialist nurse can teach you how to use this to reduce swelling.

Reflexology

Reflexology uses gentle foot massage to help the body to heal by improving energy flow and rebalancing the body. It is believed that every area of the body is reflected in corresponding areas in the feet, therefore the reflexologist can stimulate areas to improve blood flow and unblock nerve impulses.

Some studies also indicate that reflexology is useful in helping reduce pain, anxiety and depression, and that it enhances relaxation and sleep.

As always, choose a qualified reflexologist with experience in the cancer field. It may be advised not to use reflexology during chemo- or radiotherapy or immediately after surgery.

Meditation

Meditation has been used for thousands of years to bring about relaxation, but it is now known that it can affect gene expression ('turning on' a gene) too. It appears to influence inflammatory pathways by increasing antioxidant production and thus reducing oxidative stress. Mindfulness meditation (see below) has been shown to improve depressive symptoms and reduce anxiety.

Most Maggie's Centres offer stress-management programmes, tai-chi and yoga, all of which include an element of meditation.

Mindfulness

The National Institute of Clinical Excellence (NICE) recommend mindfulness as a treatment for recurring episodes of depression. However, it is becoming increasingly popular as a way of coping with the general stresses and strains of life. Many report that after a cancer diagnosis, learning to practise mindfulness has improved their ability to cope with making adjustments to this change.

Mindfulness is usually delivered as a group-based course and it teaches you to be aware of the present moment, observing details of the moment, including thoughts, feelings and emotions, and accepting them in a non-judgemental way. It is easy to go through the motions of our lives without really living it, caught up in the world of our thoughts. Mindfulness helps us to step back from our thoughts and not to brood on things. Becoming more aware of the present moment can help us enjoy the world around us more fully and understand ourselves better.

Maggie's Centres run mindfulness courses, or you may find a course within your local area; you may also find it helpful to try one of the other practices that involve the mindfulness philosophy. These include meditation (see opposite), yoga, tai-chi and qigong. What these all have in common is focusing on our breathing to bring ourselves into the present and to help us relax and heal. During times of stress we tend to take very shallow breaths. This reduces blood flow and hampers many of our body systems. Learning to breathe deeply into the abdomen improves blood flow; increases oxygen in the body; helps to pump lymph, which supports our immune system; increases 'feel-good' neurotransmitter production; and helps to heal the body.

Learning the practice of healing breath can be extremely helpful in stressful situations and can trigger many physiological benefits. If you do nothing else towards relaxation and meditation, do take time at least a couple of times a day to sit or lie comfortably and focus on your breath. Breathe deeply, allowing your chest and then your abdomen to rise gently with the breath; then breathe out slowly through your mouth or nose. You can do this anywhere, even on the bus or train on the way to work. It is also a good way to switch off your mind at night if you have trouble sleeping. Instead of counting sheep, count your breath in and out.

6 Life After Treatment

I OFTEN HEAR PEOPLE SAY that the day they finish their treatment and are told all is fine and they are in remission can actually be a challenging time. This may be hard for others to understand, but when you have had the security blanket of hospital and the knowledge that the current treatment will be killing cancer cells, you suddenly feel very vulnerable when it is taken away. This emotion often takes people by surprise because they have been longing for this day all the way through treatment.

This may well be a time when people need support of a different kind compared to the preceding months. Now is where a psychologist can help pick up the pieces, and this is part of the ongoing support that is offered at Maggie's. Many oncology centres, including Maggie's, run helpful programmes for those who are moving on from their treatment, giving them the opportunity to take stock of thoughts and feelings in a supportive group setting.

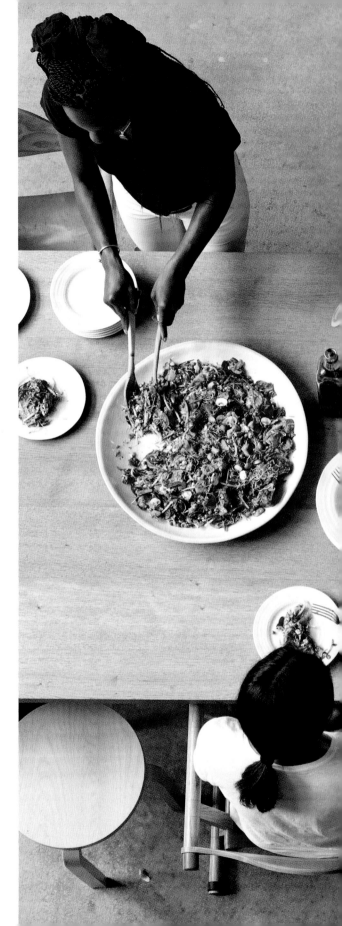

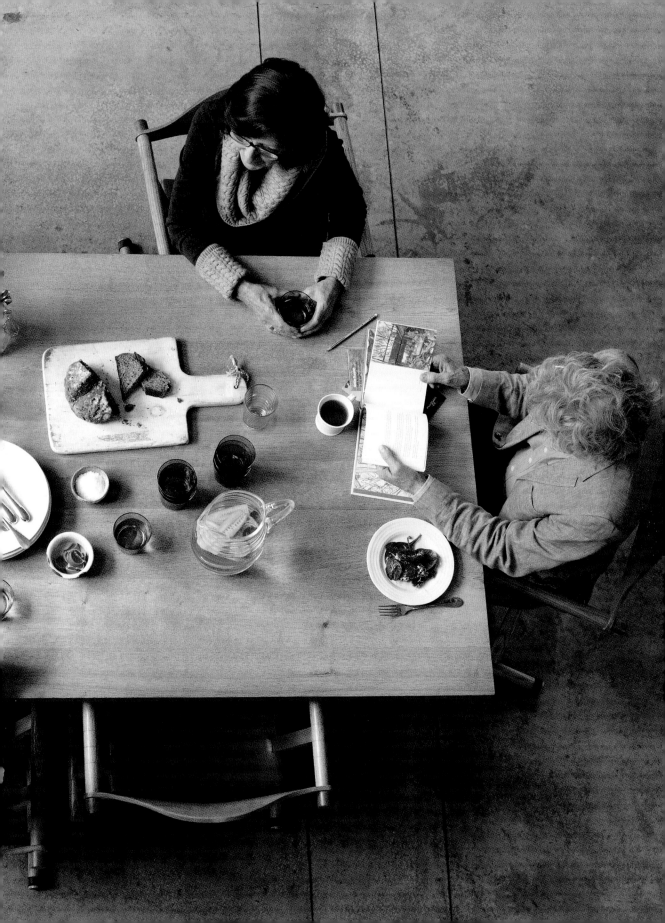

SUPPORT FOR THE FUTURE

Mary Turner, Cancer Support Specialist, Maggie's West London

A cancer diagnosis gives rise to many physical and emotional challenges that may continue well beyond treatment for the person experiencing cancer, their family and friends. Mindfulness has the potential to support people through the turbulence of a cancer diagnosis and the unexpectedness of treatment. It can also support them into their lives beyond, where a lot of adjustments may need to take place and living can be tinged with uncertainty about the future. Mindfulness instils potentially transformative ways of being, living and responding to oneself and others. It can be used as either an antidote to existing symptoms of illness and distress or as a prophylactic treatment to avoid a spiralling long-term stress reaction.

Changing Bad Habits for Good

Our lives tend to be governed by habits and learned behaviour, and reducing or eliminating unhealthy habits and establishing healthier ones in their place can be challenging. Identifying triggers that lead us to certain actions – such as eating when we are not hungry, inactivity or putting things off until tomorrow – is the first step in learning to control them. Avoiding triggers is the best strategy, but this is not always possible, so we must unlearn some of our learned behaviours.

There are two types of trigger:

• **External triggers** come from the environment around us or from our daily routine, both of which cause us to act in a certain way. These influences can trigger a response that results in an unhealthy choice or behaviour. If we understand what these influences are, we may be able to avoid or remove them and so establish a routine that encourages healthy choices instead.

• **Internal triggers** are thoughts, feelings or sensations from within which cause us to behave in a particular way. These can be complex and can interact with external influences to produce unhealthy patterns of behaviour. Learning to turn any self-defeating thoughts and feelings into positive, helpful thoughts and actions is the way to overcome negative internal triggers.

Beating the triggers:

• Avoid triggers wherever possible. For instance, not having unhealthy food in the house will eliminate one source of temptation.

• Distract yourself by taking an alternative action. If, for example, you are tempted to eat an unhealthy snack, divert yourself by going for a walk or reading a book or phoning a friend instead. Temptation often arises through boredom or craving. Cravings for food come in waves and will pass after a short time, so distracting yourself can get you through a craving whereas true hunger will not go away.

• Learn to resist. Most urges to eat when not hungry are learned – for instance eating sweets whilst watching television, or buying a chocolate bar when you fill up with petrol. The good thing is these habits can be unlearned once you recognize the difference between hunger, a craving or habit. Replace the habit with a new one, such as eating only at the table when you are at home or always keeping a healthy snack in the car.

• Stress and anxiety can lead to overeating or a lack of exercise. Learn relaxation techniques such as breathing exercises, meditation or yoga (see 'Mindfulness', page 125).

• Positive thinking – such as telling yourself you can do something rather than assuming 'I can't' – can help you build confidence in your ability to change bad habits. Small steps can lead to greater, sustained changes.

Maggie's 'Where Now?' course enables those who are post-treatment to move forward with their lives and establish some personal goals. Attendees are taught to consider the goals they hope to achieve, particularly those concerning exercise, nutrition and wellbeing. This can be invaluable in helping you to focus on what you really want to achieve and to let go of any negative patterns of behaviour. Importantly, it can lead you to feel more in charge of your own wellbeing.

Weight Management

It is at this stage that you may feel ready to address any weight-management issues. According to Cancer Research, approximately 5 per cent of cancer cases are due to being overweight or obese. It is therefore vital that you aim to keep to as healthy a weight as possible.

Excess weight is seen as a concern because fat cells promote systemic inflammation (see page 27); produce excess oestrogen and other hormones that stimulate cancer-cell growth (see page 28); and may induce insulin resistance, which increases the level of circulating insulin and insulin-like growth factor – both of which are also cancer promoters (see page 28).

At a cellular level, over-fed cells do not work as effectively. Excess insulin will be telling the cells to store more fat and grow, which will make the cells sluggish. The mitochondria (see page 25) begin to decline in number and this leads to a sick cell with increased oxidative stress. This in turn damages the DNA and can lead to the switching on of genes associated with cancer. However, eating an array of protective antioxidants from good-quality plant foods can reverse this situation.

I hear from so many people who bemoan the fact that they are eating healthily and taking lots of exercise and still they can't shift the weight. Losing excess pounds is never easy, but if you can change your body composition – in other words the fat-to-muscle ratio – and even the type of fat, you can make a real difference to your metabolism and in turn lower your risk of disease. Use a body-fat monitor rather than scales and don't get too hung up on your weight or on shifting inches initially; just be honest with yourself about your diet and lifestyle.

If you are eating a predominantly clean-food diet (fewer chemicals) consisting of sufficient protein, healthy fats, plenty of vegetables and a small amount of complex starchy carbs, along with taking enough exercise, you can feel proud of yourself and comforted that you are making a difference. If you continue to eat in this way, your body will become healthier and your body composition will change – but we need to remember that we are all individuals of different shapes and sizes who store fat cells in different areas of the body. We also have differences in our skeletal and organ weight, and in our amount of muscle, so body mass index (BMI) is not a good gauge of how overweight we are.

Fat around the middle – visceral fat – is the greatest concern and is often the hardest to shift. The body stores fat around our central and vital organs in order to protect them, but we don't want too much because then, instead of protecting them, it begins to have a detrimental impact by releasing damaging chemicals. One of the best measurements of unhealthy fat ratios is looking at the difference in size between your hips and your waist. Measure your waist at the narrowest point and your hips at the widest point. Divide the waist measurement by the hip measurement. If it is above 0.85 (woman) or 1.0 (man) you should definitely begin taking steps to change your body composition.

There are a great many weight-loss programmes and diets and some can be of great benefit, but if you are struggling with your weight you really need to address behaviour change (see pages 128–9) and introduce new habits that will last a lifetime. Diets that lead to yo-yoing weight are not the way to go; you need to find a way of maintaining a healthy weight that suits you.

Some interesting research into weight gain and breast-cancer risk has been conducted by Dr Michelle Harvie and Professor Tony Howell. This led them to write the 2-Day Diet, an approach to weight loss where you diet for two consecutive days a week and eat normally for the other five days. Maggie's run an online weight-loss programme based on this approach. The support and resources provided can be invaluable in giving you the motivation you need to change your way of eating.

Palliative Care

Palliative care is not all about end of life but is also an added layer of support or specialized care that can be accessed at any time during a serious illness. Often the side-effects of treatment take their toll on quality of life and this may be where a palliative-care team can step in and help on a more individual basis. They can provide pain relief and address other distressing symptoms, along with helping the person to live as well as possible. The specialist teams should include palliative-medicine consultants and palliative-care nurse specialists, together with a range of expertise provided by physiotherapists, occupational therapists, dietitians, pharmacists, social workers and those able to give spiritual and psychological support.

If you feel you need this extra support, ask your medical team to refer you. It is best to access the care sooner rather than later to ensure you have help when you need it. Studies have shown such support to be invaluable, improving patients' outcome and quality of life significantly.

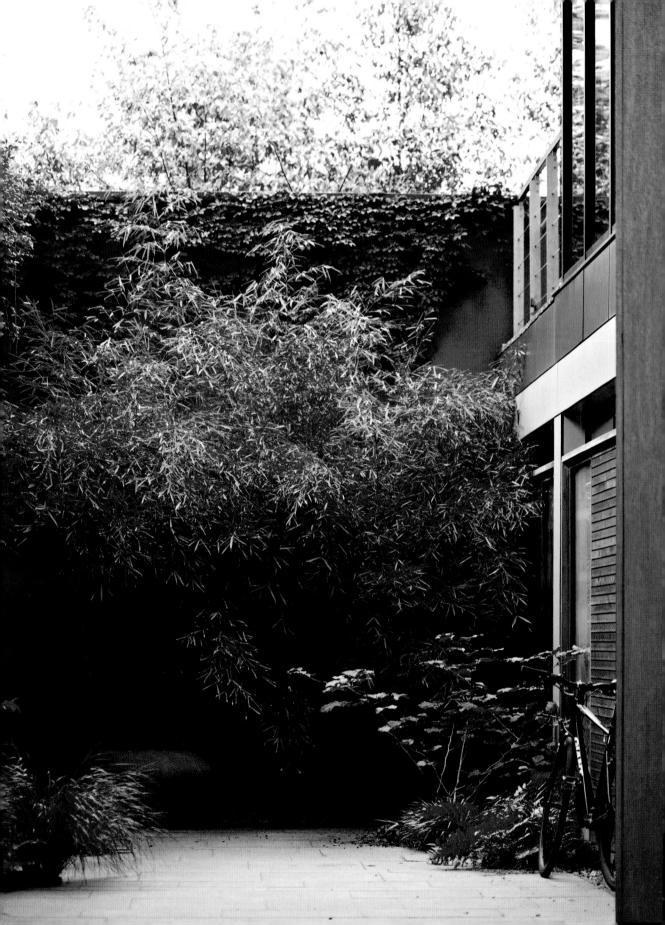

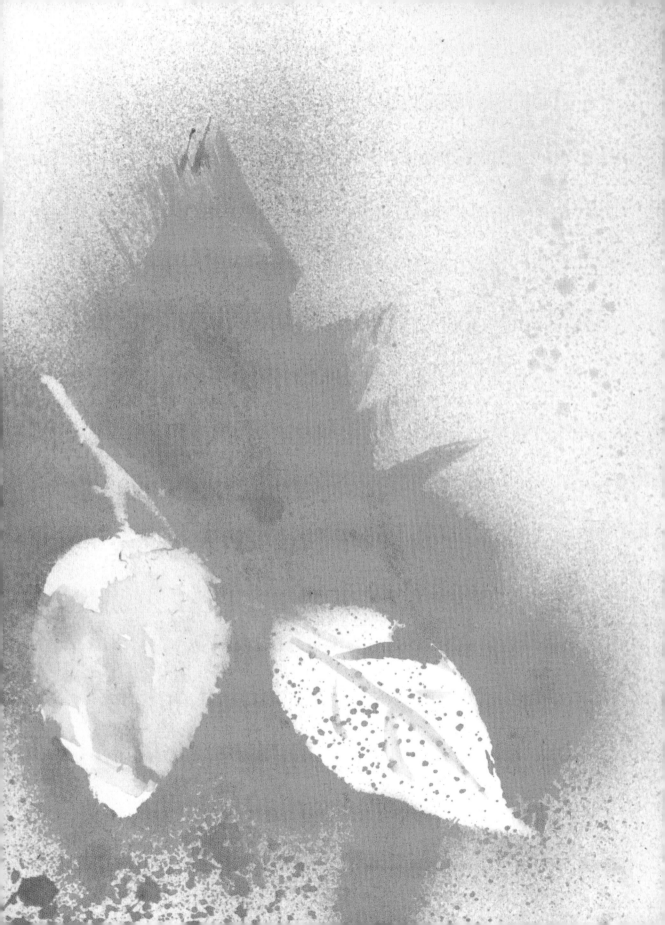

PART TWO

The Nutritional Kitchen

Preparing Your Kitchen for a Healthy Diet

BOTH CATHERINE AND I have always enjoyed good food that is well sourced and cooked from scratch, enabling us to deliver a tasty, wholesome meal to the table for our families and friends. But this book set me a new culinary challenge, demanding that every recipe be beneficial for those diagnosed with, or undergoing treatment for, cancer – not too many ingredients; not too complicated to make; all ingredients easily sourced from leading supermarkets, or from health stores such as Holland & Barrett; and finally and most importantly, both nutritionally rich in content and super-tasty for everyone to enjoy.

With all this in mind I started creating, testing, perfecting, tasting and recording each recipe. Our demands were formidable, as we wanted to offer the very best food to help cancer patients through this difficult time. During this culinary creative task I started to call my epicentre 'The Nutritional Kitchen' because with every recipe I needed to deliver on all these self-set demands.

The Nutritional Kitchen's favourite ingredients are rainbow vegetables, especially the cruciferous variety; pulses, nuts and seeds; coconut and olive oil; fruits, especially berries; spices, especially turmeric; grains, grass-fed animals, poultry and seafood; eggs and some dairy goods. Throughout the recipes you will see these healthy ingredients repeatedly being used to enrich and aid the body. You will not find refined sugar or wheat flour in any of them.

Kitchen Staples

To get started, give your kitchen cupboards and fridge a makeover and ensure they contain only foods that will enrich your health. If unhealthy, processed food is not to hand at home, you will have eliminated one source of temptation!

Here are some ideas for foods that are good to have on your regular shopping list. Many of them are included in our recipes.

Fill your kitchen cupboard and fridge with:

- virgin coconut oil

- olive oil

- almond/coconut/hemp/oat/hazelnut milks

- nuts – natural almonds/cashews/walnuts/Brazil nuts (keep in fridge)

- seeds – pumpkin/sunflower/hemp/chia/quinoa/poppy/sesame/flaxseeds (linseeds)

- fresh herbs

- spices

- berries – blueberries/raspberries/strawberries/blackcurrants/blackberries

- cruciferous vegetables – cabbage/broccoli/kale/cauliflower/Brussels sprouts/spring greens/watercress

- avocados

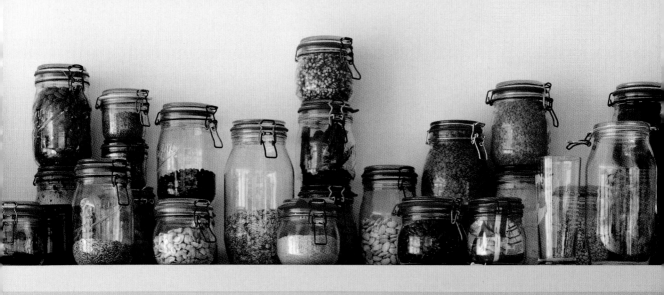

the
nutritional
kitchen

- fennel

- carrots

- sweet potatoes

- beetroot

- asparagus

- onions

- garlic

- ginger

- horseradish

- turmeric (fresh and ground)

- rocket/spinach/cucumber/tomatoes/sprouted seeds

- flours – spelt/coconut/rice/buckwheat

- beans – chickpeas/kidney beans/black beans/butterbeans

- lentils – red/green/black

- fruit – apples/pears/oranges/grapefruits/grapes/bananas/kiwis/peaches/apricots/nectarines/watermelon and all other melons/papaya/pineapple/mangos/cherries/passionfruit/figs/coconuts/dates

- almond or cashew butter

- cocoa/raw cacao/dark chocolate (85% cocoa solids)

Empty your kitchen cupboard and fridge of:

- bought biscuits, cakes, pastries

- refined cereals such as the highly sugary varieties (wholegrain types – e.g. Weetabix or Shredded Wheat – are the best of a bad bunch)

- white flour and its products – white bread, pasta, biscuits

- ready meals

- processed meats

- crisps/oven chips

- milk chocolate/chocolate spread/drinking chocolate

- fizzy drinks and concentrated juices

- chemical sweeteners – e.g. saccharin, aspartame

- alcohol (except red wine, to be drunk in moderation)

- refined oils – vegetable, corn, sunflower, rapeseed (any oil in a plastic bottle)

- anything that has an ingredients list that reads like a chemistry lesson

- anything that does not resemble real food

Useful Kitchen Gadgets

Here is a list of kitchen equipment for everyday healthy cooking, and which you'll find useful for making the recipes in this book:

- good sharp knives – small, medium, large and serrated (keep them sharp so that you enjoy using them)

- chopping board – wood is best

- hand-held stick blender – good for blending soups in the pan; helps save on washing up

- non-stick frying pan – not so much oil needed as with a standard pan and gives a good result

- pots, pans and bakeware – best are ceramic or stainless steel; cast iron is also good but it taints the flavour of the food. Line bakeware with baking parchment to stop toxic substances found in some bakeware transferring to the food; aluminium should ideally not come into contact with food

- large stock pot – also good for batch soup making

- glass Kilner jars or glass dishes for storage

- juicer or other blender for making smoothies – see below

- julienne peeler (e.g. SharpPeel by Lakeland) or more expensive spiralizer – good for making vegetable spaghetti and adding vegetables to salads

- fine sieve and muslin if making your own nut or grain milks

- stainless-steel flask and stackable lunch boxes – for transporting soups and meals when away from home

- slow cooker – I have never had one of these, but if you are working or don't have much kitchen space they are a great invention

- Electronic kitchen scales – total accuracy is essential for getting recipes right!

- mandolin – great for quickly slicing vegetables and fruits for salads

- salad spinner or tea towel – good for spinning and drying lettuce after washing

Juicers

The vast choice of juicers available can be rather daunting if you have no idea what you are looking for and you can end up spending a lot on equipment that you rarely use. If you are new to juicing and unsure how regularly you would do it, I would first go for a cheaper model so that you can assess how often you are using it.

The cheaper models are the centrifugal type, which use a cutting blade and spinning basket and extract the juice by a high-centrifugal force. This method introduces more oxygen to the juice and so it should be drunk immediately to avoid losing nutrient value. It is a quick and convenient choice, but is not efficient at juicing green leafy vegetables and will not cope with wheatgrass.

Masticating juicers are more expensive, are excellent for juicing green leafy vegetables and wheatgrass, and produce a richer juice, potentially higher in important enzymes, but they are slower and more difficult to clean. Twin-bladed machines give the best results, but less expensive and perhaps more user-friendly are the vertical single auger and horizontal single auger types.

Smoothie makers/blenders/liquidizers

Again there is quite a choice of equipment, ranging from cheap to very expensive. The power of the motor is key to efficiency, but there are some excellent small machines on the market which deliver well-blended smoothies. We recommend buying a blender initially, as it is easier and faster. Blenders may also be used for making nut butters and purées. Nutribullet has captured the market and the machines are very reliable, easy to use and fast.

Food and Kitchen Tips

Poultry and meat

It's important to know where the chicken or meat you buy comes from. Aim for organic, free-range chicken and organic, pasture-fed beef or lamb from your butcher or supermarket – or, if you are lucky enough to have a local farm shop, buy from there.

Fats

If following a dairy-free diet, replace butter with olive oil and coconut oil. Both work well, although coconut oil will adjust the flavour and may need a little time to become a healthy favourite – but it's worth it for the health benefits. Always buy raw, cold-pressed, virgin coconut oil for quality and use it if a recipe requires frying, as it is considered the best oil to heat without causing damage. Many other oils become hard for the body to digest when heated, but coconut oil is highly stable and can safely be brought to a higher temperature. It's also good for the immune system due to its antibacterial effect. Contrary to belief, although it is a saturated fat, it is good for cholesterol as it helps to raise HDL, the good cholesterol. Try it on dry skin and hair too – it works a treat!

Use cheaper virgin olive oil for cooking and better-quality, cold-pressed, extra-virgin for dressings.

Stock

We recommend that whenever possible you use homemade stocks in recipes (see Super Stocks, page 256). Alternatively, use a good organic ready-made stock, or a dried organic stock cube.

Flour

If following a wheat-free diet, do not fret: there are many good alternatives to wheat flour. Try fine cornmeal, gram flour, ground oats (you may have to grind them yourself, but it is easy to do in a blender), rice flour, coconut flour, barley flour, ground nut flour, chestnut flour, hemp flour – the list is extensive! You will need to experiment a little and a raising agent (such as baking powder) will always be needed. These flours work best in cookies, cakes and pastries. Bread really is a more technical matter, as it's hard to get a good rise from these flours – spelt and rye are probably the best alternatives.

Eggs

Eggs are a culinary lifesaver and I always have some in my kitchen. Simply boil, scramble, poach, or make an omelette or frittata, and you will have a nutritious meal. For a protein enricher, try poaching an egg in a thin soup.

Beans

If using dried beans, once soaked they will approximately double in weight. The weight of dried beans given in our recipes is the amount you need to soak.

Seeds

If you have problems with chewing or with your digestion, try soaking seeds overnight in water to soften them; this helps to remove enzyme inhibitors which can interfere with digestion and mineral absorption.

Toasted pumpkin seeds

Lightly toast seeds, roughly chop and then sprinkle on to soups, salads and casseroles to give texture and a nutritional boost. Toasting makes them more easily digestible. Pumpkin seeds contain a perfect balance of omega fatty acids; they are alkaline; high in zinc, phytosterols (which may be good for prostate health) and also tryptophan, which is a good mood enhancer and aids sleep.

Mustard seeds

On a day when you might be suffering from 'metallic mouth' due to chemotherapy, try soaking a teaspoon of mustard seeds for 24 hours, add them to a smoothie and blitz in a blender. The hot flavour of the seeds can be refreshing to the tastebuds and masks the metallic taste.

Sprouting seeds

Sprouted seeds and grains are pre-digested, making them easier to digest and absorb; also, growth increases their nutrient content, especially A, C, E and many B vitmains. Many supermarkets now sell sprouted seeds, but it is also very easy to sprout your own.

Rinse the seeds, place in a large jar in the ratio 1 part seeds to 3 parts water. Leave to soak 12–24 hours, or until they just start to sprout. Drain, rinse and then return to the jar. Lay the sprouting jar on its side, spreading the seeds out. Rinse three times a day and they should be sprouted in 2–3 days. The sprouted seeds can be used in salads and stored in an airtight container in the fridge for 2 days.

Natural protein and calorie boosters

If weight loss is a problem, try adding a little nut cream or ground seeds to soups, casseroles, salad dressings, smoothies and yoghurts for that extra calorie boost.

Herbal mouth coolers

If you are suffering from a sore mouth, try blending your favourite herb to a paste, then mix with a little water and freeze in an ice tray. Suck on the frozen cube, as you would a sweet, to calm the pain. Best for this are dill, basil, rosemary (which is quite strong in flavour) and parsley; all are very anti-inflammatory.

Seaweed

Seaweed can now be found in supermarkets and also comes in small shakers. It should be used as a seasoning along with your usual salt and pepper. Not only does it really enhance flavours, it is also rich in nutrients and adds umami flavour.

Spices that help calm metallic taste in the mouth during treatment

Suck on cloves and cardamom pods.

Juices and smoothies

For tips and ideas, see pages 69 and 156–7.

Papaya drink

Delicious and nutritious. Try scooping out the seeds from a papaya, place them in a glass, top up with water and leave in the fridge for 24 hours. Strain the seeds and drink the water. This is a refreshing, natural and delicately flavoured fruit quencher.

The Recipes

We are genuinely excited to offer and recommend over eighty innovative, delicious and easy recipes, which are set out in chapters – 'Starting the Day', 'Energizing Snacks', 'A Vegetarian Rainbow', 'Fabulous Fish', 'Satisfying Meat', 'Something Sweet' and 'Super Staples'. Each recipe begins with clear, practical nutritional information suggesting when it may help, how many people it serves or how much it makes, and how long it takes to prepare. We hope the beautiful photography that accompanies the recipes will also inspire you to get cooking.

These recipes are so delicious that in our homes we cook and enjoy them time and time again. Now you too can revolutionize the way you shop, cook and eat as you transform your diet and help yourself towards a healthier way of living.

Starting the Day

Pancakes with Fresh Fruit, Yoghurt and Honey

Makes approximately 8–10 pancakes

Takes 10 minutes

50g desiccated coconut

75g wholemeal spelt flour

1 egg

150ml milk

½ tsp baking powder

1 tsp coconut oil

To serve

bio-yoghurt

favourite seasonal fruit – berries, peaches, apricots, figs

raw honey, or for a change try maple syrup

This low-gluten pancake gets its natural sweetness from the desiccated coconut. If you want a totally gluten-free pancake, replace the spelt flour with porridge oats, which can be soaked overnight in the milk or some natural yoghurt. Pancakes can be a lovely treat at breakfast: they're tasty and visually enticing when topped with fresh fruit and a spoonful of bio-yoghurt.

Eggs are high-quality protein and contain a variety of vitamins, particularly vitamin B_2 (riboflavin), B_{12} and vitamin D. Buy the freshest eggs you can and there's no need to store them in the fridge; they cook better when used at room temperature. This is a good recipe for anyone having difficulty swallowing or suffering mouth ulcers, as it's soft and the honey and yoghurt will help soothe.

When frying pancakes or other foods on a high heat, organic coconut oil is the healthy option. Used in moderation it adds a delicious flavour and aroma to your cooking. Always choose raw, virgin organic coconut oil.

1 Place the desiccated coconut and spelt in a medium bowl and mix together.

2 Whisk the egg, add the milk and pour into the bowl, mixing with the coconut and spelt until evenly blended.

3 Finally, add the baking powder and mix through.

4 In a large non-stick frying pan melt a little coconut oil on a medium to high heat, add 2 or 3 individual spoonfuls of the mixture, but do not allow them to run into each other. Cook for 2 minutes and when set flip over with a spatula and cook for 1–2 minutes on the other side. Transfer the pancakes to a baking sheet and keep warm.

5 Repeat until all the batter is used.

6 Serve topped with yoghurt, fruits and honey, or maple syrup if desired.

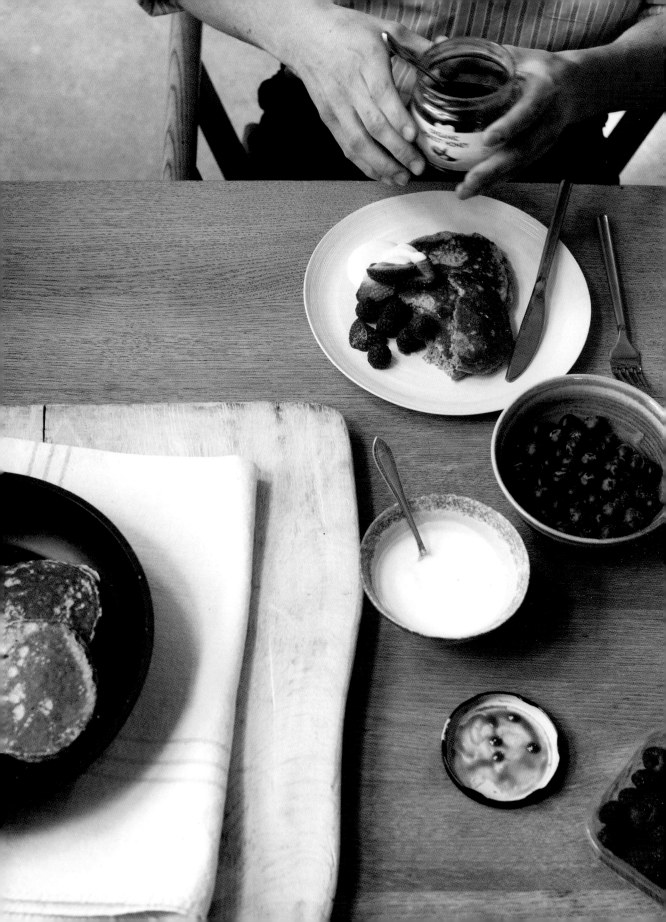

Chia Strawberry and Cashew Nut Milk Pot

Serves 2

Takes 2 hours' soaking plus 1 hour or overnight

6 cashew nuts

100ml water

200g strawberries, hulled

a drop of vanilla extract, or a pinch of vanilla seeds

2 tbsp chia seeds

Chia seeds are little grains of goodness packed with omega-3, fibre, protein and antioxidants. They may take a little while to get used to, as their taste is totally neutral and the texture is a new sensation. Enjoy this pot of low-carb goodness at breakfast; it's also perfect packed into a jar or pot and eaten when away from home.

Cashew nuts are high in magnesium and tryptophan, which can help to improve brain function and mood, so nibble on these frequently to maintain a sunny outlook.

1 Soak the cashew nuts in the water for 2 hours, then blitz in a blender until smooth and creamy.

2 Add half the strawberries, the vanilla extract or seeds and blitz again until smooth.

3 Pour into a bowl and stir in the chia seeds. Put in the fridge for 30 minutes or overnight. The seeds will swell, transforming into a rich, creamy mixture.

4 Slice the remaining strawberries and serve on top of the chia mix. If you want a fancy-looking start to your day, you can layer the remaining strawberries with the chia mix in a glass.

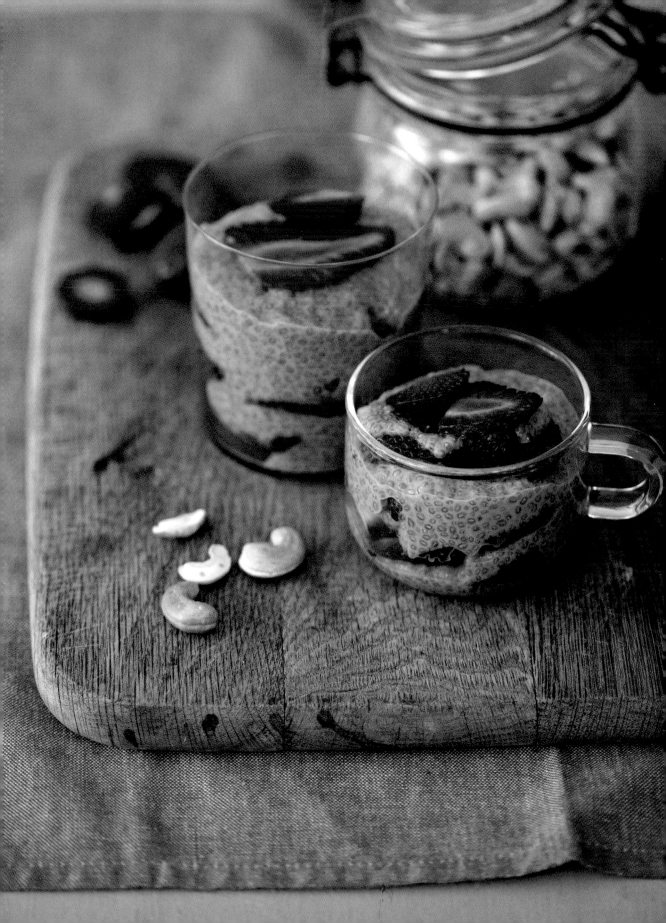

Porridge and Chia Breakfast Bowl

Serves 1

Takes 1–12 hours' soaking plus 10 minutes

1 tbsp chia seeds

50g porridge oats

a pinch of cinnamon

½ tbsp raw cacao (optional)

300ml milk (dairy, nut, seed, coconut or rice)

Winter Dried Fruit Compote or Fresh Seasonal Fruit Compote (see pages 149 and 150)

1 tsp shredded coconut (optional)

Chia seeds are renowned for their high content of plant-based omega-3 fatty acids so, if you are not a fish eater, using these may be a good way of introducing this important nutrient into your diet.

This is a very comforting bowl of goodness to start your day and ideal for anyone who has problems swallowing their food. It is low in carbs and high in soluble fibre, which encourages our healthy gut microbiota to thrive. It also binds excess hormones in the gut to stop them being re-absorbed, thus ensuring they are eliminated efficiently. If you like chocolate, add ½ tablespoon of raw cacao or cocoa. Cinnamon is very good for balancing blood sugar, but feel free to use a different spice.

You can prepare this in advance and cook as needed.

1 Put seeds, porridge oats, cinnamon and raw cacao, if using, in the milk in a non-stick pan and soak for 1 hour or overnight.

2 When ready to eat, place on a medium heat and gently bring to a simmer, constantly stirring to make sure it does not catch on the base of the pan (this is why I favour a non-stick pan, plus it makes washing up easier).

3 Adjust the consistency by adding a little extra milk if it's too stiff, and simmer for 1 minute.

4 Spoon into a bowl and add either Fresh Seasonal Fruit Compote or Winter Dried Fruit Compote and 1 teaspoon shredded coconut to sweeten, if desired.

Bircher Muesli

Serves 1

Takes 1–12 hours
or overnight

35g oats

1 tsp hemp seeds

1 tsp sunflower seeds

25g dried fruits, such
  as apricots, dates

150ml apple juice

1 apple

15g nuts, roughly
  chopped

1 tbsp bio-yoghurt

This was originally invented by the Swiss doctor and nutritionist Maximilian Bircher-Benner in the late nineteenth century. He was way ahead of his time in his aim to get more raw food and fruits into the diet. Today Bircher Muesli is made around the world with a variety of fruits, nuts and seeds and using various types of liquid – everything from dairy to juices, with some people even preferring water.

This muesli is lighter than and a great alternative to porridge (see opposite). Just like porridge, it's easy to consume when you're feeling weak and it's easy to swallow. The hemp seeds included here provide a perfect balance of omegas 6 and 3 and are rich in protein. And try coconut bio-yoghurt, made with coconut milk – it is a tasty and nutritious alternative to dairy yoghurt.

1 Place the oats, hemp seeds and sunflower seeds in a bowl.

2 Chop the dried fruit, add to the oat mix, pour in your chosen liquid and leave to soak for 1–12 hours.

3 Just before eating, grate the apple into the mixture. Add the nuts, mix well and serve with a spoonful of yoghurt.

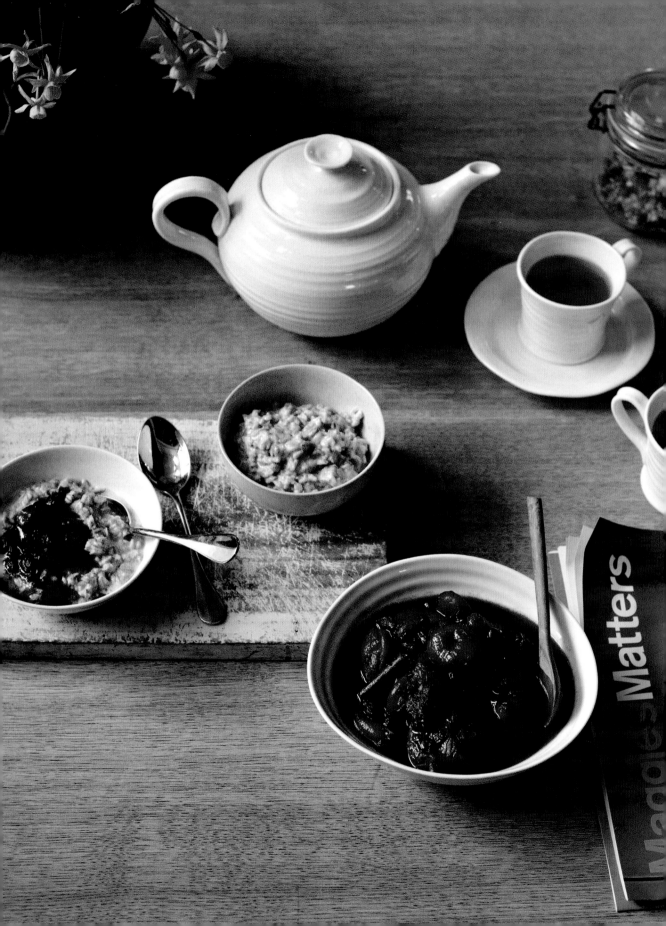

Winter Dried Fruit Compote

Makes approx. 800g

Takes 1½ hours, plus overnight soaking

200g dried apricots

200g raisins, or sultanas or dates

200g dried figs

200g stoned prunes

1 star anise

4 cloves

1 piece of cinnamon bark

When fresh seasonal fruit is not easily available this is a great alternative to help keep your fruit intake to a maximum. The richness that the dried fruits deliver offers a naturally sweet and almost 'jammy' consistency.

This compote is full of concentrated nutrients and natural sugars. Soaking dried fruit is a good way to reduce the concentration of sugars. A handful of apricots provides your daily allowance of beta-carotene, which is an antioxidant and good for boosting the immune system. And a small study showed that eating prunes can help people lose weight by increasing their fibre intake and making them feel fuller for longer.

1 Place all the dried fruits in a wide saucepan, cover with hot water, mix well and leave to soak for 1 hour or overnight.

2 Add the star anise, cloves and cinnamon and bring to the boil, then reduce the heat and simmer gently for 30 minutes. The fruit will swell and the liquid should thicken a little.

3 Serve warm or cold with porridge, bio- or Greek yoghurt, or add a spoonful to a smoothie. Honey can be added if needed, but the natural sugars in the fruits really should make it sweet enough.

4 Carefully transfer to sterilized storage jars or boxes and keep in the fridge. This will keep for up to 2 weeks.

Fresh Seasonal Fruit Compote

Makes 800g

Takes 30 minutes

200g plums

200g pears

1 stick cinnamon, or
  1 tsp ground cinnamon

100ml water

200g rhubarb, or
  strawberries or
  raspberries

200g blueberries or
  other dark berries

Use a selection of fresh seasonal fruits that suit your palate for this compote, which is wonderful when added to porridge or mixed with bio-yoghurt to produce a natural fruit yoghurt with no additives. This is a great way to incorporate fresh fruit into your diet and can be helpful for those having problems swallowing or digesting hard fruits.

Plums contain ursolic acid, which has been shown to have anti-cancer properties. Eat them fresh, or dried as prunes (see our Winter Dried Fruit Compote, page 149). To retain something of the fruits' shape, take care to simmer very gently, as they will continue to soften while cooling.

1 Stone the plums, core the pears and place in a large saucepan. Add the cinnamon and the water.

2 Gently bring to a simmer, place a lid on the saucepan and cook gently for 4–5 minutes.

3 Add the rhubarb and blueberries and bring back to a simmer for a further 2 minutes.

4 Remove from the heat, leave the lid on and allow to cool. The fruit should be soft but still holding its shape.

5 Carefully transfer to sterilized storage jars or boxes and keep in the fridge. This will keep for up to 2 weeks.

Poached Egg on Spinach and Pulse Stir-fry

Serves 2

Takes 10 minutes

1 clove garlic, crushed, peeled and chopped

½ onion, sliced

½ chilli, diced

1 tsp olive oil

100g cooked beans or lentils – haricot, butter, pinto, red or brown lentils

2 eggs

100g fresh spinach, roughly chopped

juice of ½ lemon

a bunch of oregano leaves, chopped

sea salt and freshly ground pepper

Many countries serve savoury spiced foods for breakfast and this stir-fry is also packed with goodness. Pulses are a source of complex carbohydrates, proteins and vitamins; and spinach, with its high iron content which helps the function of red blood cells, has remarkable abilities to restore energy, increase wellbeing and improve blood quality. These two superfoods, topped with a nutrient-rich poached egg, deliver a great breakfast to start the day.

Recent evidence-based research suggests garlic may be effective against high blood pressure, cardiovascular disease, cholesterol, colds and even some cancers.

Although you will need only a teaspoon of olive oil, used on a regular basis this oil has numerous health benefits. It contains antioxidants, vitamin E and is an anti-inflammatory.

1 Place the garlic, onion, chilli and olive oil in a pan and cook gently until soft.

2 Add the beans and cook for 5 minutes to heat through.

3 Heat a pan of water to poach the eggs, and when the water is just simmering, reduce the heat until the water is still.

4 Break the eggs into two small bowls, then carefully, from a low height, slide each egg into the water.

5 Simmer for 3–5 minutes, depending on how you like your yolk cooked.

6 Add the chopped spinach, lemon juice, oregano and seasoning to the bean mix, cook for a few minutes until wilted and hot and then serve on a plate, with the poached egg on top.

Energizing Snacks

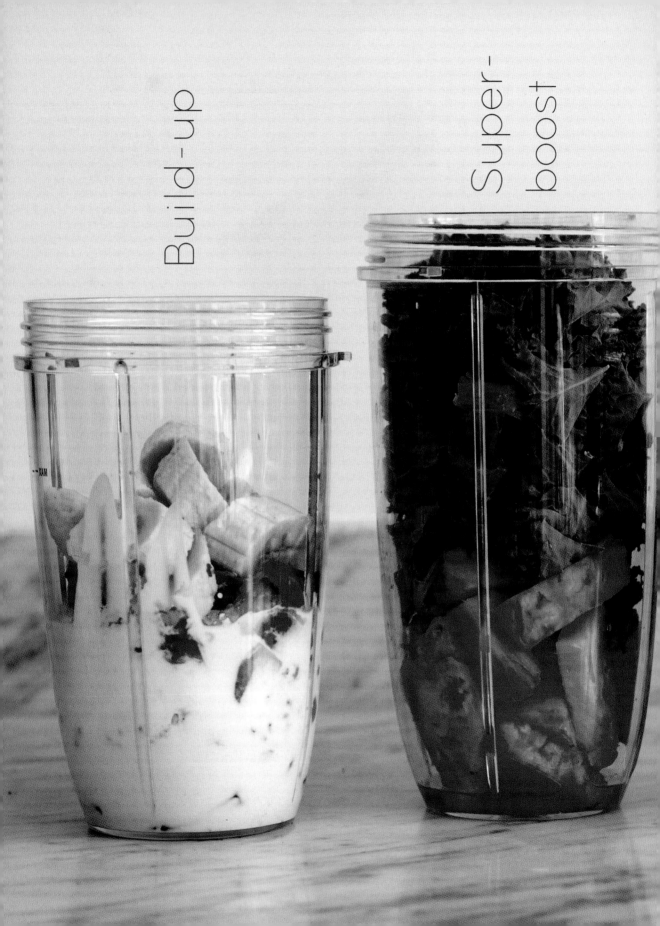

Build-up

Super-
boost

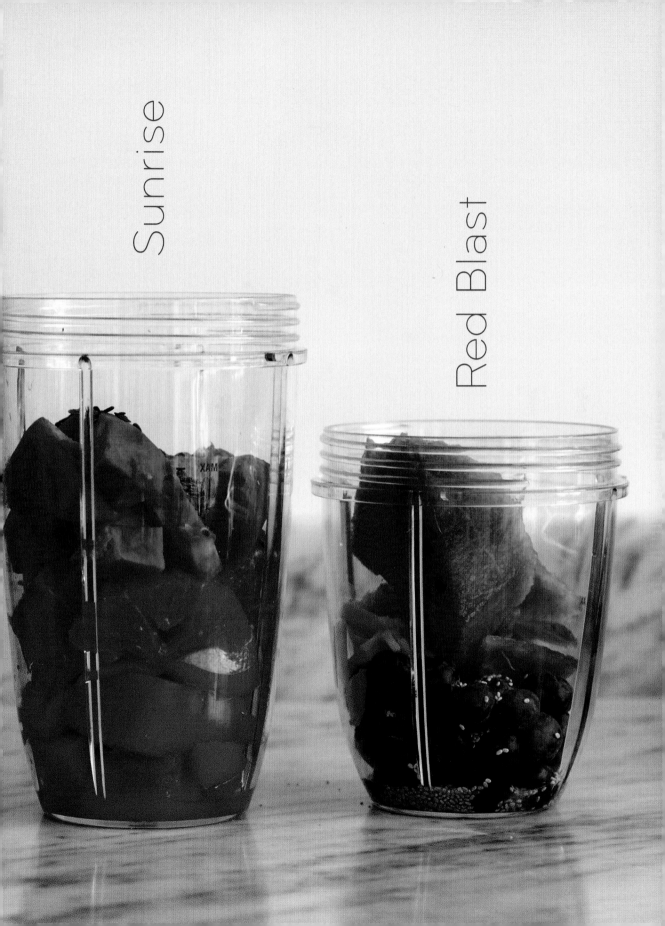

Sunrise

Red Blast

NOTE: With all these lovely drinks, if you are looking to increase your calorie intake simply add a spoonful of coconut oil, full-fat yoghurt or cream.

Build-up Smoothie

High in calories and packed with superfoods, this rich, nutritious smoothie is quick to make and easy to digest – ideal for anyone who might need to increase their body weight. If you're unable to drink this all at once, enjoy sipping it throughout the morning. Calorie intake and healthy fats can be increased by adding a teaspoon of ground seeds – see page 258.

If you have mouth ulcers, try freezing small ice-cube portions and then suck on them to ease any discomfort.

Serves 2 Takes 10 minutes

½ avocado	50g bio-yoghurt
½ banana	400ml milk – dairy, nut, seed, coconut or rice
25g dates	
25g walnuts	

1 Place all the ingredients in a blender or food processor, or cut into small pieces and use a stick blender.

2 Blitz all the ingredients until smooth, adding more liquid if necessary.

Super-boost Kale and Pineapple Juice

Smoothies are a super way to boost your intake of vegetables and fruit whilst keeping the all-important fibre content as high as possible.

Kale is one of the great superfoods. It's packed with vitamins A, B and K. Crushing or chopping cruciferous vegetables such as kale helps to release sulforaphne, a potent antioxidant. Pineapples are a rich source of both vitamin C and the trace mineral manganese, which is important for the body to function well. When you have skinned the pineapple, be sure to add the woody core, as it contains bromelain, a protein-digesting enzyme that has anti-cancer and anti-inflammatory properties.

Serves 2 Takes 10 minutes

50g kale	juice of ½ lemon
200g pineapple	400ml coconut water, or other seed, nut or dairy milk
6 mint leaves	

1 Trim any excess woody stems from the kale leaves and discard. Roughly chop the leaves.

2 Peel and chop the pineapple and place all the ingredients in a blender or food processor, or cut them into smaller pieces and use a stick blender. Blitz until smooth, adding more liquid if necessary.

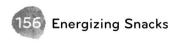 **Energizing Snacks**

Sunrise Juice

This is a sweet treat, packed with nutrients – but it includes sugars too, so it isn't something you should be drinking every day.

If the weather is hot and you're looking for a really cooling drink, try prepping the fruit the night before, freezing it and then blitzing with a strong machine for a creamy iced drink that has many nutritional benefits. The mango contains more than twenty different vitamins and minerals; the papaya aids protein digestion; and flaxseeds have the highest concentration of phytoestrogens. This drink can help to relieve constipation, as it may have a laxative effect.

For a refreshing drink using any excess papaya seeds – see page 139.

Serves 2 Takes 10 minutes

½ papaya, and a tbsp of the seeds

1 orange

1 small mango

1 tsp flaxseeds

400ml coconut water, or other seed, nut or dairy milk

1 Peel the papaya, orange and mango and remove the seeds and stone. (Reserve the papaya seeds – see above.)

2 Place all the ingredients in a blender or food processor, or cut into smaller pieces and use a stick blender. Blitz until smooth, adding more liquid if needed.

Red Blast

Enjoy this smoothie and its many benefits at the start of your day. Watermelon contains lycopene, believed to be good for prostate health; and red grape skins contain resveratrol, a powerful antioxidant. They may also help to reduce inflammation, so drink this before and after an operation to help recovery.

The red chilli adds a lovely spicy flavour and also increases metabolism, helps with blood pressure and may have anti-inflammatory benefits too.

Serves 2 Takes 10 minutes

50g red grapes

50g blueberries

75g watermelon

1 knob fresh ginger, peeled and roughly chopped

1 tsp chia seeds

½ medium/cool red chilli

juice of ½ lemon

400ml coconut water, or other seed, nut or dairy milk

1 Remove the grapes from their stalks.

2 Place all the ingredients in a blender or food processor, or cut into small pieces and use a stick blender. Blitz until smooth, adding more liquid if necessary.

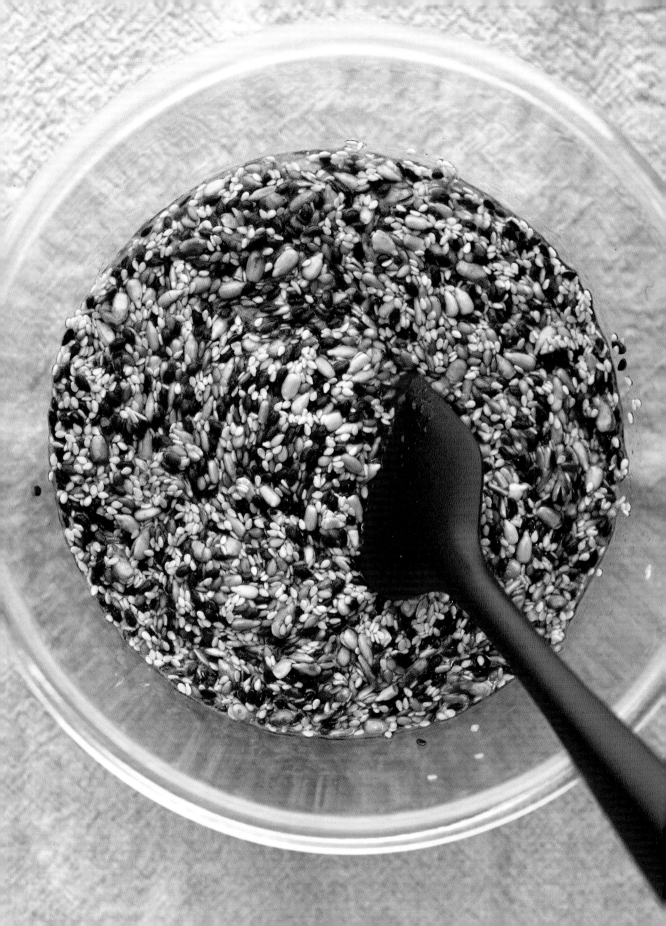

Savoury Seed Crackers

Makes approximately 20

Takes 3 hours, plus overnight soaking

100g sunflower seeds, soaked overnight

100g pumpkin seeds, soaked overnight

75g sesame seeds, soaked overnight

1 tbsp poppy seeds, soaked overnight

75g flaxseeds (linseeds)

1½ tbsp pysllium husks

½ tsp pink Himalayan salt, or sea salt

freshly ground black pepper

1 tbsp dried rosemary

1 tbsp crushed fennel seeds

250ml water

A firm favourite at Maggie's West London, this low-carb recipe was inspired by lovely volunteer Sofia. It is a deliciously tasty nibble or snack that you can enjoy with dips and cheese, and it makes a good alternative to wheat-laden bread. The crackers provide plenty of fibre and are low in carbs. Adjust the balance of seeds to suit your individual taste. Soaking them removes some of the natural compounds that can inhibit mineral absorption, making them easier to digest. All seeds are rich in omega fats; pumpkin seeds contain tryptophan, which may help to improve mood and aid sleep; flaxseeds help stabilize hormones, so are beneficial during PMS and menopause, and they may reduce the risk of prostate and breast cancer.

Low-heat methods of baking are gaining favour due to the health benefits of reducing our intake of acrylamides – see page 92. If you have an Aga these crackers can be placed in the simmering oven and cooked overnight. In fact, this method is more about drying out than cooking through.

1 Pre-heat the oven to 120°C, gas mark ½.

2 Place the sunflower, pumpkin, sesame and poppy seeds in a bowl. Generously cover with water, mix well and leave to soak (covered) overnight in a cool place.

3 The following day, drain away the excess water through a fine sieve or muslin. Add the flaxseeds, pysllium, seasoning, rosemary, fennel and water and mix well.

4 Allow the mixture to sit for 15 minutes, stirring occasionally. The pysllium will swell and make the mixture combine.

5 Line two large baking sheets with baking parchment, divide the mixture in half and place in the middle of each sheet. Gently spread the mixture out across the sheet using a palette knife. You can take it all the way to the edge of the baking sheet, as it will not expand while cooking.

6 Place in the oven and cook for 2 hours, until just golden. Cool, break into pieces and store in an airtight container.

Sardine Dip

Serves 4

Takes 15 minutes

120g sardines in olive oil

1–2 tbsp crème fraîche

2 tsp freshly grated
  horseradish, or hot
  horseradish sauce

½ lemon, zested and
  juiced

sea salt and freshly
  ground black pepper

2 tsp sunflower seeds

a bunch of parsley, finely
  chopped

Sardines are a very healthy and economical oily fish. They are rich in omega-3 fats, which have anti-inflammatory properties. Choose tinned sardines with bones included as they provide additional calcium and the vitamin D in the fish helps with the absorption of the calcium, which is essential for bone health.

Use fresh horseradish if you can as the glucosinolates contained in this fiery root vegetable have been shown to inhibit cancer cells.

1 Place the sardines and their oil in a small food processor and blend until smooth.

2 Add the crème fraîche, horseradish, lemon zest and juice, and seasoning, and whizz again until everything is evenly blended.

3 Add the sunflower seeds and parsley and stir through. Serve as a dip with vegetables, Savoury Seed Crackers (see page 159), or Spelt Soda Loaf (see page 250).

Avocado and Tofu Dip

Serves 6

Takes 15 minutes

2 avocados

1 x 300g pack silken tofu

1 red onion, finely
  chopped

1 red chilli, finely
  chopped

4 tomatoes, finely
  chopped

a large bunch of
  coriander, chopped

juice of 1 lime

sea salt and freshly
  ground black pepper

Tofu may be new to you, but do give it a try – it is an excellent source of plant protein. Select a good-quality organic variety and make this as a delicious tasty dip, or it can be served as part of a nutritious salad. Tofu, made from soya, is rich in phytoestrogens, which may help to relieve menopausal symptoms and lower the risk of some hormone-driven cancers.

Avocados are rich in healthy fats and have beneficial effects on cholesterol levels. If making this in advance, place the avocado stone on top of the dip, as miraculously it stops the avocado from browning. Coriander is nutritious and tasty and should be used frequently and liberally in the Nutritional Kitchen.

....

1 Cut the avocados in half and remove the stones. Scoop out the flesh and roughly chop or mash it together with the tofu.

2 Add the chopped onion, chilli, tomato, coriander, lime juice, salt and pepper, and mix well. Serve with Seeded Crackers (see page 159) or vegetable sticks.

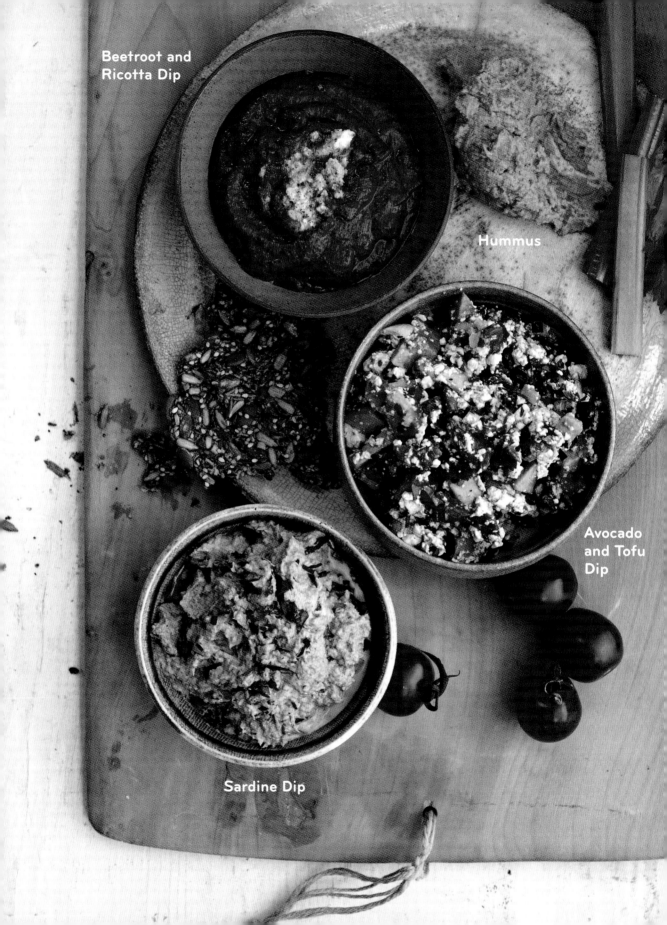

Beetroot and Ricotta Dip

Hummus

Avocado and Tofu Dip

Sardine Dip

Beetroot and Ricotta Dip

Serves 4

Takes 45 minutes

300g beetroot

175g ricotta

sea salt and freshly
  ground pepper

1 tbsp olive oil

1 tsp chopped mint
  (optional)

Beetroot is a good source of iron, folic acid, magnesium and other important antioxidants. It has pectin in its fibre, which helps to eliminate toxins in the gut that can build up during treatment. Try to increase your intake to help your digestion; it will make your stools red, but do not be alarmed. Beetroot is also good for the liver and is believed to improve stamina. Don't forget, try not to peel your vegetables (just wash them well) as all the vitamins are just below the skin.

The blended ricotta in this recipe adds extra calories for those who are looking to increase their weight.

1 Top and tail the beetroot, wash well and cut into quarters.

2 Place the beetroot in a pan and cover with water and a lid. Bring to the boil and simmer for 40 minutes or until the beetroot is soft. Drain well and leave to cool for 10 minutes.

3 Transfer the beetroot to a food processor or blender and blitz with the ricotta and seasoning until smooth.

4 Put in a bowl and drizzle with a little olive oil and, if you wish, sprinkle with chopped mint for extra zing. Serve as a dip along with vegetable sticks, toasted spelt or Savoury Seed Crackers (see page 159).

Hummus

Serves 4

Takes 30 minutes, plus overnight if soaking dried chickpeas

125g dried chickpeas, or a 250g carton prepared chickpeas

2 tbsp tahini

25ml light olive oil

juice of 1 lemon

2 cloves garlic

sea salt and freshly ground black pepper

50ml water

Beans, healthy oils and garlic are all important components of the ultra-healthy and enjoyable Mediterranean diet, which is recommended by so many health experts. Chickpeas are an excellent source of fibre and can be helpful for gut health and lowering the risk of colon cancer.

Always having something like this delicious hummus in your fridge is a really good idea for whenever you fancy a nibble. You can also take it out with you as a healthy portable snack.

1 If using dried chickpeas, place in a pan, cover generously with water and leave to swell overnight.

2 Next day, drain and rinse, cover with fresh water and bring to the boil, then simmer for approximately 1 hour or until the chickpeas are soft (cooking time will vary according to the age of the chickpeas). Skim off any residue that floats to the top while cooking. When the chickpeas are soft, drain. (If using prepared chickpeas, simply set them aside until Step 4.)

3 Place the tahini, olive oil, lemon, garlic, seasoning and water in a food processor or blender and blitz until smooth and creamy.

4 Add the chickpeas and blitz again until really smooth.

5 Adjust the seasoning according to your taste and serve with Savoury Seed Crackers (page 159) or vegetable sticks.

Quinoa Salad Pot

Serves 2

Takes 35 minutes

1 tsp olive oil

1 onion, diced

1 clove garlic, crushed, peeled and chopped

5cm fresh ginger, peeled and finely grated

1 medium red chilli, diced

1 tsp smoked paprika

100g quinoa, rinsed in water

200ml vegetable stock

50g sliced almonds, toasted

50g sultanas

1 lime, zested and juiced

a bunch of coriander, chopped

sea salt and freshly ground black pepper

This is a perfect snack to make and take with you when you are out and about, most particularly on chemo days, when your body needs lots of nourishment, preferably low-carb, to help you through tricky treatments. It contains all the essential protein amino acids needed for repairing damage to the body; the spices will help with nausea and will pep up your tastebuds. In fact, garlic, ginger, chilli and lime can help if you find the chemo gives you a nasty metallic taste in your mouth.

Enjoy this warm, or allow the mixture to cool and transfer it to a small lock-top container in the fridge.

1 Warm the olive oil in a frying pan, add the onion and garlic and gently cook for 4 minutes or until soft but not brown.

2 Add the ginger, chilli and smoked paprika to the pan, stir well and cook for 2 minutes.

3 Add the quinoa to the pan and stir well to coat.

4 Pour in the stock, bring to the boil, then reduce the heat and simmer gently for 20 minutes, stirring occasionally. When cooked, all the liquid should be absorbed and the quinoa should be fluffy.

5 Add the almonds, sultanas, lime zest and juice, coriander and seasoning. Mix well.

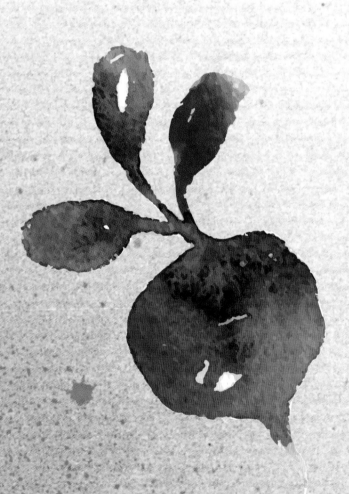

A Vegetarian Rainbow

Spiced Beetroot and Coconut Milk Soup (Happy Soup)

Serves 6

Takes 1 hour

600g beetroot

1 onion

1 tbsp coconut oil

400ml vegetable
  or chicken stock
  (see page 256)

1 tbsp red curry paste

400ml coconut milk

sea salt and freshly
  ground black pepper

a bunch of coriander,
  chopped

I call this 'Happy Soup' because the colour is so vibrant it will put a smile on anyone's face. It's rich and creamy-tasting, with subtle spices, and then there's the full-flavoured beetroot, which all blends together beautifully. Beetroot has energy-boosting properties that will help you keep going for longer, so this is a great meal for a busy day.

Put this soup in a flask and take it with you to enjoy when not at home. It freezes well and is an excellent way to nourish your body on days when you do not feel like cooking.

1 Trim and scrub the beetroots, then roughly chop them and the onion.

2 Place in a saucepan with the coconut oil and gently cook for a couple of minutes.

3 Pour in the stock, cover with a lid and simmer for 40 minutes or until the beetroot is soft.

4 Add the red curry paste, mix well, then add the coconut milk and seasoning. Simmer for 10 minutes.

5 Blend the soup until smooth, then stir through the chopped coriander before serving. Add a swirl of coconut milk to each serving to dazzle your friends!

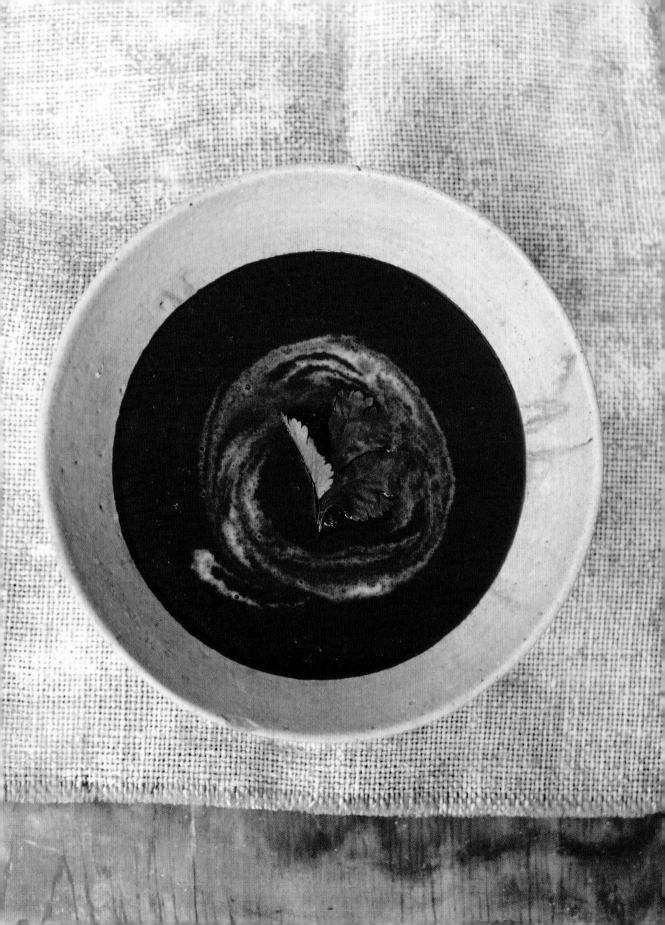

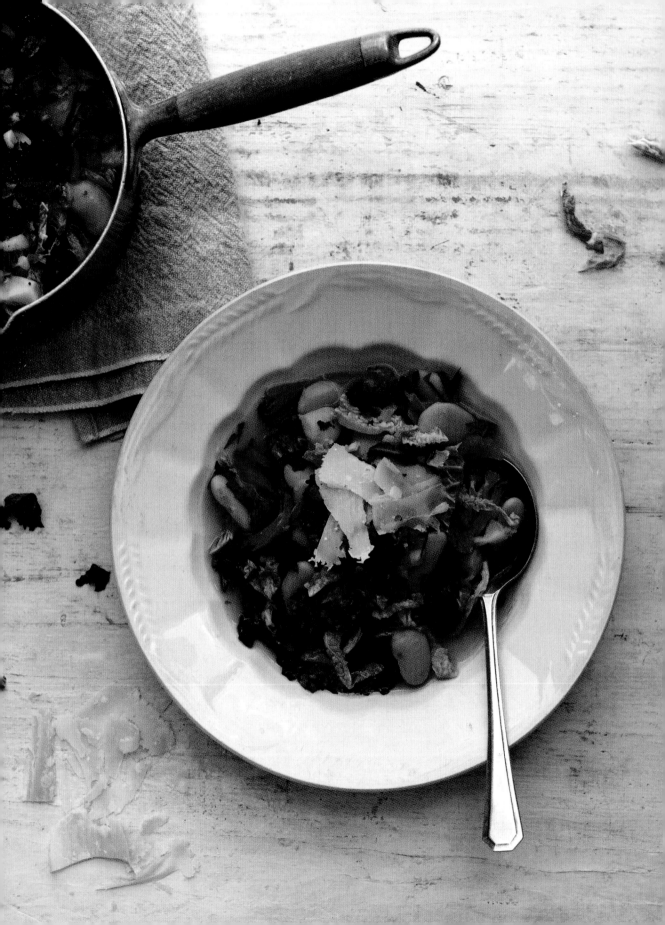

Brassica and Bean Soup with Brazil Nut Pesto

Serves 4

Takes 40 minutes, plus overnight if soaking dried beans

100g butter beans, soaked overnight, or 200g carton prepared beans

2 tbsp olive oil

1 onion, diced

1 clove garlic, crushed and peeled

1 stick celery, chopped

750ml vegetable or chicken stock (see page 256)

100g kale, finely sliced

100g Savoy cabbage, finely sliced

100g broccoli, finely diced

a bunch of parsley, chopped

sea salt and freshly ground black pepper

Brazil Nut Pesto (see page 261)

30g grated Parmesan

All brassicas are good for you, providing essential vitamins and minerals and the all-important anti-cancer phytonutrients sulforaphane and indole-3-carbinol. Sulforaphane has also been shown to help the body excrete pollutants such as petrochemicals. The vegetables are only lightly cooked, which helps to conserve the levels of phytonutrients, and a spoonful of Brazil Nut Pesto (see page 261) adds depth and a little bit of sunshine and selenium to this soup. Brazil nuts are rich in selenium, which has antioxidant properties and may help to protect cells from damage.

In other words, this is good health in a bowl. The ingredients will help to support the gut and the liver, so it is definitely beneficial to eat during treatment.

....

1 If using dried beans, soak them overnight, then drain and rinse in fresh cold water.

2 Return the beans to the pan, cover with fresh water and bring to the boil. Then reduce the heat and simmer for 1–2 hours, or until the beans are soft. Skim off any foam that accumulates on the top of the water with a slotted spoon. Drain when cooked and set aside. (If using prepared beans, simply set them aside until Step 4.)

3 Warm the olive oil in a saucepan, add the diced onion, garlic and celery, and cook gently until soft.

4 Add the beans and stock to the saucepan and simmer for 5 minutes.

5 Add all the prepared vegetables, herbs and seasoning to the pan and cook for a further 5 minutes if you like your vegetables to have a bit of crunch, or for 10 minutes if you prefer them softer. Serve topped with a large spoonful of Brazil Nut Pesto and grated Parmesan.

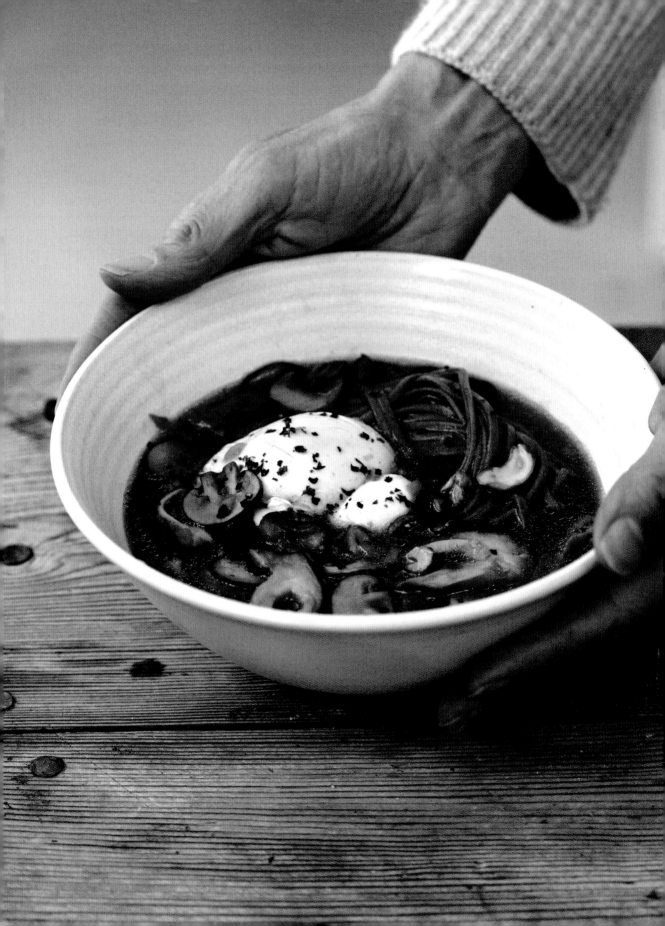

Mixed Mushroom Noodle Soup with a Poached Egg

Serves 2

Takes 30 minutes, plus 30 minutes to rehydrate the dried mushrooms

15g dried mushrooms, soaked in water for 30 minutes

1 tbsp olive oil

1 small shallot, diced

1 clove garlic, crushed, peeled and chopped

100g chestnut mushrooms, or other favourites

100g shiitake mushrooms

450ml vegetable or beef stock

¼ tsp seaweed flakes (we like Mara)

juice of ½ lemon

sea salt and freshly ground black pepper

100g buckwheat noodles

2 eggs

1 tsp soy sauce

15g chopped cashew nuts, toasted

This is the ultimate mushroom-rich, one-pot wonder. It's easy to make and gives a great boost to the immune system.

Place your mushrooms on the windowsill on a sunny day as they will make vitamin D – something we all need. The Japanese use mushrooms alongside chemotherapy to maintain white blood-cell counts and to help fight off infections. Mushrooms really are a must for cancer patients.

Seaweed is another excellent ingredient as it is high in iodine and vitamin B_{12}. We are very keen on seaweed in the Nutritional Kitchen, as it adds a salty flavour to dishes without extra salt being added. Buckwheat noodles make a healthy alternative to rice, as they are also gluten-free.

1 Drain the soaked mushrooms, reserving the liquid.

2 Warm the oil in a saucepan, add the shallot and garlic and gently cook for 3 minutes.

3 Slice all the fresh mushrooms and add to the pan, along with the soaked mushrooms. Mix well and continue to cook for a further 5 minutes or until the mushrooms are soft and golden.

4 Add the soaking liquid to the stock, bringing it to 500ml. Pour into the saucepan and bring to the boil, then simmer for 5 minutes.

5 Add the seaweed flakes, lemon juice, seasoning and noodles, stirring to submerge the noodles in the liquid and to stop them sticking together, then reduce the heat to low.

6 Carefully break two eggs into separate areas of the soup, place a lid on the pan and cook very gently for 4–5 minutes, depending on how soft you like your yolk. When cooked, ladle out the eggs and place to one side.

7 Transfer the soup to two bowls, place an egg on top of each, drizzle over the soy sauce and sprinkle with the toasted cashew nuts and an extra pinch of seaweed flakes.

Lentil and Spinach Soup

Serves 4

Takes 1–1¼ hours

125g brown lentils

2 tbsp olive oil

1 large onion, diced

2 cloves garlic, crushed,
   peeled and chopped

1 tsp cumin, ground

1 tsp grated fresh
   turmeric, or use ground

700ml chicken or
   vegetable stock

300g spinach, chopped

juice of 1 lemon

sea salt and freshly
   ground black pepper

Lentils are an excellent source of plant protein. Using them whole in this tasty recipe also provides extra fibre and flavour. (Please be aware that red lentils are slightly processed, which means they lose some of their fibre.)

Our beneficial gut bacteria love to feed on the fibre from beans and lentils, making them a healthy choice for gut health. Having said that, go easy on lentils if you have gut problems, as they can cause significant bloating and wind.

1 Wash and drain the lentils well.

2 In a large saucepan gently warm the oil, add the onion, garlic, cumin and turmeric and cook on a low heat for 5 minutes until the onion is soft and golden. Do not brown.

3 Add the washed lentils and stir well to coat them in the oil and absorb the flavours.

4 Add the stock and bring to the boil, then simmer gently for 45–60 minutes, stirring occasionally. (As with all lentils and dried beans, the cooking time varies due to the age of the ingredient, so just keep cooking until the lentils are soft.)

5 Add the chopped spinach, mix well and cover the pan with a lid. Simmer for 8 minutes.

6 Add the lemon juice and seasoning then blitz with a hand-held blender until smooth. If you like, and especially if you are looking to gain weight, add a swirl of cream, yoghurt, fromage frais or cashew cream when serving.

Amaranth Tabouli

Serves 2

Takes 45 minutes

75g amaranth

juice of 1 lemon

2 tbsp olive oil

a large bunch chopped
  mint

a large bunch chopped
  parsley

4 tomatoes, diced

½ cucumber, peeled and
  diced

25g pine nuts, toasted

sea salt and freshly
  ground black pepper

Amaranth is a gluten-free plant which has an acquired taste and texture. It is very rich in iron, calcium and amino acids, so make this ancient grain one of your store-cupboard staples.

Do not scrimp on the mint and parsley: they add great flavour and aid digestion. The toasted pine nuts add a tasty, almost butter-bursting flavour when you bite into them. This is perfect as a salad, or serve it with some grilled fish.

1 Place the amaranth in a saucepan, cover with 3 times the amount of water, bring to the boil and gently simmer for 20 minutes or until all the water is absorbed.

2 Add the lemon juice and olive oil, stir and leave to cool.

3 When cooled, add the chopped mint, parsley, tomatoes, cucumber, toasted pine nuts and seasoning. Mix together and don't worry if it is slightly sticky. Finish off with a drizzle of olive oil before serving.

Roasted Beetroot and Goat's Cheese Salad

Serves 2

Takes 50 minutes

400g beetroot

½ tbsp olive oil

freshly ground black pepper and sea salt

2 shallots, cut in half

2 tbsp balsamic vinegar

75g rocket

50g goat's cheese

25g walnuts, chopped

a bunch of oregano, chopped

Beetroot has a delicious earthy taste and roasting seems to enhance it. The combination of beetroot and goat's cheese makes a really appetizing and nutritious salad, and the balsamic vinegar adds a lovely sticky twist. The better quality your vinegar, the finer the result.

Walnuts are high in fat and a great source of omega-3, which may help with weight loss. They also contain melatonin, which can aid sleep. Rocket has a slightly bitter taste and is a great digestive aid; it is also high in vitamins, especially vitamin K, which is good for bone health.

1 Pre-heat the oven to 180°C, gas mark 4.

2 Wash and scrub the beetroot and cut it into wedges (no need to peel).

3 Place the pieces in a roasting tin, add the olive oil and seasoning and toss to coat them evenly before placing in the oven.

4 Roast the beetroot for 25 minutes, then add the prepared shallots to the tin, tossing them in the cooking juices. Cook for a further 25 minutes or until the vegetables are soft and slightly caramelized.

5 Pour over the balsamic vinegar and toss again before returning to the oven for another 8 minutes.

6 Place the rocket on a serving dish or plate, top with the roasted vegetables and spoon out any cooking juices. Crumble the goat's cheese over and scatter with the walnuts and oregano.

Raw Soft Salad with Budwig Dressing

Serves 2

Takes 20 minutes

For the Budwig dressing

juice of 1 lemon

3 tbsp cottage cheese

3 tbsp flaxseed or hemp oil

sea salt and freshly ground black pepper

For the salad

50g peas, young and tender as eaten raw

50g spinach or watercress, washed and chopped

50g sprouted seeds or beansprouts

50g mushrooms, sliced

1 avocado, chopped

1 carrot, grated

a bunch of dill, chopped

When the gut is struggling with the after-effects of treatments such as chemotherapy, this salad is easy to digest and really tasty. The creamy dressing is a take on the Budwig Protocol – see page 109. The blend of sulphurous protein and omega-3-rich oil is thought to help to deliver oxygen right to the heart of our cells.

As long as you keep to the quantities, you can replace any of the vegetables with others that you prefer. In fact, this recipe is a great way to empty your salad drawer – and remember this healthy tip: 'An avocado a day keeps cholesterol at bay!'

1 Place the lemon juice, cottage cheese, oil and seasoning in a small bowl and blend with a hand-held blender until emulsified.

2 In a large bowl combine the peas, spinach, sprouted seeds or beansprouts, mushrooms, avocado, carrot and dill. Pour the Budwig dressing over the vegetables and toss to ensure everything is thoroughly coated. Serve straight away.

Watermelon, Feta and Pomegranate Salad

Serves 2

Takes 25 minutes

½ small watermelon

100g feta

1 pomegranate,
  de-seeded

2 tbsp olive oil

a bunch of mint, leaves
  chopped

This is sunshine on a plate! On a warm summer's day this crisp, refreshing and vibrantly coloured salad is delightful on its own as a light meal or exceptionally good when served as an accompaniment to fish or lamb.

Fresh mint is a proven digestive aid and pomegranate has ellagic acid, which has been shown to be beneficial to cell health and retards the growth of cancer cells.

1 Peel and cut the watermelon into slices or chunks. If it has seeds, either remove them by hand before serving or at the table when eating.

2 Roughly chop the feta, then peel and de-seed the pomegranate, making sure you remove all the pith as it has a very bitter, dry taste.

3 To serve, I like to layer the ingredients roughly on a platter, finishing with the olive oil drizzled over and the chopped mint sprinkled on top. But you can also serve it in individual bowls, quickly tossed together, topped with the olive oil and chopped mint.

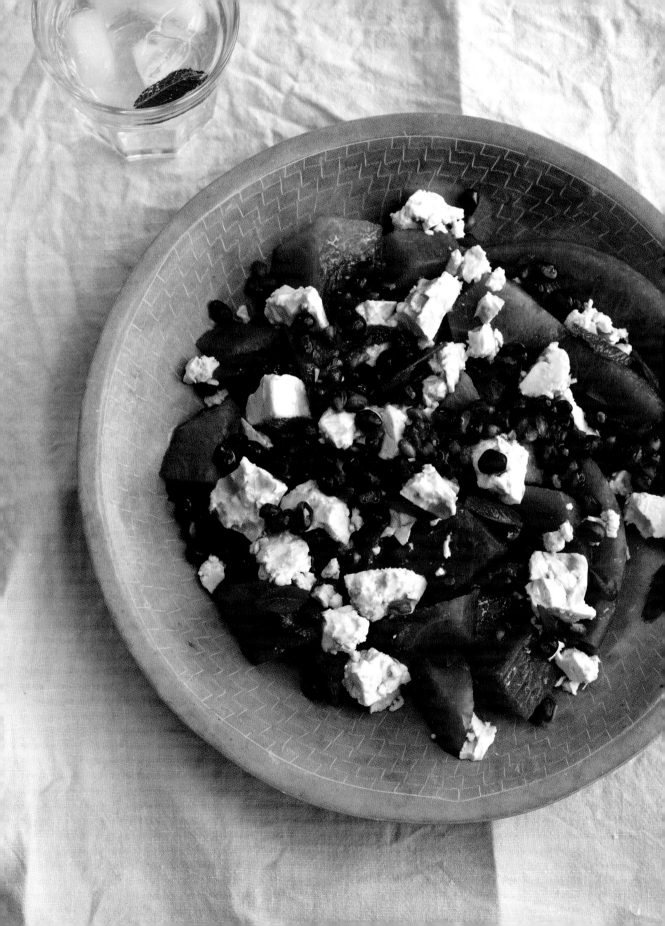

Eight Slaw

Serves 4

Takes 30 minutes

75g red cabbage

75g white cabbage

75g carrots

75g celeriac

35g apple

75g red onion

75g celery

75g broccoli

1 tsp Dijon mustard

2 tbsp cream cheese

juice of 1 lemon

2 tbsp olive oil

sea salt and freshly
  ground black pepper

We should all try to eat a diet that is high in raw vegetables, and coleslaw is a tasty and nutritious way of doing this. The cabbage alone will provide a range of vitamins and important anti-cancer phytochemicals. Remember to chew your slaw well to release their active components – see page 57.

This delicious slaw contains eight raw vegetables and fruits and comes together in a delicious tumble of creamy, crunchy goodness. You can use different vegetables, but it's a good idea to use those with a good crunch. If you like spice, try adding some fresh, finely diced chilli to the mix – just remember to remove some of the seeds if you want less heat.

1 Grate or finely slice all the vegetables and mix together in a bowl until evenly blended.

2 In another small bowl, stir together the mustard, cream cheese, lemon juice, olive oil and seasoning until smooth; if it's a little thick, adjust the consistency by adding a couple of spoons of water.

3 Add the blended mix to the vegetables and toss well. If you would prefer to serve the dressing separately, spoon a little over the vegetables and pour the remainder into a bowl so people can help themselves.

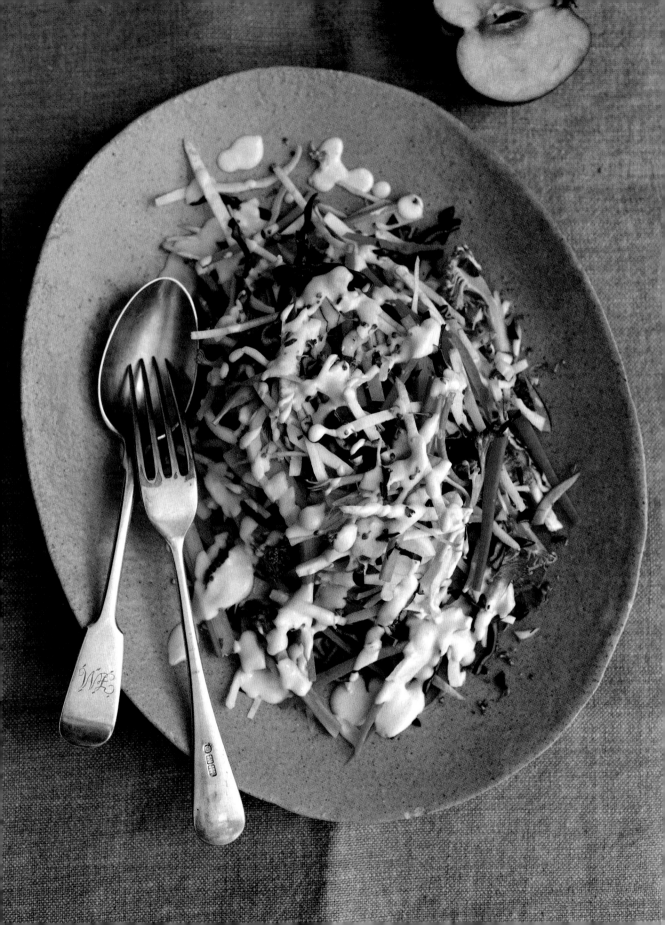

Baked Sweet Potato Stuffed with Buffalo Mozzarella

Serves 4

Takes 45 minutes

2 orange-fleshed sweet
  potatoes

1 ball buffalo Mozzarella

½ red chilli, diced

a bunch of basil leaves,
  torn

a dash of paprika

olive oil to serve

Try this quick, economical and healthy alternative to the classic baked potato.

Sweet potatoes cook far more quickly and contain high amounts of vitamins C and E, which will help to promote a healthy immune system. The orange-fleshed variety contains higher amounts of beta-carotene, which is an antioxidant the body converts to vitamin A, important for maintaining healthy cells and good vision.

The buffalo Mozzarella used here is a healthy alternative to cow's-milk cheese as it is higher in nutrients and easier to digest.

1 Preheat the oven to 180°C, gas mark 4.

2 Pierce the potato skins in several places with a small knife; this will stop them splitting and will also speed up the cooking process. Place in the oven and bake for approximately 45 minutes, depending on size. To test, insert a knife: the potato should be soft all the way through to the middle.

3 When cooked, remove the potatoes from the oven, cut almost in half and squeeze the ends together, making a space for the cheese.

4 Cut the Mozzarella in half and place a piece in each potato, then sprinkle with the chopped chilli, the basil leaves and a dusting of paprika. Finish with a splash of olive oil.

Kale, Mushroom and Egg Bake with Harissa

Serves 2–3

Takes 30 minutes

1 tsp coconut oil

300g mushrooms, sliced

100g kale, chopped

sea salt and freshly
  ground black pepper

a pinch of dried chilli
  flakes

3 eggs

75ml milk or cream

75g Parmesan, grated

Similar to a frittata, this delicious bake is packed with two beneficial vegetables – mushrooms and kale. Both are good sources of iron; mushrooms are a good source of vitamin B and minerals such as selenium and potassium. They are especially good to eat during treatment as they increase the activity of our immune system.

This would be a good recipe for anyone on a low-carb diet, or on the high-fat Ketogenic Diet (see page 106).

1 Pre-heat the oven to 180°C, gas mark 4.

2 Place the coconut oil and mushrooms in a medium ovenproof frying pan and cook for 5 minutes or until lightly browned and all the moisture has evaporated.

3 Add the chopped kale and cook for a further 4 minutes, turning frequently until the kale is soft. Season, add the chilli flakes and mix them through.

4 Whisk the eggs with the milk or cream, pour over the kale mix, then press the kale down with the back of a spoon.

5 Sprinkle with the grated Parmesan and cook in the oven for 15–20 minutes, or until the egg is set. This goes really well with a spoonful of Home-honed Harissa (see page 262).

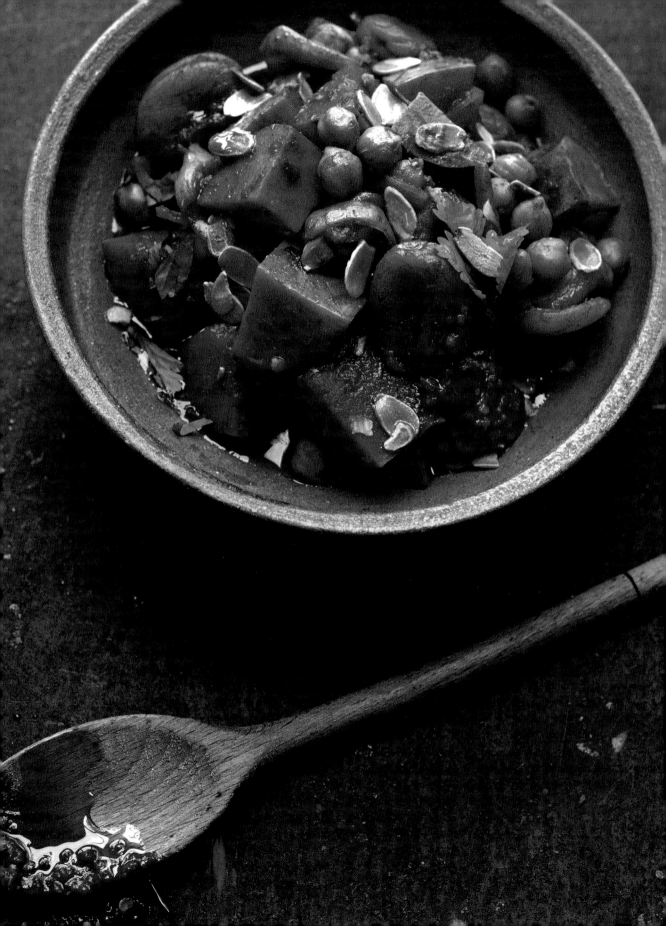

Butternut and Sweet Potato Tagine with Chermoula

Serves 4

Takes 1 hour, plus overnight if soaking dried chickpeas

100g dried chickpeas, or 200g carton prepared chickpeas

1 tsp olive oil

1 onion, sliced

2 cloves garlic, crushed, peeled and chopped

2 tsp ground cumin

2 tsp ground coriander

2–3 tbsp harissa (see page 262)

200g butternut squash

200g sweet potato

100g dried apricots

500ml vegetable stock

a large bunch of coriander, chopped

25g flaked almonds, toasted

This is good on its own as a vegetarian dish, or if you are catering for hungry carnivores you can serve it with delicious slow-roasted shoulder of lamb. If you like spice, turn up the heat by adding more harissa.

The ground cumin in this recipe will aid digestion and enhance the liver's detox enzymes. The other healthy ingredients are the butternut and apricots, which are rich in beta-carotene, and all the ingredients are high in fibre which is good for the gut.

1 If using dried chickpeas, place in a pan, cover generously with water and leave to swell overnight.

2 Next day, drain and rinse, cover with fresh water and bring to the boil, then simmer for approximately 1 hour or until the beans are soft (the cooking time will vary according to the age of the chickpeas). Skim off any residue that floats to the top while cooking. When the chickpeas are soft, drain. (If using prepared chickpeas, simply set them aside until Step 6.)

3 Heat the olive oil in a pan, add the sliced onion and cook until soft, then add the garlic, cumin and coriander, mix well and cook for 2 minutes. Next, add the harissa and mix well. Remove from the heat while preparing the other ingredients.

4 Wash the outside of the squash and sweet potato, trim and chop into equal-sized chunks. Add to the pan, return to the heat and mix well, coating the vegetables in the spice mix. Cook for 5 minutes, turning frequently.

5 Add the dried apricots and vegetable stock. Mix well, place a lid on the pan and simmer for 25 minutes or until the vegetables are soft, stirring frequently.

6 Add the prepared chickpeas, mix well and simmer for a further 15 minutes. Finally, stir in the coriander and sprinkle over the toasted almonds before serving.

Cauliflower and Asparagus Stir-fry

Serves 2

Takes 30 minutes

100g brown rice

1 tsp coconut oil

½ small head of cauliflower and young leaves

100g asparagus

25g cashew nuts, chopped

1 clove garlic, crushed, peeled and chopped

1 green chilli, chopped

1 lime, zested and juiced

sea salt and freshly ground black pepper

This super-tasty stir-fry is easy to make. The combination of the wonderfully fresh citrus flavour from the lime, a little heat from the chilli, and the fluffy rice fills a hungry stomach very nicely indeed. Serve on its own or as a vegetable side dish.

Asparagus is an excellent source of folic acid and also of phytochemicals that protect our healthy cells, and it has anti-cancer properties. Out of season, the asparagus can be changed for other green vegetables, such as Brussels sprouts cut into quarters, broccoli florets or mangetout. Cauliflower is a much overlooked vegetable, but in fact it has lots of good nutrients and fibre and is great value for money. It also grows easily and naturally in the UK, so it doesn't necessarily require spraying with many pesticides or fertilizers.

1 Place the brown rice in a saucepan, cover with water and bring to the boil. Stir, then reduce the heat to simmer for 35 minutes or until the rice is soft. Drain and set aside.

2 Heat the coconut oil in a pan and add the cauliflower florets (but not the leaves). Cook on a medium to high heat for 5 minutes, until golden. Try not to rush this stage as the golden cauliflower florets add to the flavour of the dish.

3 Trim the woody ends off the asparagus spears and discard them, then chop the spears into 5cm lengths. Reduce the heat below the pan and add the asparagus, cashew nuts, garlic, chilli, chopped cauliflower leaves and the rice. Mix well and cook for a further 4 minutes.

4 Add the lime zest and juice, and the seasoning, and cook for a further 2 minutes, constantly stirring, before serving.

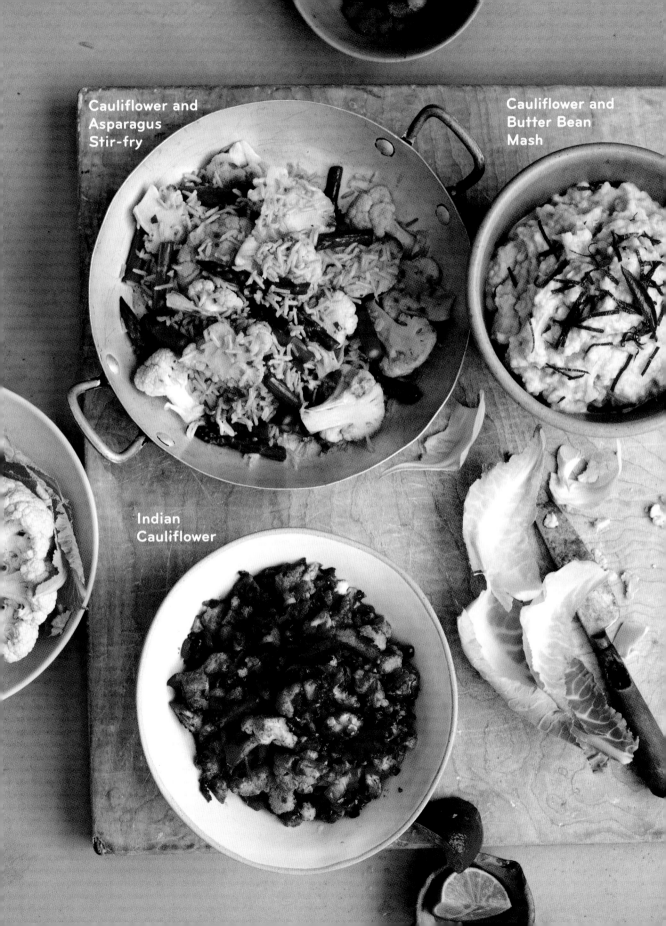

Cauliflower and
Asparagus
Stir-fry

Cauliflower and
Butter Bean
Mash

Indian
Cauliflower

Indian Cauliflower

Serves 2

Takes 25 minutes

1 tbsp coconut oil

½ head cauliflower, roughly chopped into 2cm pieces

1 onion, finely chopped

1 clove garlic, crushed, peeled and chopped

4cm grated fresh turmeric, or 2 tsp ground

1 tsp curry powder

a bunch of coriander, chopped

juice of 1 lemon

sea salt and freshly ground black pepper

The health benefits associated with turmeric are numerous: it is a powerful antioxidant and has been used in Indian and Chinese medicine for centuries as an anti-inflammatory agent – see page 58. Finely grated, turmeric adds a wonderfully subtle flavour to a dish and creates a beautifully bright, sunny colour. Fresh turmeric is available in some supermarkets and, like ginger, keeps well if stored in the fridge, but if you cannot find fresh, ground is fine. Cauliflower, meanwhile, is counted as one of the top anti-cancer foods as it is a rich source of glucosinolates.

This recipe works really well on its own or, if you want a larger meal rich in proteins, served topped with an egg cooked to your liking.

1 Heat the oil gently in a pan, add the chopped cauliflower and onion and cook on a medium heat for 10 minutes or until golden.

2 Add the garlic, turmeric and curry powder, mix well and cook for a further 2 minutes.

3 Finally, add the chopped coriander, lemon juice and seasoning. Mix well and serve at once.

Cauliflower and Butter Bean Mash

Serves 2

Takes 30 minutes, plus overnight if soaking dried beans

50g dried butter beans, or 100g carton prepared beans

¼ head cauliflower

½ clove garlic, crushed, peeled and chopped

2 tbsp cream cheese

sea salt and white pepper

2 tsp finely chopped sage leaves

This mash has great nutritional value and takes just 30 minutes to cook, unless you're using dried beans, which will need to be soaked overnight. Sage is best known for its antioxidant and anti-inflammatory properties; butter beans are a great source of protein; and the cream cheese will boost the calorie content, which is useful for those seeking to gain weight.

You can serve this either hot or cold, and it's an ideal alternative to starchy foods such as potatoes. In the winter months, serve it as an accompaniment to a warming casserole.

1 If using dried beans, place them in a saucepan and cover well with water; soak overnight and in the morning drain, rinse and then return them to the pan and cover with water again. Bring to the boil, then reduce the heat and simmer for 1 hour or until the beans are soft. Remove any residue that forms on the top of the cooking water. Test that the beans are soft, then drain and set aside. (If using prepared beans, simply set them aside until Step 3.)

2 Cut the cauliflower into florets, place in a large pan and half cover with water. Bring to the boil, then reduce the heat and simmer with a lid on for 8 minutes or until the cauliflower is soft. Drain well and return to the pan.

3 Add the drained butter beans, crushed garlic, cream cheese and seasoning, and mash together with a potato masher.

4 Finally, add the chopped sage leaves and stir through before serving.

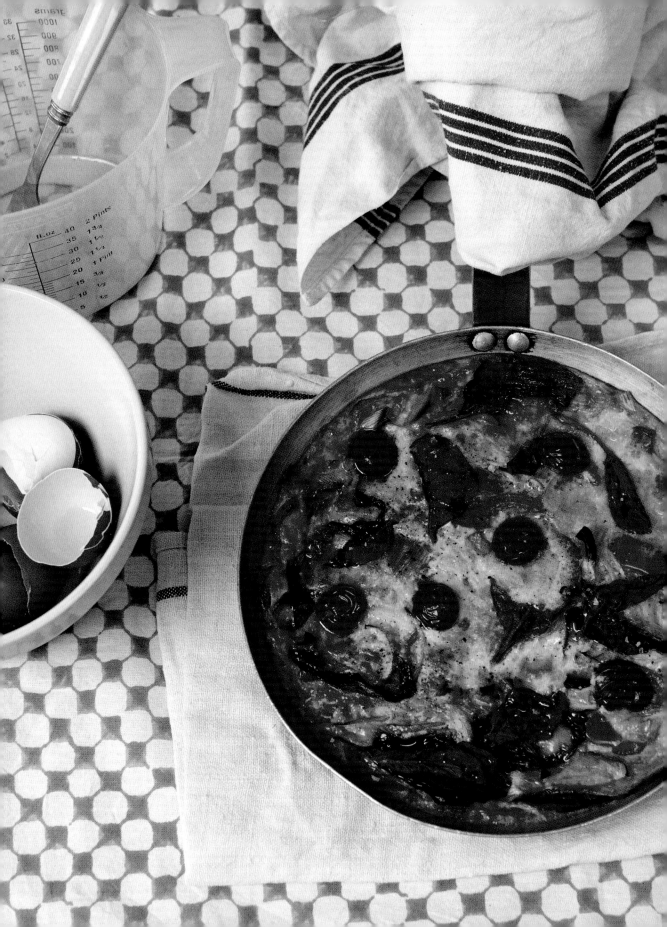

Fridge Frittata

Serves 4

Takes 45 minutes

300g of any of the
  following vegetables:
  beetroot, broccoli,
  cauliflower, kale, leeks,
  mushrooms, peas,
  peppers, potato, sweet
  potato, tomatoes

1 tbsp olive oil

1 onion, diced

1 clove garlic, crushed,
  peeled and chopped

4 eggs

150ml cream or milk

sea salt and freshly
  ground black pepper

125g cheese – Cheddar,
  Stilton, goat's cheese,
  buffalo Mozzarella, Brie,
  Emmental, Parmesan

If you have eggs, vegetables, milk or cream and a little cheese in your fridge, you have the basis of a frittata, which is why I have named this dish 'Fridge Frittata'. To clear the fridge, I often make this on the day before I go shopping.

The array of vegetables in this recipe delivers the healthy rainbow diet that contains a variety of beneficial phytochemicals, vitamins and minerals, and the eggs are a fantastic source of protein. They will help your body to heal, because protein repairs damaged tissue. Eggs are so easy to use and, contrary to reports some years ago, they do not increase your cholesterol.

1 Pre-heat the oven to 180°C, gas mark 4.

2 Cut the vegetables into even-sized pieces.

3 Warm the oil in an ovenproof, non-stick frying pan, add the onion and garlic and cook gently for 3 minutes.

4 Add the medley of vegetables and cook for a further 5 minutes, tossing to cook evenly.

5 Whisk the eggs, add the cream or milk and seasoning, and pour this over the vegetables. Gently cook for a further 5 minutes on a medium heat.

6 Scatter the cheese evenly over the top, either cut into slices or grated, and bake in the oven for 15–20 minutes. To test if the frittata is cooked, carefully press the back of a spoon into the middle of the egg. It should be firm; if not, return to the oven to cook a little longer.

7 When cooked, remove and allow to rest before cutting into wedges and serving.

Red Lentil Dhal with Grated Courgette

Serves 2

Takes 45 minutes

1 tbsp coconut oil

1 onion, finely chopped

1 clove garlic, crushed,
   peeled and chopped

1 tsp grated fresh
   turmeric, or use ground

½ tsp ground cumin

½ tsp ground coriander

½ tsp paprika

150g red split lentils

500ml chicken or
   vegetable stock

1 x 400g carton chopped
   tomatoes

sea salt and freshly
   ground black pepper

2 courgettes, grated or
   spiralized

a bunch of fresh
   coriander, chopped

Served on its own or as an accompaniment, this dhal is a warming bowl of rich goodness. Lentils are rich in protein and all these spices add flavour and complexity to this easy dish. The final addition of grated courgette and coriander will give a terrific boost to your vegetable and vitamin intake.

The spices have multiple health benefits too – see page 66. Cumin aids digestion and is a good source of iron and manganese. Paprika will provide vitamins A, E and B_6 – and although you will be using only small amounts here, they all add up to provide you with an array of extra nutrients. And let's not forget the powerhouse that is garlic. (See the recipe note for Poached Egg on Spinach and Pulse Stir-fry, page 151.)

1 Heat the oil in a saucepan and gently cook the onion for 5 minutes or until soft.

2 Add the garlic, turmeric, cumin, coriander, paprika and red lentils, and mix well to coat in all the spices.

3 Add the stock, tomatoes and seasoning, then simmer gently for 30 minutes or until the lentils are tender.

4 Finally, add the grated or spiralized courgette and mix through. Bring to a simmer for 2 minutes, stir the chopped coriander through and serve.

Stuffed Roasted Red Peppers

**Serves 2, or 4
as a side dish**

Takes 35 minutes

2 large red peppers

1 red onion, sliced

1 clove garlic, crushed,
  peeled and chopped

10 cherry tomatoes, cut
  in half

8 black olives

2 tsp capers

sea salt and freshly
  ground pepper

2–4 tbsp olive oil

1 ball buffalo Mozzarella

4 salted anchovy fillets

a bunch of basil leaves,
  torn

The Mediterranean diet is considered by many to be the healthiest of all. It is high in vegetables, fruits, nuts, whole grains, olive oil and fish, and is relatively low in dairy and red meat. If you want to enhance or enrich your diet with good, balanced, wholesome food, try the Mediterranean approach to eating – and you can begin with this delicious, colourful dish, which is rich in cancer-protective phytonutrients.

1 Pre-heat the oven to 200°C, gas mark 6.

2 Cut the red peppers in half horizontally, remove and discard the seeds and cores and place them on a non-stick ovenproof tray.

3 Mix together the prepared onion, garlic, cherry tomatoes, olives, capers and seasoning, then divide the mixture between the peppers, filling each one generously.

4 Drizzle the peppers with olive oil and place in the oven to cook for 15 minutes.

5 Cut the Mozzarella into quarters, remove the peppers from the oven and top with the Mozzarella and an anchovy fillet. Return the tray to the oven and cook for a further 5 minutes.

6 Finally, sprinkle the peppers with torn basil leaves, a further dash of olive oil and serve.

Seaweed, Mushroom and Pearl Barley Risotto

Serves 2

Takes 1 hour

200g pearl barley

600ml vegetable stock or chicken stock

400g mushrooms – a mixture, or your favourite

25g butter

1 tbsp olive oil

½ onion, diced

2 cloves garlic, crushed, peeled and chopped

1 tbsp seaweed, chopped – try Maraseaweed.com

juice of ½ lemon

a bunch of parsley, chopped

50g Parmesan, grated

sea salt and freshly ground black pepper

Seaweed is the super-vegetable of the sea. Its benefits are enormous and varied, but most importantly it boosts the immune system and aids digestion. It is also rich in iodine, iron, magnesium and calcium.

Pearl barley is a much-overlooked grain. High in fibre and selenium, it is good for the colon and it makes a tasty, more textured alternative to risotto rice. Here it marries perfectly with the beneficial seaweed and mushrooms. Try using pearl barley in other favourite risotto recipes.

1 Place the pearl barley and stock in a pan and simmer gently for 45 minutes or until the barley has swollen and is soft and most of the stock has evaporated.

2 Cut the mushrooms into quarters, which helps to add texture to the dish. Heat the butter and olive oil in a pan, add the onion and mushrooms and cook for 8 minutes, turning frequently.

3 Add the garlic and cook for a further 2 minutes.

4 Spoon the cooked pearl barley into the mushroom and onion mixture, along with the seaweed, lemon juice, parsley, half the Parmesan and the seasoning. Stir through and cook gently for a couple of minutes.

5 Sprinkle the remaining Parmesan on top and add a dash of olive oil if wished, then serve.

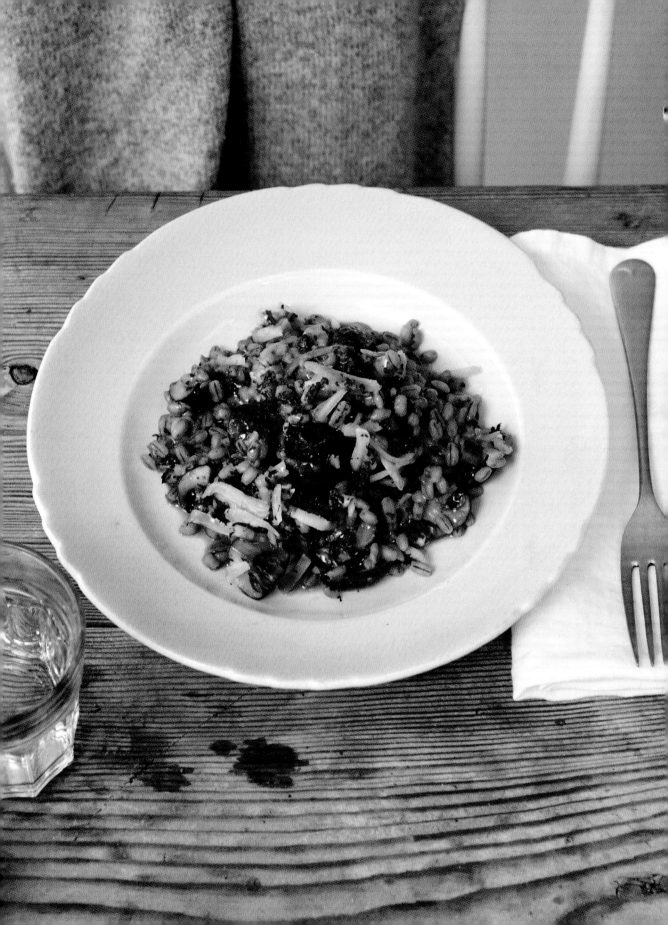

Spiced Golden Tofu with Vegetables

Serves 2

Takes 40 minutes

100g brown rice

2 eggs

1 tbsp coconut oil

1 small onion, finely chopped

1 clove garlic, crushed, peeled and chopped

1 green chilli, finely chopped

1 knob fresh ginger, grated

1 tsp curry powder

75g green vegetables – spinach, peas, broccoli, Brussels sprouts, cabbage

100g tofu, sliced

1 tsp paprika

a bunch of chives, chopped

Enjoy eating like the Japanese, who are renowned for their healthy diets. This recipe packs a real punch of nutrients and anti-cancer compounds. Tofu is made from soya-bean curd and is a good source of protein, iron and calcium, as well as containing all the essential amino acids.

This really is uncomplicated and uses a variety of store-cupboard staples and leftover vegetables, which makes it a very versatile and nutritious dish you can easily use when you don't feel up to shopping. It is also a good way of using up excess cooked rice. (If using leftover rice be sure to let it cool quickly, store it in the fridge and use within a couple of days.)

1 Place the brown rice in a saucepan, cover with water and bring to the boil. Then reduce the heat and simmer for 35 minutes or until the rice is soft. Drain and set aside.

2 Whisk the eggs, add a little oil to a large non-stick frying pan and, when just sizzling, pour in the egg and tip the pan to spread it into an even layer. Reduce the heat and continue to cook until the egg is set. Remove the cooked egg from the pan and roll it tightly into a cigar shape and place to one side.

3 Warm the coconut oil in a wok or large saucepan, add the onion and cook for 5 minutes or until soft and lightly browned. Add the garlic, chilli, ginger and curry powder and mix well. Reduce the heat, add your chosen vegetables and toss to cook.

4 Again, heat the egg frying pan with a little oil, dust the tofu with the paprika and add to the pan. Fry each slice on each side for approximately 3 minutes or until golden.

5 Chop the rolled egg into thin slices.

6 Returning to the vegetable wok, add the rolled egg, rice and seasoning, toss to mix through evenly and heat for a further 4 minutes. Serve topped with the golden tofu and chopped chives.

Braised Spiced Aubergine

Serves 4

Takes 1 hour 10 minutes

2 tbsp coconut oil

2 aubergines, chopped into 5cm cubes

1 onion, diced

2 cloves garlic, crushed, peeled and chopped

1 tsp ground cumin

1 tsp ground coriander

1 x 400g carton chopped tomatoes

sea salt and freshly ground black pepper

a bunch of fresh coriander, chopped

a bunch of fresh mint, chopped

2 tbsp natural bio-yoghurt

There are not many purple foods available to us, so the beautiful, glossy aubergine is one we should all try to include in our rainbow diet. It is a good source of vitamins B_1, B_6 and potassium, and is packed with phytonutrients that protect against free-radical damage, making it an excellent food to eat during treatment. It's also a delicious vegetable that really cannot be rushed. It needs long, slow, gentle cooking to deliver its lovely silky taste and texture. As for the coriander and mint, these herbs are not only fabulous flavour enhancers, but they deliver a bundle of essential vitamins and minerals too.

Although great to eat on the day you cook it, this dish is something you might want to make in advance, because when reheated the taste actually improves. Served at room temperature, it is an almost exotic, Middle Eastern-style salad.

1 Heat the oil in a wide-bottomed pan and add the aubergines. Toss rapidly to coat in the oil and cook for about 10–15 minutes, or until golden all over, turning frequently.

2 Add the onion and garlic, mix well and cook for a further 5 minutes.

3 Add the ground cumin, coriander, chopped tomatoes, seasoning and 100ml of water. Mix well, bring to the boil, then reduce to a simmer for 45 minutes.

4 Just before serving, add the chopped coriander and mint and stir through. Serve with a spoonful of bio-yoghurt for an extra creamy taste.

Fabulous Fish

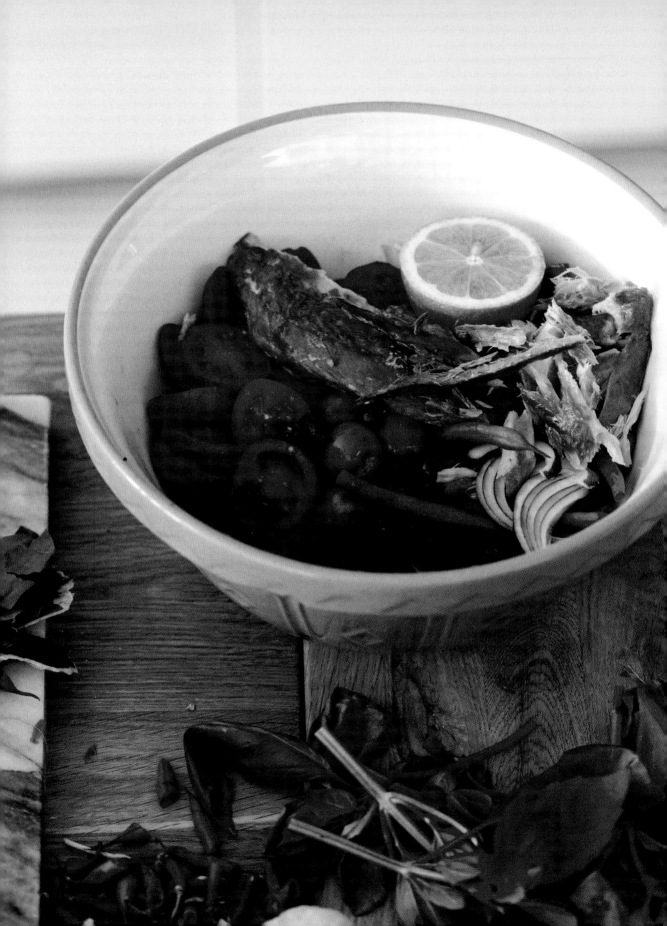

Black Bean and Mackerel Salad

Serves 4

Takes 30 minutes, plus overnight if soaking dried beans

100g dried black beans, or 1 x 200g carton prepared black beans

100g green beans

1 clove garlic, crushed, peeled and chopped

1 small red onion

4 tomatoes

75g green olives

200g smoked mackerel fillets

a bunch of basil

2 tbsp olive oil

juice of 1 lemon

sea salt and freshly ground black pepper

This is inspired by the Mediterranean diet, considered to be one of the healthiest on the planet. Mackerel is an oily fish and bursting with healthy omega-3 fatty acids. It is also good for reducing blood pressure, cholesterol and is an anti-inflammatory. If you want a change from smoked mackerel, buy fresh and try pan-frying or roasting this delicious fish to serve alongside the bean salad.

Beans are thought of as the poor man's meat, but in reality they are the healthy person's protein! They are good for gut health, as the bacteria convert the fibre to butyric acid, which in turn helps fuel our gut cells. As an added bonus, the olives are rich in omega-9 which supports the immune system.

1 If using dried beans, soak them in a pan of water overnight. Next day, drain, rinse and return them to the pan, then cover with water and simmer for approximately 1½ hours or until soft. Skim off any residue that floats to the top. When the beans are cooked through, drain and set aside. (If using prepared beans, simply set aside until Step 3.)

2 Trim the green beans and cook for 2 minutes in boiling water, drain, refresh in cold water and set aside.

3 In a large bowl, place the cold black and green beans and mix together thoroughly. Crush the garlic, finely slice the red onion, add both to the mixed beans and toss.

4 Dice or quarter the tomatoes and add to the beans, along with the olives.

5 Finally, peel away and discard the mackerel skin, then flake the fillets into the bowl with the basil leaves, olive oil, lemon juice and seasoning. Toss gently and serve.

Avocado and Salmon Open Sandwich

Serves 1

Takes 10 minutes

1 egg

1 slice rye bread

1 tomato, sliced

½ avocado, chopped

2 slices or 75g smoked salmon, or flaked cooked salmon

a pinch of dried chilli flakes

sea salt and freshly ground black pepper

a wedge of lemon

a pinch of seaweed flakes

1 tsp olive oil

This is a quick, fresh-tasting meal and, topped with a free-range egg, provides a very balanced, protein-rich meal.

Avocados are teeming with essential nutrients – potassium, B vitamins, folic acid – plus they also act as a nutrient booster, so when enjoyed with other foods they allow the body to absorb important anti-cancer nutrients. They are rich in monounsaturated fatty acids, oleic being one that may protect against breast cancer. They are so good for you that it is recommended that you try to eat half an avocado every day.

....

1 Boil the egg for 4 minutes if you like it slightly soft or 8 minutes for hard-boiled. Run it under cold water to cool and then peel when you are able to handle it.

2 Toast the rye bread, or leave it plain if you prefer. Top it with the tomato, avocado and smoked salmon.

3 Cut the peeled egg in half, then add it to the sandwich. Sprinkle with chilli, seasoning, a squeeze of lemon juice and a shake of seaweed flakes. Drizzle with olive oil and serve.

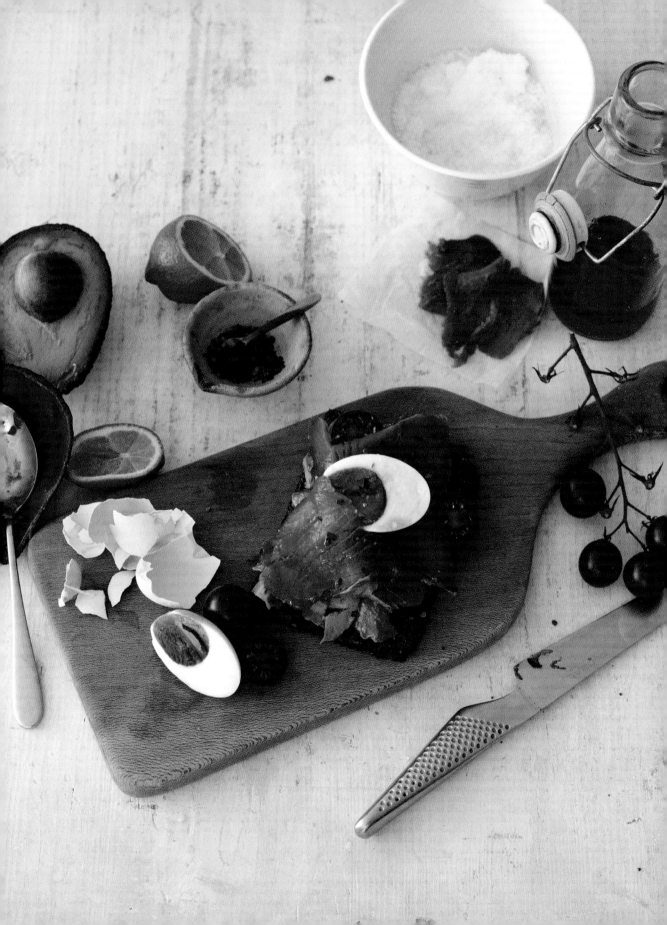

Salmon and Chia Cakes with Dill and Avocado Salad

Serves 4

Takes 25 minutes

500g skinless salmon

1 tsp cumin, ground

1 tsp grated fresh
  turmeric, or use ground

sea salt and freshly
  ground black pepper

1 tbsp chia seeds

1 tbsp sesame seeds

1 tbsp coconut oil

For the salad

2 tbsp olive oil

2 lemons, zested and
  juiced

1 tsp Dijon mustard

2 cloves garlic, crushed,
  peeled and chopped

sea salt and freshly
  ground black pepper

a large bunch of dill

1 ripe avocado

4 spring onions

Chia seeds are a great kitchen-cupboard staple and can be added to many dishes to increase our intake of important omega-3. Try using them to help thicken soups, casseroles and stewed fruits. They act as a good replacement for eggs, as they can help to bind ingredients together. As chia has no real flavour, these seeds are very adaptable.

The salmon in this dish also delivers extra omega-3, and is an excellent source of high-quality protein, vitamins and minerals, including potassium, selenium and vitamin B_{12}. This recipe is a great way of increasing your raw vegetable intake too. Avocados are a dream food, rich in good fats and an array of vitamins, calcium and phosphorus amongst other minerals, whilst the dill is carminative and good for digestive disturbance. As dill also promotes detoxification reactions in the liver, which helps to rid the body of toxic chemicals, it is a great cleansing herb to eat during treatment. This would be a good choice for those following the Ketogenic Diet.

1 Place the salmon, cumin, turmeric and seasoning in a food processor and pulse until chopped. Transfer to a mixing bowl. Add the chia and sesame seeds, mixing together by hand for an even blend.

2 Divide the mixture into four and shape into patties about 3cm thick. Set aside.

3 In a bowl, mix together the olive oil, lemon zest and juice, Dijon mustard, garlic and seasoning, and whisk together with a fork until blended.

4 Chop the dill, avocado and spring onions and add to the dressing, tossing it all together again to coat thoroughly. Set aside.

5 Heat the coconut oil in a large non-stick pan, add the salmon cakes and cook for 4 minutes on each side, or 3 minutes if you prefer a pink centre. Serve with the dill and avocado salad.

Oven-Baked Trout and Kale with Millet

Serves 1

Takes 40 minutes

1 tsp coconut oil

50g millet

a bunch of parsley, chopped

3 tbsp olive oil

50g kale

4 cherry tomatoes

2 trout fillets – ask your fishmonger to fillet them for you

juice of ½ lemon

1 tsp capers, chopped

sea salt and freshly ground black pepper

Rather unfairly, trout are often overlooked. They are delicious, sustainable, affordable and nutritiously rich in omega-3, so we really should try to eat them more often.

Millet is gluten-free and rich in magnesium, protein and fibre – another ancient grain we recommend as a store-cupboard staple; when cooked like this, it delivers a fluffy and tasty result.

....

1 Pre-heat the oven to 180°C, gas mark 4.

2 Warm the coconut oil in a saucepan, add the millet and gently toast over a medium heat for 5 minutes, stirring constantly. This will release a lovely toasty aroma.

3 Add 150ml of water, bring to the boil and simmer gently for 15 minutes. (It's important to cook gently to retain the texture of the grain.) Once cooked through, drain, add the chopped parsley and a dash of olive oil, mix and keep warm.

4 Place the kale and cherry tomatoes in a small roasting dish, add the remaining olive oil and mix well, coating all over. Lay the trout fillets on top, skin side down, and cook in the oven for 12 minutes.

5 Finally, add the lemon juice, capers and seasoning to the millet and mix. Serve topped with the oven-cooked vegetables and trout.

Fish Soup

Serves 2

Takes 40 minutes

1 tbsp olive oil

1 stick celery, chopped

½ onion, chopped

½ fennel, chopped

1 medium potato, chopped into cubes

½ leek, chopped

1 clove garlic, crushed, peeled and chopped

½ tsp grated fresh turmeric, or use ground

500ml vegetable stock

400g carton chopped tomatoes

¼ tsp seaweed flakes

sea salt and freshly ground black pepper

a bunch of dill, chopped

2 tbsp crème fraîche

100g cod fillet, skinned

100g peeled prawns

a bunch of parsley, chopped

½ red chilli, diced (optional)

Fish offers many vitamins, minerals and proteins, and when combined with all the other ingredients in this recipe, you will have a really hearty, delicious, nutrient-dense meal.

Fennel is excellent for the digestion and is packed with vitamin C, and the crème fraîche adds a wonderfully creamy richness and a touch of style to this simple and easy-to-prepare dish.

. . . .

1 Warm the olive oil in a saucepan, add the chopped celery, onion, fennel, potato and leek, and cook gently for 5 minutes.

2 Add the garlic, cook for a further 2 minutes, then add the turmeric, vegetable stock, chopped tomatoes, seaweed and seasoning. Bring to the boil, then reduce to a simmer and cook for 20 minutes with a lid on.

3 Mix the chopped dill and crème fraîche together and set aside.

4 Cut the cod into chunks and place on top of the soup, along with the prawns. Replace the lid and simmer again for 5–8 minutes or until the fish is cooked.

5 Sprinkle with the chopped parsley and chilli, and ladle into bowls, topped with a spoonful of the crème fraîche and dill mix.

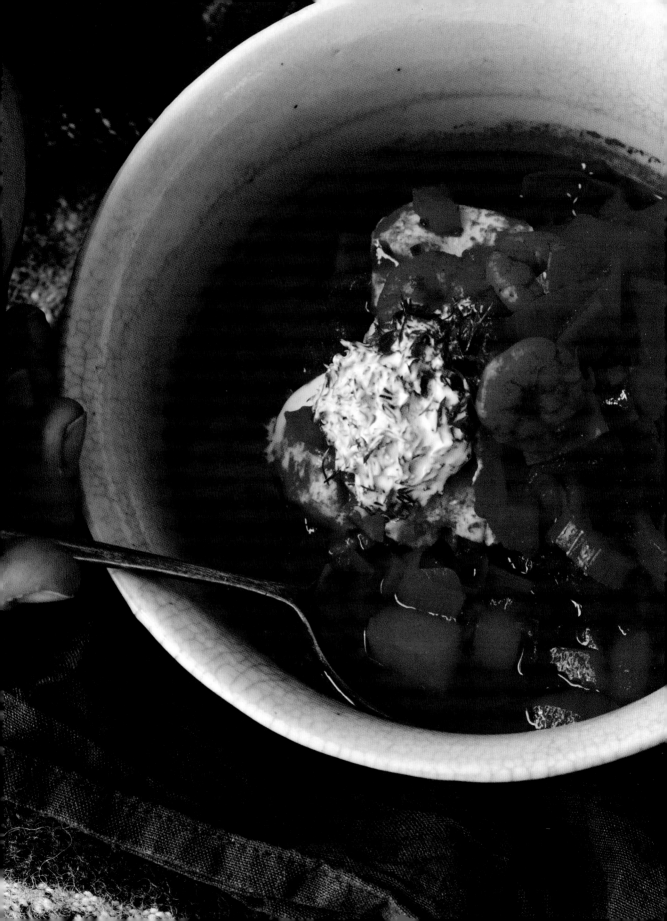

Kedgeree with Leafy Greens

Serves 4

Takes 50 minutes

300g brown basmati rice

350g undyed smoked haddock, cut into 4 pieces

200g cold freshwater prawns, peeled

2 eggs

1 tbsp coconut oil

2 shallots, diced

1 tsp grated fresh turmeric, or use ground

1 tsp curry powder

100g favourite leafy greens, chopped – e.g. kale, spinach, Savoy cabbage

a bunch of parsley, chopped

1 lemon, zested and juiced

sea salt and freshly ground black pepper

Kedgeree was brought to the UK by returning colonials who had enjoyed it in India during the days of the British Empire. It was served at breakfast by the staff, who would add spices to the dish to give it an exotic twist. The rice was sometimes replaced with beans or lentils. Today, kedgeree should be enjoyed as a meal at any time of the day as it is has terrific nutritious value. The brown rice increases the complex carbohydrates, providing even more fibre, vitamins and minerals, and the fish and vegetables offer another host of vitamins and minerals. It is a great dish for adding turmeric, as the vibrant yellow pigment enhances the colour and brings a whole host of anti-cancer effects.

Buy cold, freshwater prawns if you can, as they are the healthiest and most ethical option.

1 Rinse the rice in cold water and place in a saucepan. Cover with water, bring to the boil, then reduce the heat and simmer for 35 minutes or until the rice is just cooked. Drain well and set aside.

2 In a non-stick frying pan, heat 2cm of water, add the smoked haddock and put a lid on. Reduce the heat to a simmer and cook for 8–10 minutes. Halfway through, add the prawns. Retaining the water, remove the haddock and the prawns from the pan and keep warm.

3 Place the eggs in a saucepan, cover with warm water and bring to a gentle simmer. Cook for 6 minutes for a soft centre, or for 8 minutes if you prefer your eggs to have a firmer yolk. Drain, cool under a running tap and peel.

4 Heat the coconut oil in a medium pan, add the shallots and cook for 5 minutes or until soft. Then add the turmeric and curry powder, mix well and cook for a further 2 minutes.

5 Add the cooked rice to the shallots, your chopped chosen greens, parsley, lemon juice and 4 tablespoons of the liquid that the fish was cooked in. Season, mix well and cook on a medium heat for 5 minutes, or until the greens just start to wilt.

6 Add the warm cooked fish and prawns, and mix gently. Serve with half a boiled egg and some extra chopped parsley on top.

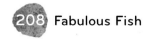

Salmon and Puy Lentils with a Coriander Sauce

Serves 2

Takes 40 minutes

1 tbsp coconut oil

1 onion, diced

1 clove garlic, crushed, peeled and chopped

100g puy lentils

450ml vegetable or fish stock

4 tbsp coriander, finely chopped

1 tomato, finely chopped

1 tsp cumin, ground

1 tsp curry powder

1cm fresh ginger, grated

1cm grated fresh turmeric, or 1 tsp ground

2 tbsp bio-yoghurt

sea salt and freshly ground black pepper

2 x 125g skinless salmon fillets

75g peas

1 lime, zested and juiced

Puy lentils are a speciality from France, favoured for their great texture, pretty marbled outer layer and light peppery flavour. They also have a high protein, mineral and vitamin content, as do all pulses. The spices and herbs in this recipe are all beneficial too. Try to use ginger and coriander as much as possible in your kitchen as they deliver both flavour and many healthy nutrients.

This recipe can have a calming effect on the digestive tract. The ginger is anti-inflammatory, the bio-yoghurt helps to increase all the healthy microbes in your gut and the omega-3 found in fish oils is anti-inflammatory.

1 In a wide pan, heat the coconut oil, add the onion and gently cook for 4 minutes.

2 Add the garlic and cook for a further minute before adding the lentils. Cover with the stock, stir well and cook for 25 minutes.

3 Place the chopped coriander, tomato, cumin, curry powder, ginger, turmeric, yoghurt and seasoning in a bowl and mix. Set aside.

4 Carefully place the salmon fillets on top of the lentil mix and cover with a lid. Simmer gently for a further 8–10 minutes, or until the salmon is cooked to your liking. Then remove the lid and continue cooking gently to evaporate any excess liquid.

5 Add the peas and simmer for a further 3 minutes. Add the lime juice and zest, then serve the lentils and salmon with the coriander sauce.

Seed-crusted Cod Loin

Serves 1

Takes 30 minutes

125g loin of cod, skinned

1 tsp olive oil

2 tbsp pumpkin seeds

1 clove garlic, crushed,
  peeled and chopped

1 tbsp chopped dill

1 lemon, zested and
  juiced

a pinch of seaweed flakes

2 tbsp cream cheese

sea salt and freshly
  ground black pepper

This is an easy, one-person meal which can be served with some steamed brassica, such as spring greens, broccoli, Savoy cabbage, purple sprouting broccoli or kale. You can replace the cod with any other fillet of fresh fish available. The seed topping in this recipe adds a delicious crunch and texture to the cod.

Fish is easy to digest, which may be an important factor for some, and it's a good source of many nutrients. It is often regarded as a brain-protective food. Fish also has good levels of iodine, which helps support the thyroid. Many of us are deficient in iodine, so when not eating fish try having a shaker of seaweed flakes at your table to add to all meals. A good addition to a ketogenic meal.

. . . .

1 Pre-heat the oven to 200°C, gas mark 6.

2 Dry the excess moisture from the cod loin with kitchen paper and place on a lightly oiled non-stick baking sheet.

3 Roughly chop the pumpkin seeds, reserving a few, and place in a small bowl together with the chopped garlic, dill, lemon zest and juice, seaweed flakes, cream cheese and seasoning. Combine well before spreading this mixture over the top of the fish. Sprinkle with the reserved pumpkin seeds.

4 Place in the oven and cook for 8–12 minutes, depending on the thickness of the cod. The seed topping should be lightly browned.

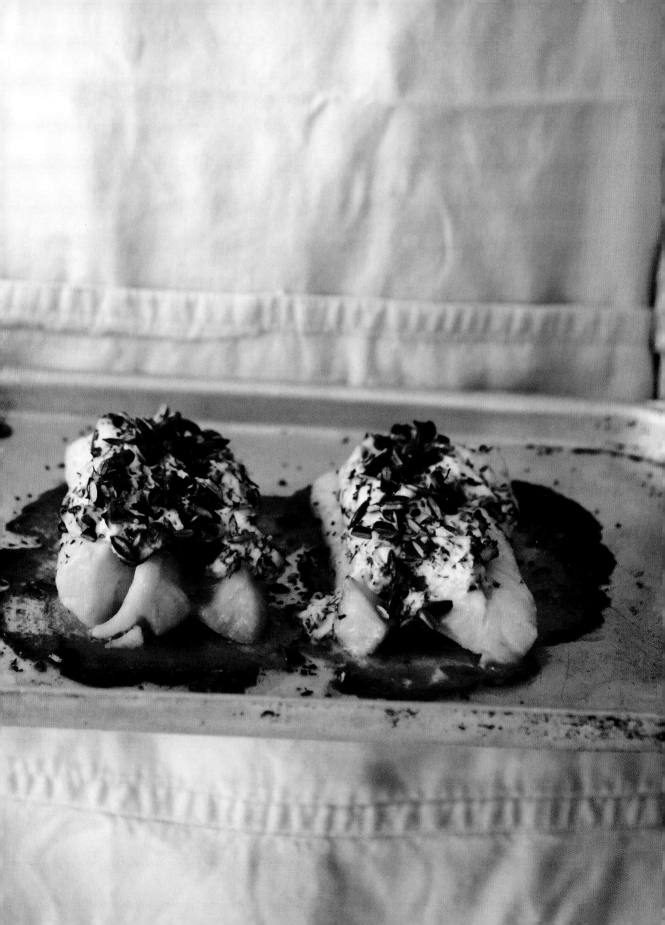

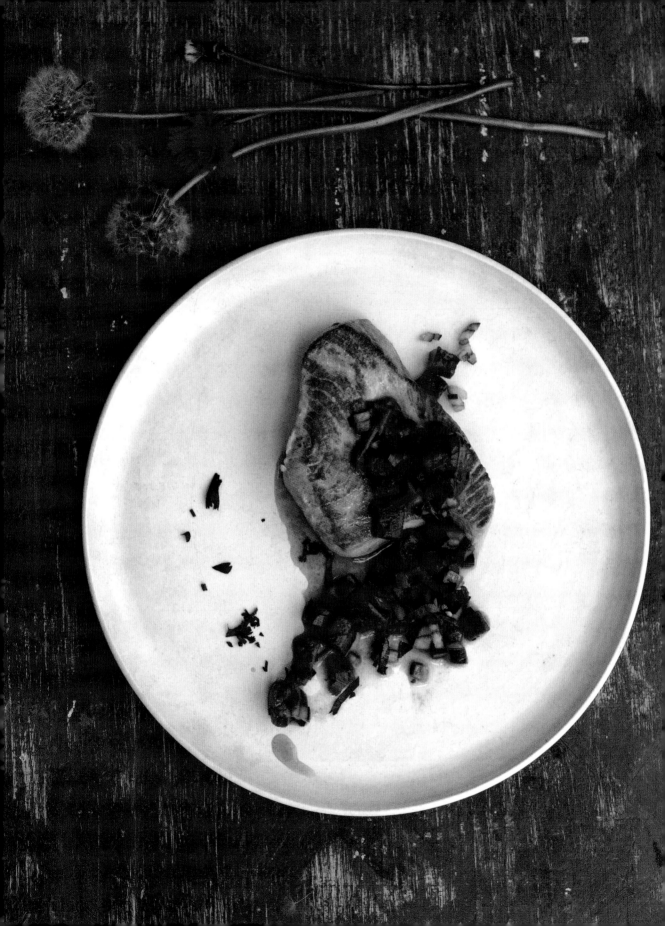

Grilled Fish and Papaya Salad

Serves 2

Takes 30 minutes

1 papaya, finely chopped

½ red onion, finely
   chopped

½ red pepper, finely
   chopped

½ red chilli, finely
   chopped

juice of 1 lime

a bunch of coriander,
   chopped

2 x 125g fillets of
   favourite fish – cod,
   halibut, salmon, tuna,
   trout, bream

Papaya flesh is rich in papain, a powerful digestive enzyme that helps break down proteins and toxins. It has antioxidant properties such as carotenes and vitamin C which can support the immune system. Do try to include papaya in your weekly shop when they are in season. See page 139 for information on how to make a refreshing drink using papaya seeds.

. . . .

1 Make the salsa by combining the chopped papaya, onion, red pepper, chilli, lime juice and coriander in a bowl, then set aside.

2 Grill your chosen fish fillet on a lightly oiled baking sheet. The timing will vary according to the thickness of the fillets, but aim for approximately 6–10 minutes. This should deliver beautifully juicy fish.

3 Serve with a generous spoonful of the papaya salad.

Crab with Courgette Spaghetti

Serves 1

Takes 20 minutes

2 courgettes (approx. 200g)

1 tbsp olive oil

1 clove garlic, crushed, peeled and chopped

a bunch of oregano

juice of 1 lemon

200g crab meat

sea salt and freshly ground black pepper

This is an ideal low-carb supper dish and spiralized courgettes are a wonderfully healthy alternative to wheat-laden pasta. Courgette spaghetti works really well with a variety of sauces – Bolognaise, mushroom, Neapolitan – or simply tossed in harissa or pesto (see pages 261 and 262).

When you try this fresh, light alternative you will boost your vegetable intake and the crab will provide a multitude of minerals, including copper, zinc and selenium, along with some essential B vitamins.

1 Prepare the courgettes according to the equipment you have. A spiralizer is best for making spaghetti, or you can use a mandolin/vegetable peeler for ribbons, or simply grate.

2 Warm the olive oil in a pan, add the garlic and oregano and fry gently for a minute.

3 Add the lemon juice, crab meat and seasoning, toss the ingredients and cook for a further 2 minutes.

4 Finally, add the prepared courgettes and carefully toss for 3 minutes if you like a bit of crunch, or 5–8 minutes if you prefer them soft.

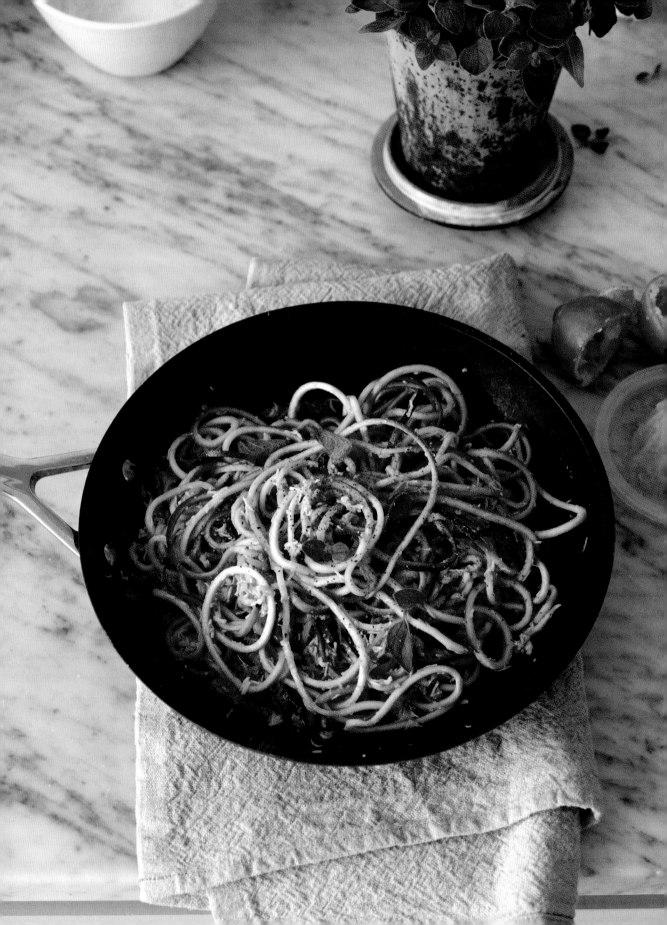

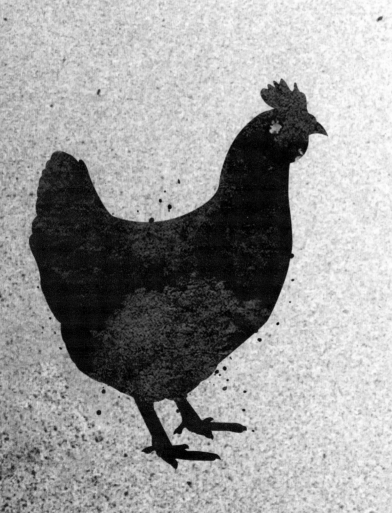

Satisfying Meat

Fragrant Herb and Almond Chicken with Quinoa

Serves 2

Takes 35 minutes

1 tbsp olive oil

2 chicken breasts, boneless

1 shallot, diced

1 clove garlic, crushed, peeled and chopped

80g quinoa, red or plain

400ml chicken stock (see page 256)

1 bay leaf

sea salt and freshly ground black pepper

2 tbsp mascarpone

a bunch of dill, chopped

a bunch of parsley, chopped

20g almond slivers, toasted

juice of ½ lemon

This dish is brimming with fresh herbs that are high in nutrients, vitamins and minerals. It is made in a similar way to risotto, but instead of rice, we're using quinoa – a complete protein, containing all the essential amino acids.

This dish is delicate in flavour and easy to prepare, making it a great meal to eat when you are feeling under the weather. If you want something with a more robust flavour, add more herbs, such as rosemary, chives or wild garlic.

1 Heat the oil in a medium shallow pan and fry the chicken and shallot gently for 5 minutes on a medium heat. Add the garlic and continue cooking for an extra minute.

2 Wash and rinse the quinoa several times, drain, then add to the chicken and mix well.

3 Pour in the stock, bay leaf and seasoning and bring to the boil. Then reduce the heat and simmer for 15 minutes.

4 In a small bowl mix the mascarpone, dill and parsley, adding a little stock from the quinoa pan to thin the juices.

5 Remove the pan from the heat, cover and leave to sit for 5 minutes or until all the stock has been absorbed by the quinoa.

6 Finally, take out the chicken breasts and slice them evenly. Serve the quinoa and spoon the herb mix over it. Top this with the chicken slices and finish off with a sprinkling of toasted almonds and lemon juice.

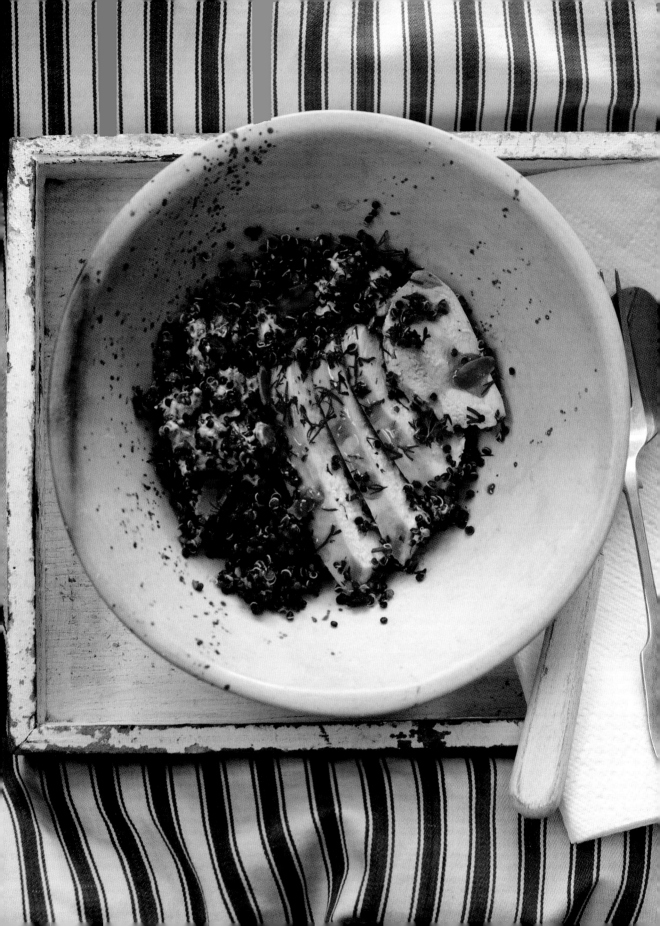

Thai Chicken Stir-fry

Serves 2

Takes 40 minutes

200g chicken meat, brown or white

2 tsp coconut oil

2 cloves garlic, crushed, peeled and chopped

2 sticks lemongrass, finely sliced

1 green chilli, diced

5cm knob fresh ginger, grated

1 red pepper, sliced into strips

100g mangetout

100g beansprouts

2 limes, zested and juiced

a bunch of coriander, chopped

sea salt and freshly ground black pepper

Either white (breast) meat or brown (leg and thigh) meat is suitable for this dish. Brown is generally cheaper and also tastier, making it a good way of keeping down the cost of buying better-quality organic meat. Breast can be expensive but is more tender in texture and more delicate in flavour. So, choose according to your personal preference and budget when cooking this healthy Asian dish, which can be served on its own or with rice noodles.

Lemongrass contains citral, which gives the plant its lemony taste and aroma. It has been shown to have anti-cancer properties; while receiving treatment, or when you're under the weather, try infusing sliced lemongrass in hot water to drink.

1 Remove the skin from the chicken, trim off any excess fat and cut into small strips.

2 Heat the coconut oil in a large pan or wok, add the chicken and cook for 6–8 minutes or until browned on the outside.

3 Add the garlic, lemongrass, chilli and ginger and continue cooking for a further 2 minutes, continually tossing.

4 Add the red pepper and mangetout, toss and cook for 2 minutes.

5 Finally, add the beansprouts, lime zest and juice, coriander and seasoning. Toss well and cook for a further 2 minutes before serving on its own or with rice noodles.

Turkey, Kale and Black-eyed Bean Broth

Serves 2

Takes 45 minutes, plus overnight if soaking dried beans

100g dried black-eyed beans, or 1 x 200g carton prepared beans

1 tbsp coconut oil

200g turkey, cut into strips

1 onion, chopped

1 clove garlic, crushed, peeled and chopped

1 tsp paprika

sea salt and freshly ground pepper

500ml homemade chicken stock (see page 256)

200g kale

2 fresh tomatoes

ground seeds (optional; see page 258)

This rich, nourishing broth is perfect as a main meal. It contains three key ingredients – tryptophan-rich turkey, iron-rich kale and fibre-packed beans, a low glycaemic food which aids blood-sugar control. Turkey is an economical, lean meat, but do try to use organic or free-range turkey if you can; chicken also works well in this recipe.

....

1 If using dried beans, place in a pan, cover with water and leave to soak overnight. Next day, drain and rinse, cover with fresh water, then bring to the boil and simmer for 1–1½ hours or until the beans are soft. While cooking, skim off any cooking residue that may float to the top. When cooked, drain and use as below. If not using immediately, keep the beans covered with water otherwise they will start to dehydrate. (If using prepared beans, simply set aside until Step 4.)

2 Heat the oil in a pan, add the turkey and onion and cook gently for 5 minutes.

3 Add the garlic and cook for a further 2 minutes.

4 Add the prepared beans, paprika and seasoning, pour in the chicken stock and simmer for 20 minutes.

5 Cut the kale into thin ribbons, dice the tomato and add to the pan. Stir and simmer for 4 minutes, then serve. This is really delicious topped with a teaspoon of ground seeds or with Cashew Cream mixed through (see page 261).

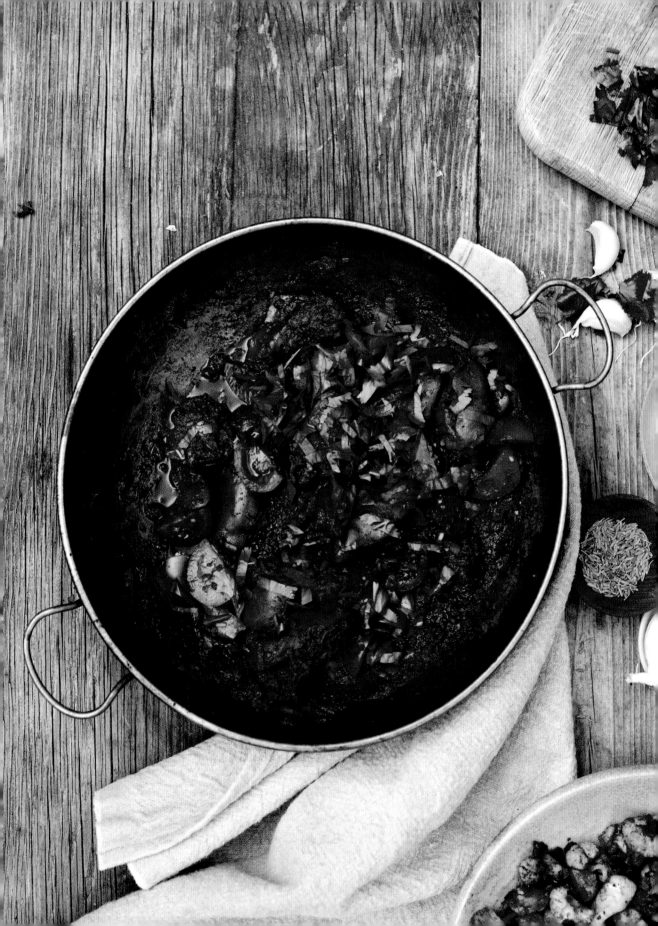

Keralan Chicken Liver Curry

Serves 4

Takes 30 minutes, plus 1 hour for marinading

400g trimmed chicken livers (organic if possible)

1 tbsp grated fresh turmeric, or use ground

1 tsp ground cumin

3 cardamom pods, crushed and seeds removed

5cm fresh ginger, peeled and chopped

2 cloves garlic, peeled

1 green chilli

1 red onion, chopped

sea salt and freshly ground black pepper

1 tbsp coconut oil

2 curry leaves

4 tomatoes, roughly chopped

a bunch of coriander, chopped

A tasty south Indian dish using economical chicken livers, which are bursting with iron and vitamins A and B_{12}. Offal has become less popular nowadays, but it is a good choice for its many health-promoting properties. Try to buy organic if possible, which is very reasonably priced.

This dish contains a host of healthy spices, such as cumin, cardamom and ginger, which will aid digestion and blend really well to deliver a super-tasty dish. You can serve this curry with boiled brown rice, or it goes really well with Indian Cauliflower (see page 188).

1 Trim the chicken livers of any sinewy parts and rinse well in cold water. Place in a colander, drain well, then transfer to a bowl.

2 In a small food processor place the turmeric, cumin, cardamom seeds, fresh ginger, garlic, chilli, red onion and seasoning, and blitz into a rough paste. Add a little water to help blend if needed.

3 Add this paste to the chicken livers, mix well and leave to marinade for 1 hour or overnight in the fridge.

4 When the livers have marinaded, heat the coconut oil in a wok or pan, add the livers and curry leaves, then cook, turning frequently, for 5–7 minutes or until the chicken livers are browned.

5 Add 100ml water to the chicken livers, bring to the boil and simmer for a further 5 minutes, stirring frequently.

6 Finally, add the chopped tomatoes and coriander, stir through and cook for a further 2 minutes.

Asian Broth Bowl with Duck, Buckwheat Noodles and Greens

Serves 2

Takes 45 minutes

1 duck breast, large

1 tbsp coconut oil

1 knob fresh ginger, peeled and diced

2 cloves garlic, crushed, peeled and chopped

1 red chilli

1 litre homemade chicken stock (see page 256)

sea salt and freshly ground black pepper

200g buckwheat or soft rice noodles

50g spinach leaves

1 head pak choi, chopped

4 spears asparagus, trimmed

1 tsp seaweed flakes

a bunch of coriander, chopped

1 tsp sesame seeds

A bowlful of gluten-free goodness, and all made in one saucepan. To add variety you can substitute chicken, pork, prawns, fish or tofu in place of the duck. (Remember to adjust the cooking times depending on the main ingredient you use.)

Duck meat is a good source of protein, vitamins and minerals such as iron, selenium and calcium – essential nutrients that will promote good health. It has a higher fat content than most meats but is a tasty alternative to chicken. Choose a good flavoursome duck, such as Gressingham, and buy organic if you can. Pak choi can be counted as a cruciferous vegetable and is one of those top anti-cancer foods.

1 Using a sharp knife, carefully score the skin of the duck breast in a criss-cross pattern.

2 Heat a non-stick frying pan and place the duck skin-side down on a medium heat and cook for 5–8 minutes. The skin will become crisp and golden. Turn and cook for a further 3–4 minutes if you like your duck pink; if you prefer to have it cooked all the way through, cook for an extra 8 minutes.

3 Once cooked, remove the duck from the heat. Keep it warm and leave to rest, which will help the meat to relax and retain its juices.

4 In another pan, heat the coconut oil, add the ginger, garlic and chilli, then fry for 2 minutes, stirring frequently.

5 Pour in the chicken stock and seasoning, bring to the boil and reduce to a simmer. Add the rice noodles and stir for a few seconds before quickly adding the spinach, pak choi, asparagus and seaweed flakes. Place a lid on the pan and bring to a simmer for 1 minute.

6 To serve, ladle out into two bowls, dividing the noodles and vegetables equally, and add the chopped coriander. Slice the duck thinly and place on top of the soup. Add a sprinkling of sesame seeds to finish off this delicious dish.

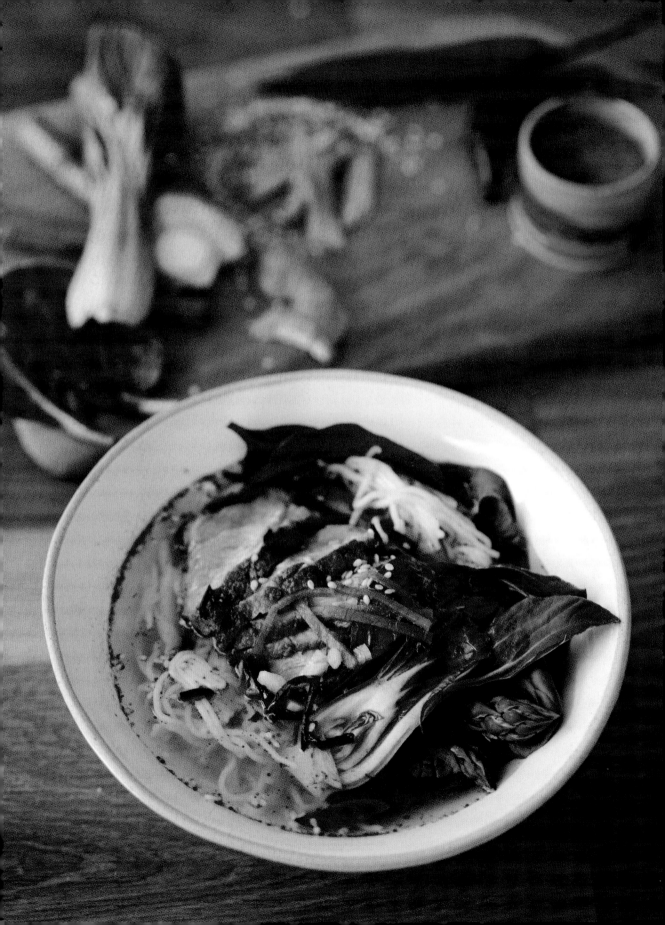

Lamb Shepherd's Pie with Mash and Greens Topping

Serves 2

Takes 1–1¼ hours

½ tbsp coconut oil

1 small onion, finely chopped

1 carrot, finely chopped

1 stick celery, finely chopped

½ small swede, finely chopped

250g minced lamb

400ml lamb or beef stock

sea salt and freshly ground black pepper

1 bay leaf

For the topping

375g potatoes, peeled

1 egg, beaten

100g Savoy cabbage, or kale

25g Cheddar cheese

sea salt and freshly ground black pepper

Treat yourself to this healthy version of a classic favourite. It has added green vegetables, which are the most nutrient-dense of all the vegetables we can use in the Nutritional Kitchen.

A stick of celery can often be popped into a recipe with other vegetables to enhance nutrient value – especially important phytonutrients which are anti-inflammatory.

1 Pre-heat the oven to 180°C, gas mark 4.

2 Warm the oil in a small ovenproof saucepan/casserole dish, add the chopped onion, carrot, celery and swede, and cook for 5 minutes or until soft.

3 Add the mince, mix well and cook for a further 5 minutes.

4 Pour in the stock, add the seasoning and bay leaf, bring to the boil, then reduce the heat and simmer with the lid on for 30 minutes, stirring occasionally.

5 Meanwhile, place the potatoes in a pan of hot water and simmer for 20 minutes, or until soft. Drain them well (reserving the cooking liquid) and return to the pan. Mash until smooth, add beaten egg and quickly mix.

6 Boil the reserved potato water in a pan, shred the cabbage or kale into thin ribbons and add to the boiling water. Mix and cook for 1 minute, then drain well.

7 Add the vegetables to the mashed potato, along with the grated cheese and seasoning, and mix well.

8 Finally, carefully spoon the mashed potato mix in a layer over the lamb mix, then put in the oven and cook for 30 minutes, so that the potatoes are just brown and the juices are bubbling up around the edges.

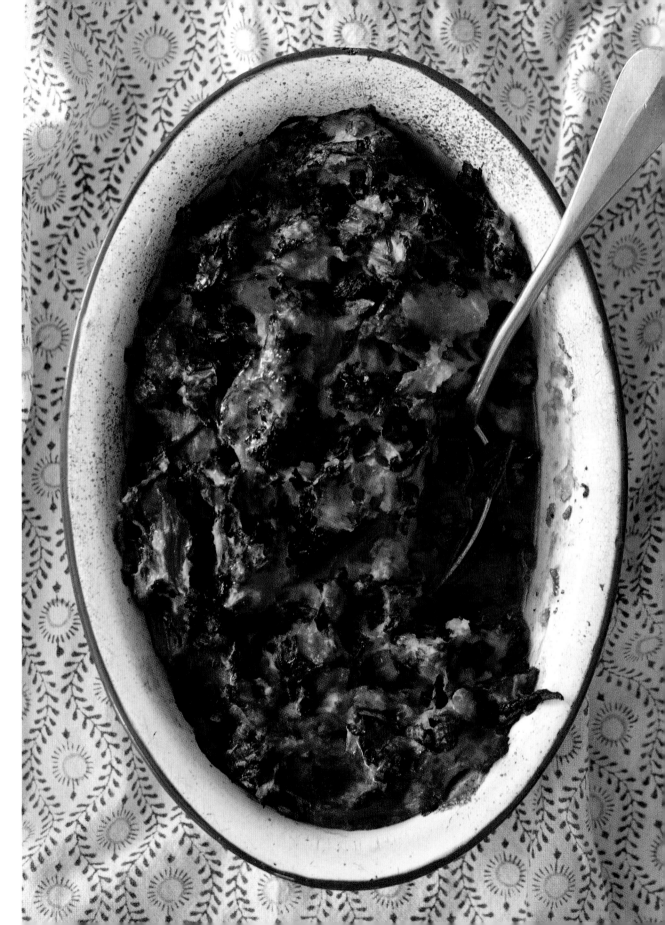

Lamb Tagine

Serves 4

Takes 2 hours, plus overnight marinating

1 onion, finely chopped

2 cloves garlic, crushed, peeled and chopped

2 tbsp olive oil

3cm fresh ginger, grated

a pinch of chilli flakes

½ tsp paprika

1 tsp ground cumin

a pinch of saffron flakes, or ¼ tsp grated fresh or ground turmeric

sea salt and freshly ground black pepper

500g braising lamb, cut into cubes – shoulder or neck fillet

1 x 400g carton chopped tomatoes

1 tsp grated orange zest

juice of 1 orange

1 cinnamon stick, or 1 tsp ground cinnamon

10 dates, stoned and chopped

2 tbsp honey, raw or locally produced

a bunch of coriander, chopped

50g whole almonds, toasted

This is a really hearty tagine that is naturally enriched and sweetened with dates and honey, giving it a velvety texture and fruity flavour. Lamb has a healthier nutrient profile than some meats, such as beef, as cattle are frequently given extra feed (protein nuts, for example) before slaughter to boost their weight. Usually, the only time sheep are given supplementary food is in winter when the ground is covered with snow; then they may be fed hay, which is also a natural product. It's a good idea to be a little more inquisitive about the source of your produce and how it has been raised.

The ginger used in this dish also has an abundance of health benefits, including aiding blood-sugar control by increasing insulin sensitivity.

1 Pre-heat the oven to 160°C, gas mark 3.

2 In a bowl, place the onion, garlic, olive oil, ginger, chilli flakes, paprika, cumin, saffron or turmeric and seasoning. Stir together well, add the lamb and coat it in the mix. Cover and leave in the fridge overnight.

3 Heat the oil in a large ovenproof pan, add the lamb and cook on a medium to high heat, or until the lamb cubes are evenly browned.

4 To this pan, add the tomatoes, orange zest, juice, cinnamon, dates and honey, mix well and bring to the boil. Add just enough water to cover the meat (this will depend on the size of saucepan that you use). Cover with a tight-fitting lid and place in the oven to cook for 1 hour 40 minutes.

5 Add the chopped coriander and stir through before returning to the oven with the lid on for 15 minutes. Remove from the oven, sprinkle with the toasted almonds and serve.

Beef Stock and Herb Restorative Soup

Serves 2

Takes 15 minutes with pre-prepared stock

500ml homemade beef stock (see page 256)

3 sprigs parsley

3 sprigs oregano

3 sprigs marjoram

1 sprig mint

a small bunch of chives

50g watercress

This wonderful soup is something that can be made from your pre-made, frozen Super Stocks (see page 256). All you need to do is defrost it, finely chop all the herbs, heat and stir. Then sit back and just let the simple soup gently nourish and heal your body. All the goodness is easily absorbed and because it is really tasty, it's ideal to eat if your tastebuds are playing up during treatment.

1 Bring the stock to the boil. Meanwhile, finely dice all the herbs and watercress.

2 When the stock is boiling, add the herbs and stir thoroughly. Serve at once.

Simple Steak with Asian Power Butter

Serves 2

Takes 15 minutes, plus 30 minutes to chill

20g macadamia nuts

50g butter, room temperature

1 tsp wasabi

1 lime, zested and juiced

1 green chilli, finely chopped

1 tsp olive or coconut oil

2 x 125g beef (rib eye, fillet, sirloin, bavette or onglet) or tuna steaks

This is a great way of adding extra fats to a diet for those concerned about weight loss. Every now and again our bodies crave protein, making this an easy and very tasty option. The hot, spicy, nutritious power butter works with both a beef or tuna steak; they are cooked in similar ways and can be served rare, medium or well done, so choose whichever you like. Any leftover butter can be stored in the freezer for another day.

1 Place the macadamia nuts in a food processor and blitz until finely ground.

2 Cut up the butter and add to the macadamia nuts in the processor, along with the wasabi, lime juice and zest, and the chilli. Blitz until blended. (This can also be done by hand: finely dice all the ingredients, place in a bowl and use a fork to mix in the butter until blended.)

3 Transfer the butter mix to a sheet of baking parchment and roll into a cigar shape. Wrap the paper around and twist each end. Place in the fridge for 30 minutes to firm the butter.

4 In a non-stick frying pan, heat the oil, add the beef or tuna steaks and cook according to your preference: 3–4 minutes each side for rare, 4–6 minutes each side for medium, 7–8 minutes each side for well done. Remove from the heat once cooked and, if using beef steaks, keep them warm while they rest for 3 minutes; if using tuna steaks, they can be served at once.

5 Remove the butter from the fridge and slice into 4 discs. Put the steaks on plates and lay the power butter slices on top.

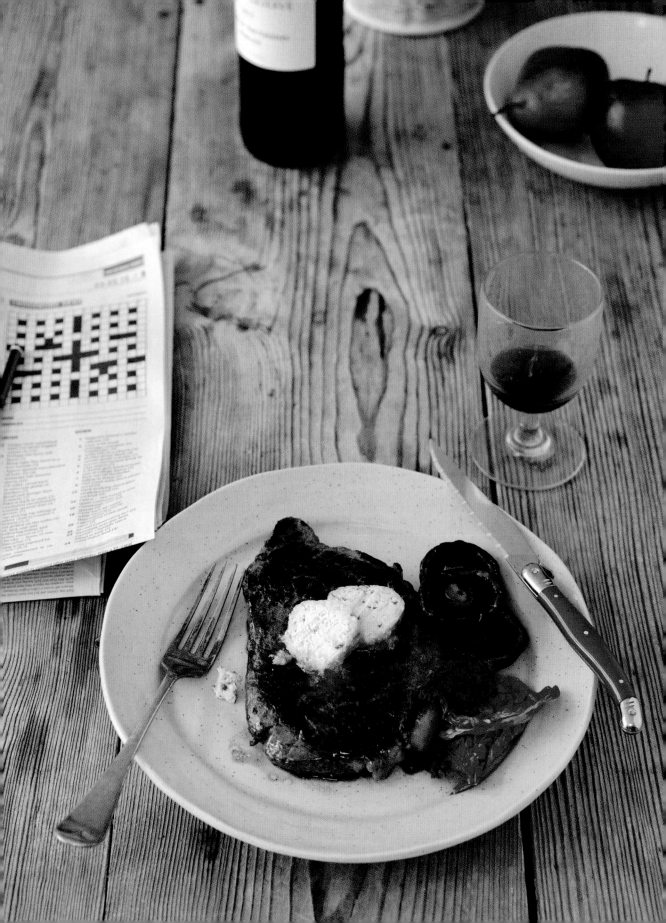

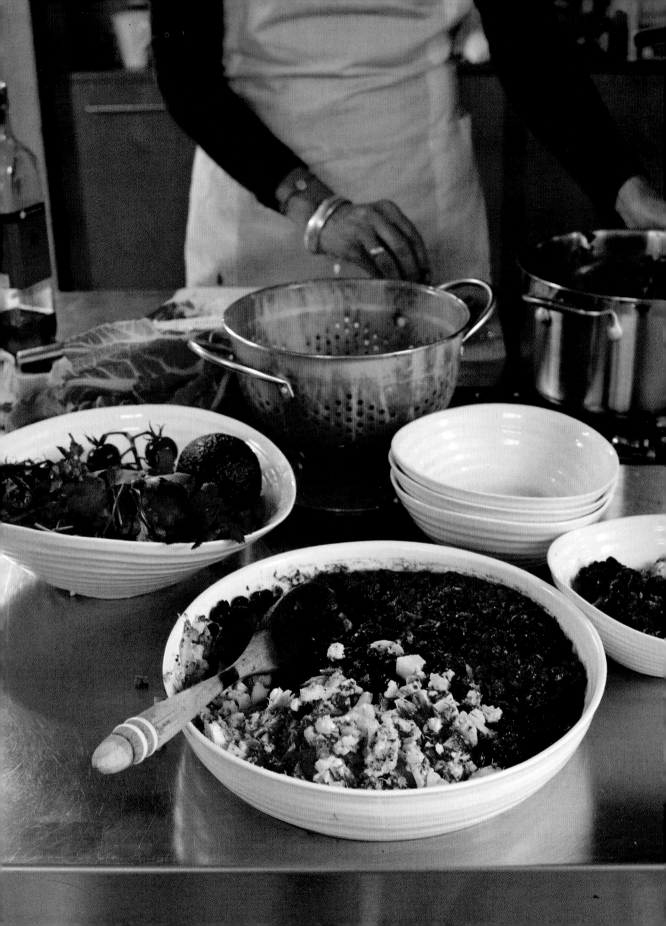

Chilli con Carne with Beans and Green and White Vegetable Rice

Serves 4

Takes 1½ hours, plus overnight if soaking dried beans

50g dried red kidney beans, or 100g carton prepared kidney beans

50g dried black beans, or 100g carton prepared black beans

1 tbsp coconut oil

1 onion, diced

2 cloves garlic, peeled, crushed and diced

1 red chilli, diced

400g minced lean beef

2 tsp ground paprika

1 tsp ground cumin

1 tsp ground coriander

1 cinnamon stick, or 1 tsp ground cinnamon

sea salt and freshly ground black pepper

2 tbsp tomato purée

500ml passata, or 1 x 500ml carton chopped tomatoes

500ml beef stock

200g cauliflower

200g broccoli

a bunch of coriander, chopped

This protein-dense recipe gives a healthy twist to traditional chilli con carne and is an economical dish to serve at a gathering. I've used a mix of black beans and kidney beans to add variety, colour and lots of fibre. Beans are a very healthy, low-glycaemic-index food which can help to boost your serotonin levels too.

Replacing the rice with cruciferous superfood vegetables such as broccoli and cauliflower enriches this dish and offers a lighter, more colourful alternative to the usual chilli. If you're looking to add extra calories, serve this topped with a spoonful of soured cream or natural bio-yoghurt.

....

1 If using dried black beans and kidney beans, soak them overnight in separate pans of cold water. Next day, drain, return the beans to the pans and cover generously with water. Bring to the boil and simmer for 1–1½ hours or until they are soft. Skim off any residue that may rise to the surface while cooking. Drain the beans when soft and ready for use. (If using prepared beans, simply set aside until Step 4.)

2 Warm the oil in a pan, add the onion, garlic, chilli and minced beef and cook on a medium heat for 8 minutes, stirring frequently.

3 Add the paprika, cumin, coriander, cinnamon, seasoning, tomato purée, passata and stock, and mix well. Bring to the boil and simmer for 30 minutes, stirring frequently.

4 Add the prepared kidney and black beans and simmer for a further 30 minutes, adding a little stock if needed.

5 Roughly chop the heads of the cauliflower and broccoli and grate the stems. Place the vegetables in a large pan with 200ml of boiling water, then reduce the heat to a simmer, stirring constantly, until the vegetables are just soft – approximately 3 minutes.

6 Add the chopped coriander to the chilli mixture, spoon the vegetables into a bowl and top with a ladleful of the chilli.

Turmeric Beef and Sweet Potato Pot

Serves 4

Takes 2½ hours, plus overnight if soaking dried chickpeas

100g dried chickpeas, or 200g carton prepared chickpeas

2 tbsp coconut oil

300g braising beef, cubed

1 onion, diced

2 cloves garlic, crushed, peeled and chopped

1 x 400g carton chopped tomatoes

2 tsp grated fresh turmeric, or use ground

1 tsp paprika

500ml vegetable or beef stock

sea salt and freshly ground black pepper

300g sweet potatoes

a bunch of coriander, chopped

This recipe is best made with a cheaper, richer braising cut such as shank, clod or flank, which is packed with protein, vitamin B_{12} and zinc, an important mineral for healthy hair, skin, eyesight and cognitive functions. As always, use organic beef if you can.

Turmeric contains curcumin and research shows that this versatile spice has beneficial anti-inflammatory and anti-cancer properties. As for the sweet potato, it is rich in nutrients, especially beta-carotene which supports the immune system. Use sweet potatoes as a regular alternative to ordinary potatoes. Despite their name they contain fewer sugars (in the form of starches) and more nutrients.

1 If using dried chickpeas, soak them overnight in a pan of cold water. Next day, drain, return to the pan and cover generously with water. Bring to the boil and simmer for 1–1½ hours or until they are soft. Skim off any residue that may rise to the surface while cooking. Drain the chickpeas when soft and ready for use. (If using prepared chickpeas, simply set aside until Step 4.)

2 Heat the oil in an ovenproof dish, add the beef and brown all over.

3 Add the onions and garlic and cook for a further 5 minutes, stirring frequently.

4 Next add the tomatoes, chickpeas, turmeric, paprika, stock and seasoning to the pan. Stir well, bring to the boil, then reduce the heat and simmer gently for 2 hours with a lid on.

5 Wash the sweet potato and chop into good-sized chunks, add to the beef, mix well and cook for a further 30 minutes without the lid on. The juices should be rich and should coat the back of your spoon. If need be, increase the heat, but be sure to stir frequently.

6 Finally, add the chopped coriander, mix and serve.

Pork Tenderloin with Sage and Lemon Cream Sauce

Serves 2

Takes 40 minutes

20g butter

1 tbsp olive oil

200g pork tenderloin

16 sage leaves

100ml white wine

100ml double cream

juice of 1 lemon

sea salt and freshly
   ground black pepper

This enriching treat is high in fats – an important factor for those troubled by weight loss. However, unlike other cuts of pork, tenderloin is relatively lean. It offers important minerals, including phosphorus and selenium, which help to regulate metabolism and protect blood vessels from damage. If you prefer you can use chicken instead of pork.

Sage is rich in antioxidants, aids digestion and has anti-inflammatory properties. It was used to make the medieval 'Four Thieves Vinegar', a potent mixture that was believed to help prevent the plague.

This dish goes really well with the Cauliflower and Butter Bean Mash (see page 189).

1 Pre-heat the oven to 180°C, gas mark 4.

2 In a pan, heat half the butter and olive oil, cut the tenderloin into two equal pieces and add to the pan. Cook until lightly browned on the outside, approximately 8–10 minutes.

3 Place the meat in an ovenproof dish and cook in the oven for 12–15 minutes, by which time the pork should be cooked through.

4 Put the sage leaves in the pan you used to cook the pork, adding a little extra butter if needed. Fry the leaves on each side for a couple of minutes, remove and set aside.

5 Add the wine to deglaze the pan and quickly simmer to reduce by half. Reduce the heat, then add the cream. Mix well and simmer again until the sauce thickens. If it is too thin, increase the heat and stir until it reaches the consistency you want.

6 Remove the pork from the oven and let it rest for a few minutes. Add any juices from the ovenproof dish to the cream sauce, along with the lemon juice and seasoning. Mix thoroughly.

7 Slice the pork and serve with the sauce spooned over. Scatter with the fried sage leaves and serve.

Something Sweet

Peaches Poached in Green Tea with Honey and Almond Yoghurt

Serves 4

Takes 1 hour

4 peaches

1 tsp green tea

3 slices fresh ginger

6 tbsp natural bio-yoghurt

3 tbsp ground almonds

2 tsp flaked almonds, toasted

4 tsp honey, raw or locally produced

This is a pretty, elegant and unusual dessert which uses beneficial green tea for poaching the fruit. Green tea has potent anti-cancer properties, particularly in its enhancement of liver detoxification. Animal research into breast-cancer cells has also found that a compound in peaches can kill cancer cells without affecting normal cells so may inhibit the spread of the disease.

The rich, creamy almond yoghurt is high in proteins yet gentle on the mouth and easy to swallow. Aim to use raw or good-quality local honey whenever possible.

1 Find a pan that the peaches will fit into snugly, then remove them and set aside.

2 Add 500ml water to the pan, the green tea and ginger, and bring to a boil, then reduce the heat to a simmer.

3 Add the peaches, put a lid on the pan and simmer for 6 minutes, turning the peaches halfway through cooking.

4 Remove from the heat, take off the lid and leave the peaches to cool. Carefully peel the peaches, revealing their beautiful, soft, velvet flesh. They can be left whole, halved or cut into slim wedges.

5 Mix the yoghurt and ground almonds until thoroughly blended. Serve with the prepared peaches, a sprinkling of toasted almonds and the honey drizzled over.

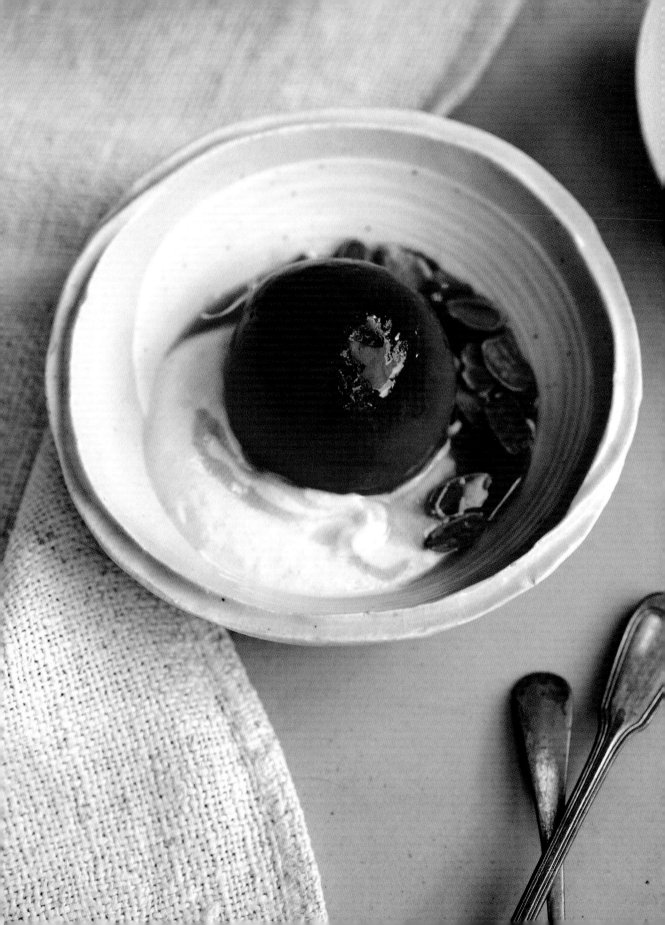

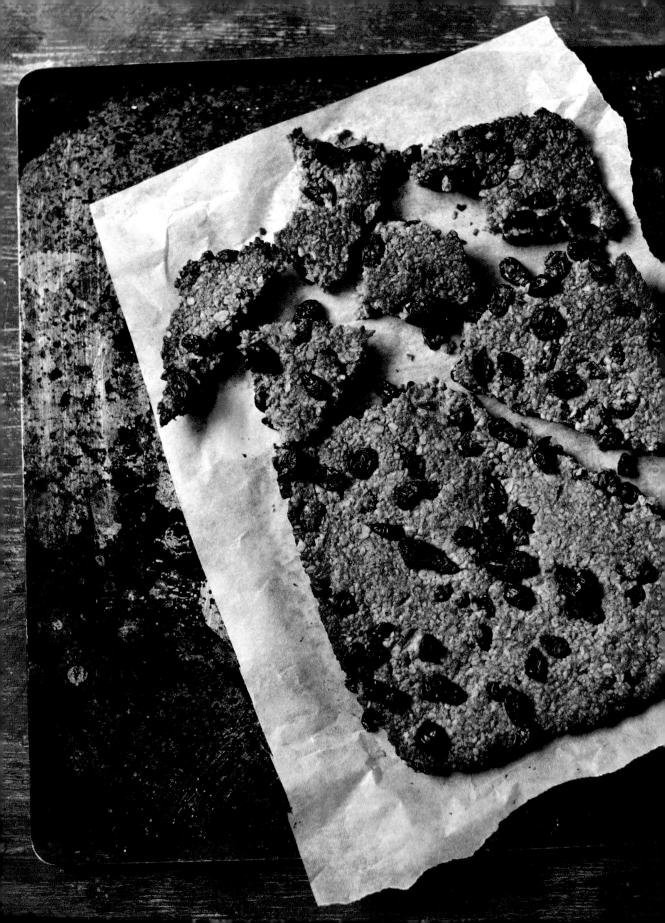

Oats and Dried Berry Bars

Makes 1 tray

Takes 45 minutes

150g oats

100g Brazil nuts

75g coconut oil

50g honey, raw or locally
   produced

100g dried berries –
   blueberries, cherries

1 egg

Enjoy these biscuits when you want something in your diet that's sweet but free from refined sugars.

1 Pre-heat the oven to 160°C, gas mark 3. Line a 28 x 18cm baking tray with baking parchment.

2 Place the oats and Brazil nuts in a food processor and blitz until roughly ground.

3 Gently heat the coconut oil and honey, then remove from the heat and blend in the ground oats and nuts, the berries and egg. Mix together well, then transfer to the prepared tray, spreading it evenly and scattering with a few extra berries if desired.

4 Place in the oven and cook for 20 minutes. Leave to cool in the tray before cutting or breaking into pieces.

Chocolate Walnut Brownies

Makes 1 tray (approx. 16 brownies)

Takes 45 minutes

150g butter

200g dark chocolate (at least 75% plus)

100g molasses

3 eggs

100g desiccated coconut, or coconut flour

1 tsp baking powder

110g walnuts, chopped, or other favourite nut

Everyone deserves a tasty, indulgent treat now and then, and small amounts of good-quality dark chocolate (85 per cent cocoa solids) is actually beneficial as it contains polyphenols (plant chemicals, which have been shown to kill cancer cells in labs).

Using coconut flour makes this a gluten-free recipe and therefore even healthier. Indulge, but in the knowledge that this comfort food is doing you good.

1 Pre-heat the oven to 180°C, gas mark 4. Line a 28 x 18cm baking tray with baking parchment.

2 Melt the butter in a saucepan, break the chocolate into pieces, add to the warm butter and mix on a very low heat until melted.

3 Add the molasses, mix and gently warm to loosen. Remove from the heat and allow to cool for 5 minutes.

4 Beat the eggs and quickly blend them into the chocolate mix along with the desiccated coconut or coconut flour, baking powder and nuts. Ensure that all the ingredients are folded in well before transferring the mixture to the lined baking tray. Place in the oven and cook for 20 minutes.

5 Allow the brownies to cool for about 10 minutes before cutting into 16 equal pieces. Enjoy with ice cream, dairy cream or a non-dairy option of your choice.

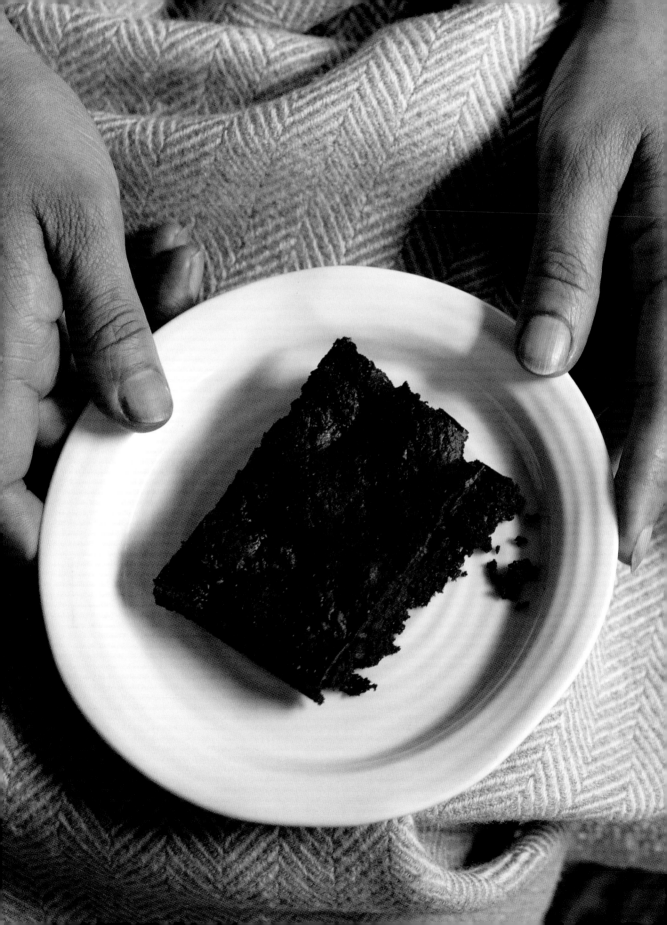

Banana and Date Loaf Cake

Makes 1 loaf

Takes 1 hour, plus overnight soaking

200g dates

2–3 ripe bananas

3 eggs, beaten

100g butter, melted

150g cornmeal, fine

1½ tsp baking powder (gluten-free)

This flour- and sugar-free cake is practically guilt-free too, but it's still packed with nutritious bananas and dates, making it a tasty sweet treat for anyone who wants to avoid gluten and refined sugar.

Bananas are one of the most widely consumed fruits in the world and are a great source of magnesium and potassium; they are thought to be a good-mood food too.

The soaked dates are not only easy to digest and high in fibre, but they are also a good source of vitamins A and K. This is an excellent nutritional snack – particularly if you are looking to add calories to your diet.

1 Place the dates in a bowl and just cover with boiling water, then leave to soak overnight.

2 Next day, pre-heat the oven to 180°C, gas mark 4 and line a 500g loaf tin with baking parchment. Place the dates and any excess soaking liquid, the bananas and eggs in a food processor or blender and blitz until smooth.

3 Melt the butter, add to the banana mix along with the cornmeal and fold in until evenly blended.

4 Mix the baking powder with a couple of tablespoons of water and add to the cake mix. Stir through until blended, pour into the prepared cake tin and bake for 50 minutes. To test if the cake is cooked, insert a knife into the centre. It should come out clean; if not, return to the oven for a little longer and re-test.

5 Remove from the oven when cooked through, leave to cool for 10 minutes in the tin, then turn out and cool on a wire rack. Once cool, if you are not eating immediately, wrap in foil or greaseproof paper and store in an airtight container.

Energy Bombs

Makes 20

Takes 30 minutes

150g dates, stoned

1 tbsp sunflower seeds

100g ground almonds

1 tbsp raw cacao

1 tbsp tahini

½ tsp cinnamon

30g desiccated coconut

These are super-healthy truffles that can be enjoyed at the end of a meal; they also make great snacks to have with you on days when you are away from home and want a little treat to get you through the day. These small but efficient power balls of energy are easily digested and absorbed into the body. You can adapt them by swapping the dates for prunes, apricots or raisins and changing the ground almonds for another favourite ground nut if you prefer.

The coconut added at the end gives these truffles a pretty coated finish. A word of warning: these balls may be small but they are very rich and it's much better to eat two dainty little bombs than one or two large ones!

1 Place the dates and sunflower seeds in a food processor and blend until smooth.

2 Add the ground almonds, raw cacao, tahini and cinnamon. Blend until smooth.

3 Divide the mixture into 20 equal-sized pieces and roll into small balls.

4 Place the coconut on a plate, slightly dampen each ball under a running tap and roll them in the coconut so that they are evenly coated. Store in an airtight container in the fridge until needed.

Mixed Fruit, Seed and Nut Cake

Makes 1 cake

Takes 2 hours, plus overnight soaking

50g sultanas

50g pitted prunes

50g figs

50g dried cranberries

50g dried apricots

50g dates

50g pumpkin seeds

50g sunflower seeds

50g sesame seeds

1 teabag of your choice, plus water to cover fruit

100g molasses

50ml olive oil

50g Brazil nuts, chopped

50g ground almonds

50g walnuts, chopped

25g coconut flakes, or desiccated coconut

100g gram flour

1 tsp nutmeg, grated or ground

1 tsp mixed spice

2 eggs

This cake is another of the Nutritional Kitchen's flour- and refined-sugar-free recipes. It's a healthy option because it is packed with a variety of fruits, seeds and nuts and has a rich, dense texture. It will improve with age, so make it in advance, wrap it in foil or greaseproof paper and keep it in an airtight container.

Just a small slice with a cup of tea is all you need, especially on days when you're receiving treatment and want something tasty, healthy and uplifting. As long as the total weight of dried fruit is 300g, you can adjust the selection to include your favourites.

1 Place the sultanas, prunes, figs, cranberries, apricots and dates, the pumpkin, sunflower and sesame seeds in a bowl with the teabag and molasses. Cover with boiling water, mix well and leave to soak overnight.

2 Next day, pre-heat the oven to 180°C, gas mark 4 and line a 20cm-deep push-up-bottom cake tin with baking parchment.

3 Remove the teabag and discard. Add the olive oil, Brazil nuts, ground almonds, walnuts, coconut, gram flour, nutmeg, mixed spice and eggs. Mix well until evenly blended.

4 Place the cake tin in the middle of the oven and bake for 2 hours, checking and turning occasionally to ensure an even bake. To test if cooked, insert a knife into the centre and it should come out clean. If it isn't quite cooked, bake for a further 5–10 minutes, then turn out the cake and cool on a wire rack.

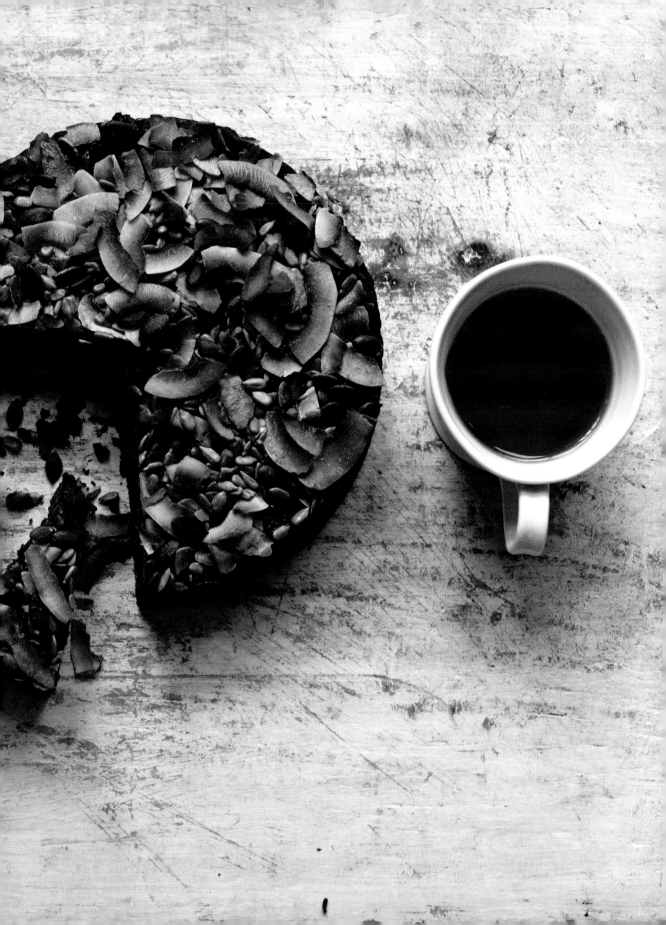

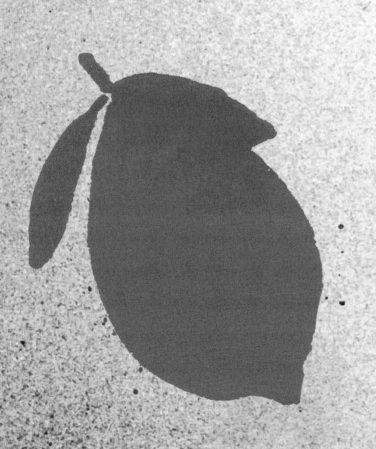

Super Staples

Seeded Spelt Soda Loaf

Makes 1 loaf

Takes 1 hour

300ml whole milk

1 tbsp freshly squeezed
   lemon juice

450g spelt flour

50g sunflower seeds

50g pumpkin seeds

2 tsp bicarbonate of
   soda

a pinch of salt

This golden loaf is bursting with goodness. Spelt is ancient wheat grain but, unlike modern hybridized wheat, it has a lower, more fragile gluten content that is far more easily broken down and digested by the body. It's thought that as much as 80 per cent of the population has a problem digesting gluten, so if you sometimes feel bloated after eating normal wheat, do give spelt a try. The use of bicarbonate of soda as a raising agent can give the body a nudge towards a more alkaline state (see pages 87–8). An increase in the intake of these foods, however small, can have a positive impact on the body.

1 Pre-heat the oven to 200°C, gas mark 6.

2 Measure the milk into a jug, add the lemon juice and mix. Leave for 5–10 minutes, after which time you will find that it will split and become ready for use.

3 Place the spelt flour, sunflower and pumpkin seeds, bicarbonate of soda, salt, milk and 50ml water in a large bowl and mix together by hand until evenly blended.

4 Dust the kitchen worktop with a little spelt and knead the dough for 3 minutes.

5 You can shape the dough into a ball or loaf. For a ball, place on a spelt-dusted baking sheet and make a cross on the top with a sharp knife; for a loaf, use a 500g loaf tin brushed with melted coconut oil and scatter the sides of the tin with the sesame seeds. Shape the loaf to fit the tin and transfer to the oven.

6 Bake in the middle of the oven for 40 minutes. Check if the bread is cooked through by tapping the base – it should sound hollow.

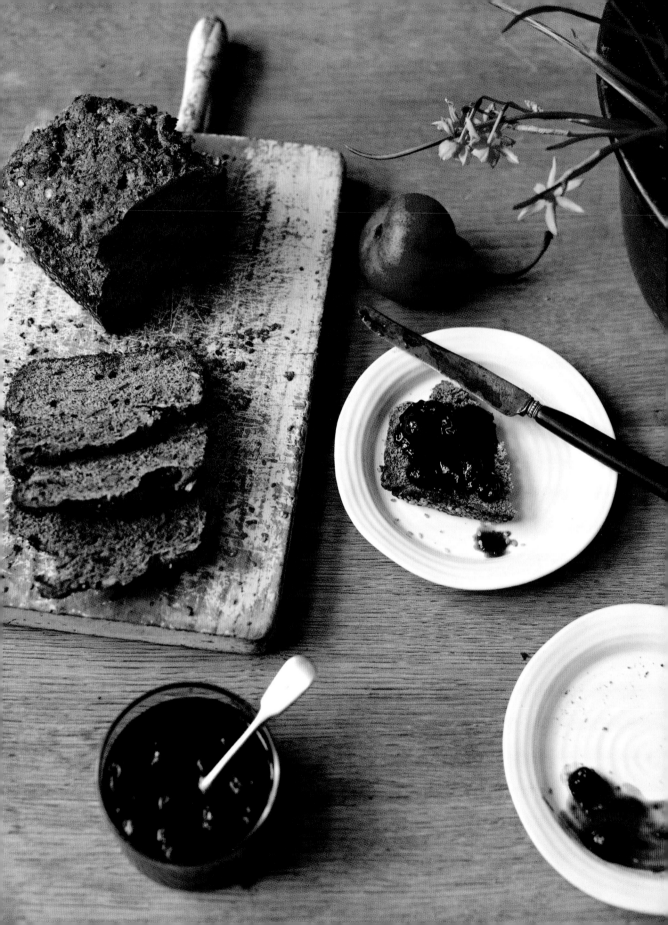

Sauerkraut

Makes 1 jar

Takes 40 minutes,
plus up to 7 days
to ferment

½ red or white cabbage

1 tbsp sea salt

1 tsp mustard seeds

1 tsp caraway seeds

Sauerkraut is a neglected accompaniment in the UK, but the health benefits are multiple. Fermented foods such as this give a great boost to the colony of microbiota that live in the gut, aiding not only digestion but the immune system too.

You can make this with red or white cabbage; I like the rich, deep colour of red, but it tastes just the same as white. Serve with simply grilled or roasted meats, or it's really delicious added to an open sandwich made with something wholesome, like the Seeded Spelt Soda Loaf (see page 250), and topped with cheese.

1 Trim the cabbage base and peel away the outside leaves, reserving one.

2 Cut the cabbage into quarters and remove the hard central core. Slice very finely by hand, in a food processor or on a mandolin. Place in a bowl, add the salt, mustard and caraway seeds and mix with a wooden spoon, or massage the cabbage by hand for 5 minutes until it softens to become moist, naturally producing salted juices. (This may sound odd, but the salt and the mixing action tenderize the cabbage.)

3 Transfer the cabbage and its juices to a sterilized jar (a dishwasher hot-wash is the easiest way of sterilizing) and pack down firmly. Place the reserved leaf on top, wedge it in and weight it down with a small jar that has also been sterilized. You want to ensure that all the cabbage is submerged in the natural salted juices. (Add a small amount of water if needed.) Leave at room temperature for up to 7 days, mixing each day, then replacing the leaf and submerging the mixture as above. This timing varies according to the ambient temperature – the warmer your kitchen, the faster it will start to ferment.

4 When small bubbles start to rise in the jar it is then ready to store in the fridge. It will keep for 6 weeks. We like to serve it as a side pickle so that it is eaten in small amounts and regularly to constantly help the gut.

Kim-chi

Makes 1 jar

Takes 40 minutes, plus up to 7 days to ferment

1 head Chinese leaf, finely sliced

6 cloves garlic, grated

5cm knob fresh ginger, grated

1 mooli, or 8 red radishes, finely sliced

½ onion, finely sliced

1–2 red chillis, finely sliced

1 tbsp sea salt

1 tsp fish sauce

Originating from Korea and served with all meals as a healthy side dish and pep-up condiment, this hot and vibrant pickle can be adjusted to suit your edible thermometer! As with Sauerkraut (opposite), the beneficial microflora that are produced during the fermentation process will aid digestion. Enjoy Kim-chi as you would Sauerkraut, and you can also serve it with Asian meals as a delicious pickle that adds extra punch.

1 Keep one complete leaf from the outside of the Chinese leaf and very finely slice the rest by hand, or with a mandolin, into a bowl.

2 Finely slice the garlic, ginger, mooli/radish, onion and chillis, mix well, then add the sea salt and fish sauce. Mix with a wooden spoon or by hand for about 5 minutes, or until the vegetables soften and it produces natural salty juices.

3 Transfer to a sterilized jar (a dishwasher hot-wash is the easiest way of sterilizing) and pack down firmly. Place the reserved leaf on top and then wedge it in and weight it down with a small jar that has also been sterilized. You want to ensure that all the cabbage is submerged in the natural salty juices. (Add a little water if needed.)

4 Leave at room temperature for up to 7 days; this varies according to the ambient temperature – the warmer your kitchen, the faster it will ferment.

5 When small bubbles start to rise, it is ready to store in the fridge. It will keep for 6 weeks.

Fruit and Turmeric Chutney

Makes 1 kg

Takes 50 minutes

1 tsp coconut oil

½ red onion, chopped

2 cloves garlic, crushed, peeled and chopped

½ red chilli, diced

4cm knob grated fresh turmeric, or 2 tsp ground

4cm knob fresh ginger, grated

2 apples

2 pears

1 lemon, zested and juiced

1 tsp cider vinegar

2 cloves

1 piece cinnamon bark

sea salt and freshly ground black pepper

The food scientists are in agreement that turmeric is *the* anti-cancer spice due to its anti-inflammatory properties. Fresh root turmeric is more widely available in supermarkets these days; it looks similar to ginger but the cut flesh is bright orange. It should be finely grated before adding to dishes – use gloves when you handle it or you will end up with Day-Glo fingers! If you can't find fresh turmeric, ground is good too.

If you really love your chutney and don't want to eat too much sugar, you can enjoy this subtle fruit and spice version *without* the addition of sugar. It makes a jar packed with anti-inflammatory goodness. It's also very versatile and goes well with most meals – hot or cold.

1 Heat the oil in a large shallow pan and gently cook the onions, garlic, chilli, turmeric and ginger for 5 minutes.

2 Peel and core the apples and pears, then chop into even-sized pieces. Add to the pan along with the lemon zest and juice, cider vinegar, cloves, cinnamon bark and seasoning. Mix well, add 50ml water and simmer gently for 25 minutes, stirring gently.

3 Transfer into sterilized jam jars or other glass containers (putting them through a hot-wash cycle in the dishwasher is the easiest way to sterilize them), leave to cool, then store in the fridge, where it will keep for up to 1 week.

10-Vegetable Tomato Sauce, Smooth or Coarse

Makes 1 litre

Takes 1 hour

1 tbsp coconut oil

1 onion, diced

1 clove garlic, crushed, peeled and chopped

1 leek, diced

1 carrot, diced

1 courgette, diced

50g mushrooms, diced

1 stick celery, diced

1 red pepper, diced

1 red chilli (optional)

1 x 400g carton tomatoes, chopped

500ml vegetable stock or water

sea salt and freshly ground black pepper

100g spinach, chopped

A very versatile, super-healthy sauce that can be made in advance and frozen in small pots to use when you may not feel up to cooking. Use as a sauce, or to enrich other dishes such as soups, casseroles, pasta, risotto, baked vegetables, etc. Remember, we love it when you are able to eat a rainbow of vegetables at any one meal and there is certainly a colourful selection here!

1 Heat the oil in a large saucepan and cook the onion for 5 minutes on a medium heat but do not brown.

2 Add the garlic, leek, carrot, courgette, mushrooms, celery, pepper and chilli, if using. Mix well and cook for 10 minutes or until soft, stirring frequently.

3 Pour in the tomatoes and stock or water, bring to the boil and simmer for 35 minutes.

4 Season, then add the chopped spinach. Cook for a further 5 minutes.

5 If you like a textured sauce, leave it as it is; if you prefer a smoother sauce, whizz it through a blender until you reach the right consistency.

Super Stocks

Makes approximately 2 litres

Takes 12 hours for beef or lamb, 6 hours for chicken, 30 minutes for fish, 1½ hours for vegetable

2kg bones – beef, lamb, chicken, fish – or this weight in vegetables

2 bay leaves

1 onion, chopped

1 leek, sliced

1 carrot, sliced

1 stick celery, sliced

1 tsp black peppercorns

juice of ½ lemon

Nutritious and flavoursome, all savvy cooks need a good stock. Although readily available in shops and supermarkets, if you have the time there's nothing quite like homemade stock and the nutritional benefits are abundant.

This recipe forms a basis for all stocks, with the addition of roasting meat for brown stocks. Do not mix species of bones when making stock, as it will deliver a confusing result. The slow cooking of bones ensures that all the nutritious elements are extracted, making a super-healthy, restorative liquid. It is great for healing the gut and so is particularly beneficial if consumed in soups or drunk as a warming broth during treatment.

....

1 If making a beef or lamb stock, you should aim for a rich brown colour. To achieve this, heat the oven to 180°C, gas mark 4, place all the bones and vegetables in a large roasting pan and roast for 1 hour or until golden brown, then continue as below.

2 For all stocks, place all the ingredients in a large pan, cover with water and bring to the boil, then reduce the heat and simmer: beef/lamb 12 hours, chicken 6 hours, vegetable 1½ hours, fish 30 minutes.

3 When cooked, carefully strain off the stock and discard the bones/vegetables. Pass the stock through a fine sieve/chinois, or a sieve lined with muslin.

4 Use fresh, or place into containers and freeze until needed.

goodness

nutritious

depth

flavour

tasty

Ground Mixed-seed Boost Powder

Makes 80g

Takes 5 minutes

1 tbsp sesame seeds

1 tbsp pumpkin seeds

1 tbsp sunflower seeds

1 tbsp flaxseeds
(linseeds)

1 tbsp hemp seeds

Seeds have a highly concentrated supply of nutrients because these are needed to help them grow. Therefore eating seeds frequently can give your nutrient levels an extra boost.

This is best used when fresh because grinding seeds exposes their high levels of fats to the air, causing them to become rancid fairly quickly. We recommend keeping this for a maximum of 3 days in an airtight container in the fridge. Sprinkle on porridge, salads, soups, casseroles and smoothies, or add to soups, casseroles and pasta sauces to enrich and thicken them and give them an amazing creamy texture.

1 Place a mixture of your chosen seeds in a blender and blitz until evenly chopped. The more you blitz, the finer the seeds will become, making them great for adding to soups and casseroles. A coarser chop may be preferred for salads.

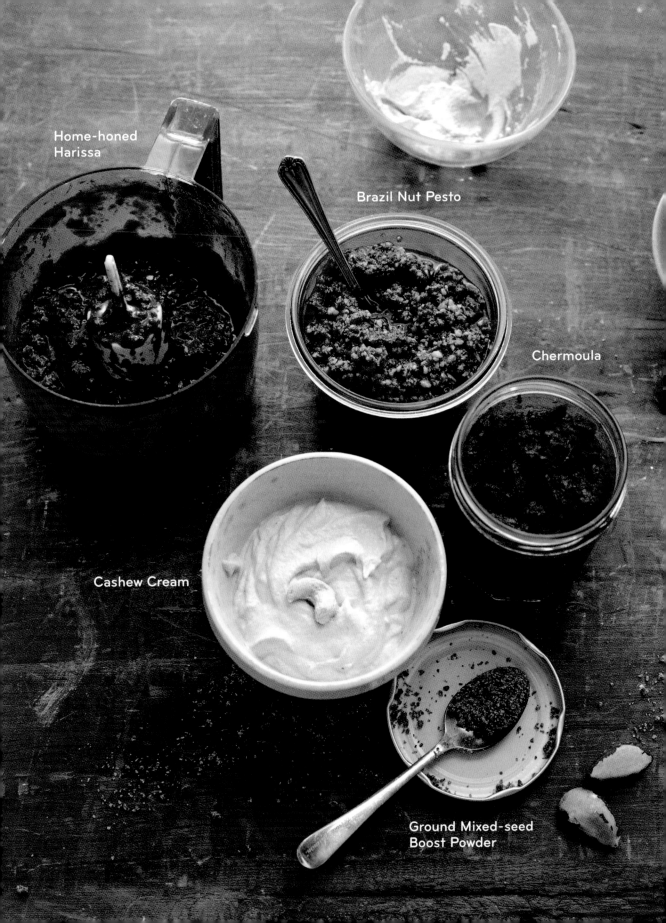

Home-honed
Harissa

Brazil Nut Pesto

Chermoula

Cashew Cream

Ground Mixed-seed
Boost Powder

Chermoula

Makes 150g

Takes 20 minutes

2 cloves garlic, peeled

2 green chilli

2cm knob fresh ginger, peeled

a large bunch of coriander, roughly chopped

1 tbsp smoked paprika, ground

1 tsp cumin, ground

1 tsp coriander, ground

1 tsp grated fresh turmeric, or use ground

a pinch of saffron threads (optional)

juice of 1 lemon

100ml olive oil

sea salt and freshly ground black pepper

This is a tasty green sauce from north Africa, where it is used to marinate meat, fish and vegetables, but we like it served as a relish with baked vegetables, oily fish, chicken or meat. Just a simple accompaniment like this can add an array of extra nutrients and anti-inflammatory compounds to a dish. It will keep in the fridge in a lidded jar or airtight container for 2 weeks.

1 Place all the ingredients in a blender and blitz until you have a rough paste. Put in a lidded jar or airtight container and store in the fridge until needed.

Brazil Nut Pesto

Makes 250g

Takes 25 minutes

40g Brazil nuts

40g basil

40g Parmesan

4 cloves garlic, crushed
   and peeled

100ml olive oil

juice of ½ lemon

freshly ground black
   pepper

A couple of Brazil nuts a day is all you need to top up your anti-cancer selenium levels – important in the UK where we tend to be deficient in this mineral.

This pesto is a great, nutritious addition to many savoury dishes. Serve with a simple grilled fish, poached chicken, baked sweet potato, or you can thin it down with olive oil and add to salad dressing.

1 Place all the ingredients in a food processor and blitz until smooth. Alternatively, you can make a rough pesto by chopping all the ingredients by hand.

2 Place in a lidded jar or airtight container and store in the fridge until needed.

Cashew Cream

Makes 1 x 200g jar

Takes 30 minutes

100g plain cashew nuts

100ml warm water

a pinch of salt

This is the one recipe that all the Maggie's nurses at Charing Cross Hospital said *must* be included in this cookbook! When eating is difficult, this cream can be spooned into soups or casseroles, adding not only a lovely creamy texture to the dish but healthy fatty acids, protein and important minerals. You can replace the cashews with other raw or unprocessed nuts, such as Brazil nuts or almonds, to create your very own favourite nut cream.

1 Place the cashews and warm water in a blender, leave for 30 minutes to soften and then blend rapidly until you achieve a smooth, creamy consistency. Add a little extra water for a thinner cream.

2 Always store in an airtight container in the fridge, where it will keep for up to 5 days.

Home-honed Harissa

Makes 250g

Takes 25 minutes

1 red pepper

1 tbsp coriander seeds, or ground

2 tbsp caraway seeds, or ground

1 tbsp cumin seeds, or ground

4 cloves garlic, crushed, peeled and chopped

3 red chillies, with seeds

1 tsp tomato purée

200ml olive oil

sea salt and freshly ground black pepper

I call this 'home-honed' as you can adjust the spice and heat to your particular liking. Use this to add to the Butternut and Sweet Potato Tagine (page 185), as a side sauce with some simple grilled fish, or thin it down with a little olive oil and add to a dressing to increase complexity and flavour. Try it also with courgette spaghetti for a very simple, tasty light lunch.

1 Grill the pepper until the skin blisters and is blackened all over, taking care not to burn it too much.

2 Place it in a bowl and cover with cling film to capture the heat and enable it to continue cooking. When cool, peel the skin off, remove the core and stem and chop.

3 Place in a food processor and, if using seeds, toast them in a frying pan gently, grind them and then add to the red peppers, along with the garlic, red chillies, tomato purée, olive oil and seasoning.

4 Blitz according to your preference, rough or smooth, place in a sealed jar or airtight container and store in the fridge until needed (it will keep for up to 2 weeks).

Grape and Blueberry Spread

Makes 500g

Takes 20 minutes, plus
1 hour cooling/setting

250g seedless red
  grapes

a small sprig of rosemary,
  finely chopped (optional)

250g blueberries

1 tbsp chia seeds

It's beneficial to eat these fruits frequently as they are rich in anthocyanidins, which come from the blue and red colour in the blueberries and grapes and contain amazing antioxidant properties. This delicious spread works a treat to replace sugar-laden jam; it contains enough natural sugars to make it sweet without the need for added refined ones. Enjoy it as a spread or spooned on to porridge, bio-yoghurt or ice cream.

1 Place the grapes and rosemary (if using) in a small pan and add a few drops of water. Stirring frequently, heat through and then reduce to a gentle simmer until the grapes have broken down. This will take approximately 12 minutes.

2 Add the blueberries and cook for a further 3 minutes, or until the berries have collapsed.

3 Check the consistency, and continue to cook until excess liquid has evaporated and you have a rich 'jammy' consistency.

4 Add the chia seeds, stir through and leave to cool. They will swell and thicken the mixture, making this into our super-healthy jam.

5 Store in the fridge in an airtight container; it will keep for up to a week. Alternatively, divide into smaller portions and freeze.

Almond Milk

Makes 300ml

Takes 30 minutes, plus overnight soaking

100g almonds

300ml water

This is an unbelievably easy, healthy and natural alternative to dairy and has none of the additives of shop-bought almond milk.

Try this method using other nuts, seeds, grains such as oats or hemp seeds to suit your own dietary requirements and likes. You could also try warming through with a pinch of turmeric, black pepper and cinnamon for a calming, restorative drink.

1 Soak the almonds in water overnight.

2 Next day, transfer the almonds and their soaking liquid to a blender and blitz repeatedly until broken down and milky white in colour.

3 Line a sieve with muslin and place it over a bowl/jug. Pour the blended almond mix in and allow it to pass through.

4 When all the milk has passed, draw the corners of the muslin together and twist to extract all the milk.

5 Store in the fridge and use within 2 days.

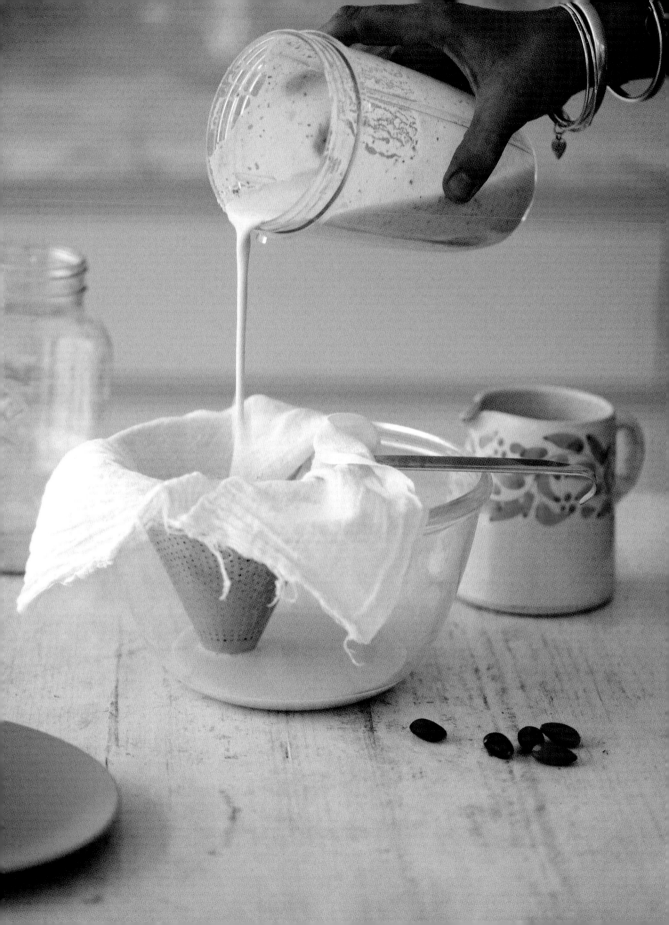

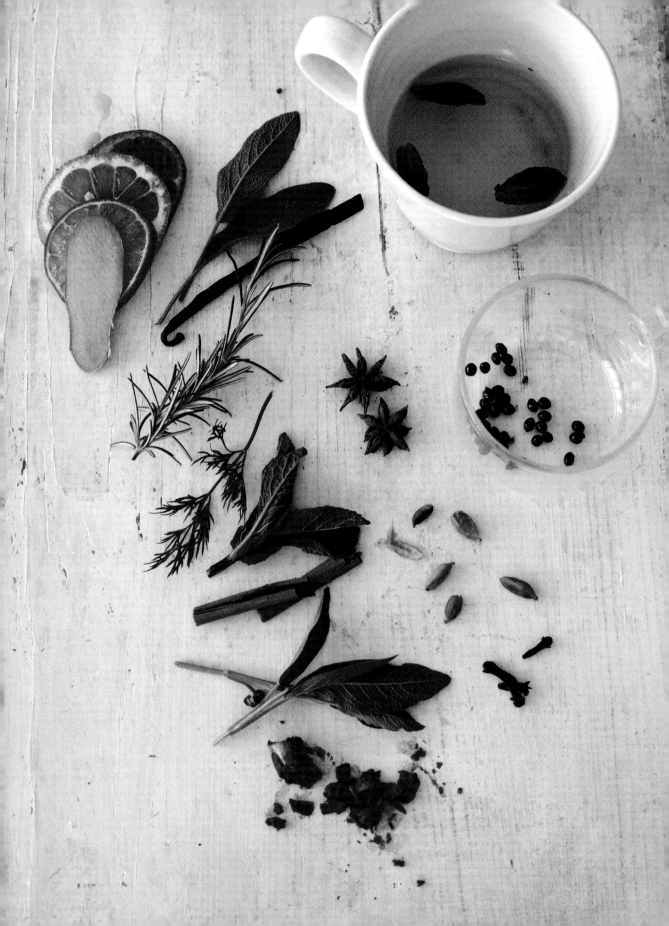

Homemade Teas and Infusions

Serves 2

Takes 5 minutes

1 tbsp mint leaves

1 tbsp lemon verbena
   leaves

½ tbsp sage leaves

2 sprigs rosemary

½ tbsp fresh ginger,
   grated or sliced

1 tsp turmeric root,
   grated or sliced

1 tbsp citrus fruits, sliced

1–2 star anise

1 stick cinnamon bark

2–3 cloves

3 crushed cardamom
   pods

1 stick licorice root

½ stick vanilla pod

1 stick chopped
   lemongrass

raw or locally produced
   honey

Quick, easy and nutritious, you can drink these either hot or chilled. They are made from fresh, natural ingredients and are good for their restorative and refreshing taste as well as for giving you a reason to sit down, relax and increase your liquid uptake.

Choose any of the ingredients listed that suits your tastebuds.

1 Place your chosen infusion in a heatproof glass or mug, pour on boiling water, cover the receptacle and leave to infuse for 5–10 minutes.

2 In summer, make a stronger infusion and allow to cool, then serve with ice cubes.

Miso Soup

Serves 2

Takes 15 minutes

400ml of your favourite fresh stock – see page 256

2 tbsp miso paste

1 tbsp seaweed flakes

100g firm tofu

2 spring onions

1 tsp sesame seeds, ground

A great staple to use on days when you are not feeling up to eating a full meal or a hearty soup. It is highly nutritious due to the fresh stock, miso paste, seaweed and tofu, all of which are easily and quickly digested. This is a good soup for putting into a flask and taking with you to enjoy when you're away from home and need to keep your food intake up, or if feeling weak or nauseous. Just try taking small sips every 20 minutes or so; it's amazing how much you will consume without realizing. It's very important to keep up your food intake during difficult times, so just try to think small and frequent.

Miso is produced by fermenting soy, rice, barley, hemp or buckwheat with salt and the fungus aspergillus oryzae; the different types of miso are made from individual grains or a combination. This creates a thick paste that can be used for soups or sauces. Think Oriental Marmite. This fermented food adds microbiota in our gut, which have so many disease-prevention properties. The seaweed will provide iodine for thyroid health.

1 Heat the stock and boil for 1 minute. Remove from the heat, add the miso paste and seaweed, then stir until the miso has dissolved.

2 Return the pan to a low heat; do not boil as it changes the flavour.

3 Cut the tofu into cubes, slice the spring onions and add to the soup. Heat gently for 1 minute.

4 Spoon into bowls and sprinkle with sesame seeds.

Quick Cupboard Salad (Pulses, Nuts and Avocado)

Serves 2

Takes 10 minutes

200g cooked chickpeas or other beans (kidney, butter, black, haricot, etc.)

60g pistachios, hazelnuts or cashews

75g basil, parsley, rocket or spinach

2 tbsp olive oil

juice of ½ lemon

sea salt and freshly ground black pepper

1 ripe Hass avocado

2 tsp Ground Mixed-seed Boost Powder (see page 258) or a sprinkling of your favourite seeds

It is possible to make this quick salad out of a reasonably stocked kitchen, using pre-cooked or soaked pulses, nibbling nuts and sprinkling seeds, a cluster of soft green leaves or herbs from the fridge and an avocado. Whenever I go shopping I buy a good avocado, as it will make the basis of a healthy meal, be it on toast with tomatoes and a poached egg or as here.

Nutritionally, this dish contains proteins in the pulses and vitamins in the green herbs or leaves, the avocados are rich in healthy fats and antioxidants, and the seeds contain healthy oils and minerals. It works as a side dish or on its own when your appetite is not so needy.

1 Drain the beans and place in a bowl.

2 Roughly chop the nuts and herb or salad leaves and add to the beans.

3 Add the olive oil, lemon juice and seasoning and toss. Divide the salad between two bowls.

4 When you are ready to eat, cut the avocado in half, remove the stone, and peel and slice the flesh. Place on top of the beans and sprinkle each with a teaspoon of the ground or whole seeds.

Food Diary

When attempting to make changes to your diet a food diary can be a very useful tool. It gives a good overview of how you are doing and you can clearly assess the balance of your diet – do you have a sufficient intake of vegetables and fruit, an adequate supply of healthy fats and protein, or are you overdosing on starchy carbohydrates and sugar? Always be honest when recording your intake and complete the diary throughout the day as later on it is easy to forget what you ate earlier.

This version has a column for recording symptoms and emotions that could be related to food intake. This can be invaluable if you suspect you have any intolerances or blood-sugar control issues. If you keep a food diary for at least two to three weeks, a pattern of symptoms may emerge which flags up potential problematic foods, especially those related to gut issues such as excessive wind and bloating.

Use goal-setting to help you change unhealthy habits to healthy ones over a period of time.

Date	Goal for the day *				
	Example: 'I will swap my sweet biscuit with my morning tea for a healthy seeded cracker.' Make this your goal until you have succeeded in changing your sweet-biscuit habit!				

	Foods eaten	Serving size	Time	Drinks (water/tea/ coffee,etc.)	How you feel (emotions/ symptoms)
Breakfast					
Lunch					
Dinner					
Snacks					

Glossary

Adjuvant therapy
Additional therapy given after primary treatment to lower the risk of the cancer coming back.

Angiogenesis
The development of new blood vessels.

Antibodies
Specialized cells of the immune system which can recognize organisms – such as bacteria, viruses and fungi – that invade the body.

Antioxidant
A substance that inhibits *oxidation*.

Apoptosis
The death of cells which occurs as a normal and controlled part of an organism's growth or development.

Autophagy
The cleaning-up process within cells through the digestion of damaged or dysfunctional cellular components by enzymes within that cell.

Benign
A *tumour* that does not have the ability to migrate away from the site of origin.

Bioavailability
The extent to which a substance is absorbed and reaches the circulation intact.

Cachexia
Weakness and wasting of the body due to chronic illness.

CAM
Complementary and alternative medicine.

Carcinogenic
Any substance or agent that tends to produce cancer.

Carminative
A herb which prevents the formation of gas in the gastrointestinal tract, or helps with its expulsion.

Compounds
Something that is composed of two or more separate elements.

Cytokines
Chemicals such as interferon, interleukin and growth factors which are secreted and have an effect on other cells.

Detoxification
The process of removing toxic substances.

Differentiation
The specialization of cells. In cancer it describes how much or how little *tumour* tissue resembles the normal tissue from which it came.

Epigenetics
The study of changes in organisms caused by the modification of *gene expression* by external or environmental factors rather than the alteration of the genetic code itself.

Free radical
An atom or group of atoms which has at least one unpaired electron, making it unstable and highly reactive.

Gene expression
The process by which the information contained within a gene becomes a product.

Glycaemic index
A figure representing the relative ability of a carbohydrate food to increase the level of glucose in the blood.

Gut flora
The bacteria living within the gut.

Hormone
A regulatory substance produced in an organism and transported in tissue fluids, such as blood, to stimulate specific cells or tissues into action.

Hypoxia
Lack of oxygen.

Integrative oncology
The combination of conventional cancer treatment with complementary and alternative therapies.

Ketones
Chemicals that are produced by the liver from fatty acids during periods of low food intake (fasting), or carbohydrate restriction, for cells to use as energy instead of glucose.

Ketosis
A metabolic state where most of the body's energy supply comes from *ketones* in the blood.

Malignant
Cancer that has the ability to spread from the primary site to secondary sites.

Metastasis
The development of secondary *malignant* growths at a distance from the primary site.

Microbiome
The collection of the genes of the microbes within the human body.

Microbiota
A collection of microbes (gut bacteria).

Mitochondria
An organelle found in large numbers in most cells, in which the biochemical processes of *respiration* and energy production occur.

Mucositis
Inflammation and ulceration of the mucous membranes lining the digestive tract.

Mutation
A permanent change to a DNA sequence as a result of DNA copying mistakes made during cell division.

Necrosis
Death of cells through injury or disease.

Neurotransmitter
A chemical released from the end of a nerve fibre by the arrival of a nerve impulse, which then causes the impulse to spread.

Neutropenia
The presence of abnormally few neutrophils (a type of white blood cell) in the blood, leading to increased susceptibility to infection.

Nutraceutical
A food or part of a food which may provide medicinal or health benefits.

Oncogene
A gene which has the potential to cause cancer.

Oxidation
A chemical reaction that involves the loss of electrons, as when a material combines with oxygen.

Peripheral neuropathy
Damage to those nerves outside the central nervous system which causes pain, tingling or burning, usually to the extremities of the body.

Polyphenols
Abundant micronutrients in plants which are generally involved in the plants' defence mechanism against ultraviolet radiation or pests.

Prebiotics
Promoting the growth of beneficial *microbiota* in the intestines.

Probiotics
Micro-organisms that are believed to exert health benefits when consumed.

Protocol
A set of detailed instructions to guide the care of a patient.

Receptor
A structure on the surface of a cell that selectively receives and binds a specific substance.

Respiration
The process within cells of oxidizing food molecules, like glucose, to carbon dioxide and water to create energy.

Stem cells
A master cell within the body which has the ability to grow into any cell type.

Stoma
An opening, either natural or surgically created, which connects a portion of the body cavity to the outside environment.

Systemic
Relating to, or affecting, the entire body.

Tumour
A lump formed from cancer cells.

Tumour-suppressor gene
A gene that protects a cell from becoming cancerous.

Vascular endothelial growth factor (VEGF)
A signalling protein that promotes the growth of *angiogenesis*.

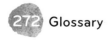

Bibliography

Introduction: Becoming an Active Partner

Turner, Dr Kelly A., *Radical Remission: Surviving Cancer Against All Odds – the Nine Key Factors that Can Make a Real Difference*, HarperCollins, London, 2014

1 Why Food Matters

Anand, P., *et al.*, 'Cancer is a Preventable Disease That Requires Major Lifestyle Changes', *Pharmaceutical Research*, Vol. 25, No. 9, 2008: 2097–116

Goldacre, B., and Heneghan, C., 'How Medicine Is Broken, and How We Can Fix It', *British Medical Journal*, 350, 23 June 2015: h3397

Heaney, R. P., 'Nutrients, Endpoints, and the Problem of Proof', *The Journal of Nutrition*, 138(9), 2008: 1591–5

Parkin, D. M., and Boyd, L., 'Cancers Attributable to Overweight and Obesity in the UK in 2010', *British Journal of Cancer*, 105 Suppl. (S2), 2011: S34–7

Vrieling, A., *et al.*, 'Dietary Patterns and Survival in German Postmenopausal Breast Cancer Survivors', *British Journal of Cancer*, 108(1), 2013: 188–92

Wicki, A., and Hagmann, J., 'Diet and Cancer', *Swiss Medical Weekly*, 141, September 2011: p.w. 13250

World Cancer Research Fund/American Institute for Cancer Research, *Food, Nutrition, Physical Activity, and the Prevention of Cancer: A Global Perspective*, AICR, Washington, DC, 2007

2 The Science Behind Cancer

Ahmad, A. S., Ormiston-Smith, N., Sasieni, P. D., 'Trends in the Lifetime Risk of Developing Cancer in Great Britain: Comparison of Risk for Those Born from 1930 to 1960', *British Journal of Cancer*, 112, 2015: 943–7

Arends, J., 'Metabolism in Cancer Patients', *Anticancer Research*, 30(5), 2010: 1863–8

Baker, S. G., 'Recognizing Paradigm Instability in Theories of Carcinogenesis', *British Journal of Medicine and Medical Research*, 2014, 4(5), 2014: 1149–63

Balkwill, F. R., and Mantovani, A., 'Cancer-related Inflammation: Common Themes and Therapeutic Opportunities', *Seminars in Cancer Biology*, 22(1), 2012: 33–40

Baniyash, M., Sade-Feldman, M., Kanterman, J., 'Chronic Inflammation and Cancer: Suppressing the Suppressors', *Cancer Immunol. Immunother*, 63(1), 2014: 11–20

Bhui, K., *et al.*, 'Bromelain Inhibits Nuclear Factor Kappa-B Translocation, Driving Human Epidermoid Carcinoma A431 and Melanoma A375 Cells Through G(2)/M Arrest to Apoptosis', *Molecular Carcinogenesis*, 51(3), 2012: 231–43

Bissell, M. J., and Hines, W. C., 'Why Don't We Get More Cancer? A Proposed Role of the Microenvironment in Restraining Cancer Progression', *Nature Medicine*, 17(3), 2011: 320–9

Bremnes, R. M., *et al.*, 'The Role of Tumor Stroma in Cancer Progression and Prognosis', *Journal of Thoracic Oncology*, 6, 2011: 209–17

Brown, J. M., and Attardi, L. D., 'The Role of Apoptosis in Cancer Development and Treatment Response', *Nature Reviews Cancer*, 5, 2005: 231–7

Cheng, I., *et al.*, 'Common Genetic Variation in IGF1 and Prostate Cancer Risk in the Multiethnic Cohort', *Journal of the National Cancer Institute*, 98(2), 2006: 123–34

Choi, S. W., and Friso, S., 'Epigenetics: A New Bridge Between Nutrition and Health', *Advances in Nutrition*, 1, 2010: 8–16

Clayton, P. E., *et al.*, 'Growth Hormone, the Insulin-like Growth Factor Axis, Insulin and Cancer Risk', *Nature Reviews Endocrinology*, 7, 2011: 11–24

Fidler, I. J., 'The Pathogenesis of Cancer Metastasis: 'The "Seed and Soil" Hypothesis Revisited', *Nature Reviews Cancer*, 3, 2003: 453–8

Fraisl, P., *et al.*, 'Regulation of Angiogenesis by Oxygen and Metabolism', *Developmental Cell*, 16 (2), 2009: 167–79

Grivennikov, S. I., Greten, F. R., and Karin, M., 'Immunity, Inflammation, and Cancer', *Cell*, 140(6), 2010: 883–99

Hanahan, D., and Weinberg, R. A., 'Hallmarks of Cancer: The Next Generation', *Cell*, 144(5), 2011: 646–74

Harris, A. L., 'Hypoxia – A Key Regulatory Factor in Tumour Growth', *Nature Reviews Cancer*, 2, 2002: 38–47

Indran, I. R., *et al.*, 'Recent Advances in Apoptosis, Mitochondria and Drug Resistance in Cancer Cells', *Biochimica et Biophysica Acta*, 807(6), 2011: 735–45

Jackson, C. L., *et al.*, 'Pectin Induces Apoptosis in Human Prostate Cancer Cells: Correlation of Apoptotic Function with Pectin Structure', *Glycobiology*, 17(8), 2007: 805–19

Jung, U. J., and Choi, M. S., 'Obesity and Its Metabolic Complications: the Role of Adipokines and the Relationship Between Obesity, Inflammation, Insulin Resistance, Dyslipidemia and Non-alcoholic Fatty Liver Disease', *International Journal of Molecular Sciences*, 15(4), 2014: 6184–223

Kim, Y. S., *et al.*, 'Cancer Stem Cells: Potential Target for Bioactive Food Components', *Journal of Nutritional Biochemistry*, 23, 2012: 691–8

Klement, R. J., and Kämmerer, U., 'Is There a Role for Carbohydrate Restriction in the Treatment and Prevention of Cancer?', *Nutrition and Metabolism*, 8, 2011: 75

Koppenol, Willem H., Bounds, Patricia L., and Dang, Chi V., 'Otto Warburg's Contributions to Current Concepts of Cancer Metabolism', *Nature Reviews Cancer*, 11(5), 2011: 325–37

Kundu, Joydeb Kumar, and Surh, Y., 'Emerging Avenues Linking Inflammation and Cancer', *Free Radical Biology and Medicine*, 52(9), 2012: 2013–37

Lamy, Sylvie, Gingras, Denis, and Béliveau, Richard, 'Green Tea Catechins Inhibit Vascular Endothelial Growth Factor Receptor Phosphorylation Advances in Brief', *Cancer Research*, 62, 2002: 381–85

Li, Y., *et al.*, 'Sulforaphane, A Dietary Component of Broccoli/Broccoli Sprouts, Inhibits Breast Cancer Stem Cells', *Clinical Cancer Research: An Official Journal of the American Association for Cancer Research*, 16(9), 2010: 2580–90

López-Lluch, G., *et al.*, 'Calorie Restriction Induces Mitochondrial Biogenesis and Bioenergetic Efficiency', *Proceedings of the National Academy of Sciences of the United States of America*, 103(6), 2006: 1768–73

Lord, Richard S., Bongiovanni, Bradley, and Bralley, J. Alexander, 'Estrogen Metabolism and the Diet-Cancer Connection: Rationale for Assessing the Ratio of Urinary Hydroxylated Estrogen Metabolites', *Alternative Medicine Review*, 7(2), 2002: 112–29

Lowe, S. W., and Lin, A. W., 'Apoptosis in Cancer', *Carcinogenesis*, 21, 3, 2000: 485–95

McMillan, D. C., 'The Systemic Inflammation-based Glasgow Prognostic Score: A Decade of Experience in Patients with Cancer', *Cancer Treat. Rev.*, 39, 2013: 534–40

Menshikova, E. V., *et al.* 'Effects of Exercise on Mitochondrial Content and Function in Aging Human Skeletal Muscle', *The Journals of Gerontology. Series A, Biological Sciences and Medical Sciences*, 61(6), 2006: 534–540

Mimeault, M., and Batra, S. K., 'Potential Applications of Curcumin and its Novel Synthetic Analogs and Nanotechnology-based Formulations in Cancer Prevention and Therapy', *Chinese Medicine*, 6(1), 2011: 31

Morris, Patrick G., *et al.*, 'Inflammation and Increased Aromatase Expression Occur in the Breast Tissue of Obese Women with Breast Cancer', *Cancer Prevention Research*, 4(7), 2011: 1021–9

Müller, Silke, *et al.*, 'Placebo-Controlled Randomized Clinical Trial on the Immunomodulating Activities of Low- and High-Dose Bromelain after Oral Administration – New Evidence on the Antiinflammatory

Mode of Action of Bromelain', *Phytotherapy Research*, 27(2), 2013: 199–204

Pandey, P. R., *et al.*, 'Resveratrol Suppresses Growth of Cancer Stem-like Cells by Inhibiting Fatty Acid Synthase', *Breast Cancer Research and Treatment*, 130(2), 2011: 387–98

Renehan, Andrew G., *et al.*, 'Insulin-like Growth Factor (IGF-1), IGF Binding Protein-3, and Cancer Risk: Systematic Review and Meta-Regression Analysis', *Lancet*, 363(9418), 2004: 1346–53

Romano, Barbara, *et al.*, 'The Chemopreventive Action of Bromelain, from Pineapple Stem (Ananas Comosus, L.), on Colon Carcinogenesis is Related to Antiproliferative and Proapoptotic Effects', *Molecular Nutrition and Food Research*, 58 (3), 2014: 457–65

Seyfried, T. N., *Cancer as a Metabolic Disease: On the Origin, Management and Prevention of Cancer*, John Wiley & Sons Inc., New York, 2012

Seyfried, T. N., *et al.*, 'Cancer as a Metabolic Disease: Implications for Novel Therapeutics', *Carcinogenesis*, 35(3), 2014: 515–27

Stubbs, M., *et al.*, 'Causes and Consequences of Tumour Acidity and Implications for Treatment', *Molecular Medicine Today*, 6(1), 2000: 15–19

Tsoli, M., and Robertson, G., 'Cancer Cachexia: Malignant Inflammation, Tumorkines, and Metabolic Mayhem', *Trends in Endocrinology and Metabolism*, 24(4), 2013: 174–183

Vesely, M. D., *et al.*, 'Natural Innate and Adaptive Immunity to Cancer', *Annual Review of Immunology*, 29, 2011: 235–271

Visconti, R., and Grieco, D., 'New Insights on Oxidative Stress in Cancer', *Current Opinion in Drug Discovery and Development*, 12(2), 2009: 240–245

Zhang, G., *et al.*, 'Epoxy Metabolites of Docosahexaenoic Acid (DHA) Inhibit Angiogenesis, Tumor Growth, and Metastasis', *Proceedings of the National Academy of Sciences*, 110(16), 2013: 6530–5

3 Nourishing Your Body

Abdelmalek, Manal, F., *et al.*, 'Increased Fructose Consumption Is Associated with Fibrosis Severity in Patients with Nonalcoholic Fatty Liver Disease', *Hepatology*, 51(6), 2010: 1961–71

Aggarwal, Bharat B., and Bokyung, Sung, 'Pharmacological Basis for the Role of Curcumin in Chronic Diseases: An Age-Old Spice with Modern Targets', *Trends in Pharmacological Sciences*, 30(2), 2009: 85–94

Albini, A. et al. 'Exogenous hormonal regulation in breast cancer cells by phytoestrogens and endocrine disruptors', *Current Medicinal Chemistry*, 21, 2014: 1129–1145

Altenburg, J. D., *et al.*, 'A Synergistic Antiproliferation Effect of Curcumin and Docosahexaenoic Acid in SK-BR-3 Breast Cancer Cells: Unique Signaling Not Explained by the Effects of Either Compound Alone', *BMC Cancer*, 11(1), 2011: 149

Arisi, Maria F., *et al.*, 'All Trans-Retinoic Acid (ATRA) Induces Re-differentiation of Early Transformed Breast Epithelial Cells', *International Journal of Oncology*, 44(6), 2014: 1831–42

Avci, B., *et al.*, 'Oxidative Stress Induced by 1.8 GHz Radio Frequency Electromagnetic Radiation and Effects of Garlic Extract in Rats', *International Journal of Radiation Biology*, 8 (11), 2012: 799–805

Baranski, M., *et al.*, 'Higher Antioxidant and Lower Cadmium Concentrations and Lower Incidence of Pesticide Residues in Organically Grown Crops: A Systematic Literature Review and Meta-analyses', *British Journal of Nutrition*, 112, 2014: 794–811

Bindels, L. B., *et al.*, 'Gut Microbiota-derived Propionate Reduces Cancer Cell Proliferation in the Liver', *British Journal of Cancer*, 107(8), 2012: 1337–44

Bley, K., *et al.*, 'A Comprehensive Review of the Carcinogenic and Anticarcinogenic Potential of Capsaicin', *Toxicologic Pathology*, 40(6), 2012: 847–73

Block, G., Patterson, B., and Subar, A., 'Fruit, Vegetables, and Cancer Prevention: A Review of the Epidemiological Evidence', *Nutrition and Cancer*, 18, 1992: 1–29

Bode, A. M., and Dong, Z., 'Epigallocatechin 3-Gallate and Green Tea Catechins: United They Work, Divided They Fail', *Cancer Prevention Research*, 2, 2009: 514–17

Boffetta, P., and Hashibe, M., 'Alcohol and Cancer', *Lancet Oncology*, 7(2), 2006: 149–56

Bourn, Diane, and Prescott, John, 'A Comparison of the Nutritional Value, Sensory Qualities, and Food Safety of Organically and Conventionally Produced Foods', *Critical Reviews in Food Science and Nutrition*, 42(1), 2002: 1–34

Bradbury, K. E., *et al.*, 'Organic Food Consumption and the Incidence of Cancer in a Large Prospective Study of Women in the United Kingdom', *British Journal of Cancer*, 110(9), 2014: 2321–6

Büchner, F. L., *et al.*, 'Fruits and Vegetables, Consumption and the Risk of Histological Subtypes of Lung Cancer in the European Prospective Investigation into Cancer and Nutrition (EPIC)', *Cancer Causes and Control: CCC*, 21(3), 2010: 357–71

Buck, K., *et al.*, 'Meta-analyses of Lignans and Enterolignans in Relation to Breast', *American Journal of Clinical Nutrition*, 92, 2010: 141–53

Bulathsinghala, P., Syrigos, K. N., and Saif, M. W., 'Role of Vitamin D in the Prevention of Pancreatic Cancer', *Journal of Nutrition and Metabolism*, 2010: 721365

Cardenas, E., and Ghosh, R., 'Vitamin E: A Dark Horse at the Crossroad of Cancer Management', *Biochemical Pharmacology*, 86(7), 2013: 845–52

Castrellon, A. B., and Gluck, S., 'Chemoprevention of Breast Cancer', *Expert Review of Anticancer Therapy*, 8(3), March 2008: 443–52

Chan, D. S. M., *et al.*, 'Red and Processed Meat and Colorectal Cancer Incidence: Meta-analysis of Prospective Studies, *PloS One*, 6(6), 2011: e20456

Chen, Jianmin, *et al.*, 'Dietary Flaxseed Enhances the Inhibitory Effect of Tamoxifen on the Growth of Estrogen-Dependent Human Breast Cancer (MCF-7) in Nude Mice', *Clinical Cancer Research*, 10(22), 2004: 7703–11

Chen, Shaohua, *et al.*, 'Fucoidan Induces Cancer Cell Apoptosis by Modulating the Endoplasmic Reticulum Stress Cascades', *PloS One*, 9(9), 2014: e108157

Chiang, Emily C., *et al.*, 'Defining the Optimal Selenium Dose for Prostate Cancer Risk Reduction: Insights from the U-Shaped Relationship Between Selenium Status, DNA Damage, and Apoptosis', *Dose-response: A publication of the International Hormesis Society*, 8(3), 2009: 285–300

Chlebowski, R. T., 'Vitamin D and Breast Cancer: Interpreting Current Evidence', *Breast Cancer Research*, 13(4), 2011: 217

Colomer, Ramón, *et al.*, 'N-3 Fatty Acids, Cancer and Cachexia: A Systematic Review of the Literature', *British Journal of Nutrition*, 97(5), 2007: 823–31

Conklin, K. A., 'Coenzyme Q10 for Prevention of Anthracycline-induced Cardiotoxicity', *Integrative Cancer Therapies*, 4, 2005: 110–30

Constantinou, A. I., *et al.*, 'The Soy Isoflavone Daidzein Improves the Capacity of Tamoxifen to Prevent Mammary Tumours', *European Journal of Cancer*, 41(4), 1990: 647–54

Crew, K. D., *et al.*, 'Effects of a Green Tea Extract, Polyphenon E, on Systemic Biomarkers of Growth Factor Signalling in Women with Hormone Receptor-negative Breast Cancer', *Journal of Human Nutrition and Dietetics*, 28(3), 2015: 272–82

Crous-Bou, M., *et al.*, 'Mediterranean Diet and Telomere Length in Nurses', Health Study: Population-based Cohort Study, *British Medical Journal*, 6674, 2014: 1–11

Curl, C. L., *et al.*, 'Estimating Pesticide Exposure from Dietary Intake and Organic Food Choices: The Multi-Ethnic Study of Atherosclerosis (MESA)', *Environmental Health Perspectives*, National Institute of Environmental Health Sciences, 2015

Daley, Cynthia A., *et al.*, 'A Review of Fatty Acid Profiles and Antioxidant Content in Grass-Fed and Grain-Fed Beef', *Nutrition Journal 9*, 2010: 10

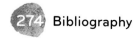

Derr, R. L., *et al.*, 'Association Between Hyperglycemia and Survival in Patients with Newly Diagnosed Glioblastoma', *Journal of Clinical Oncology: Official Journal of the American Society of Clinical Oncology*, 27(7), 2009: 1082–6

Dikshit, A., *et al.*, 'Flaxseed reduces the pro-carcinogenic micro-environment in the ovaries of normal hens by altering the PG and oestrogen pathways in a dose-dependent manner', *British Journal of Nutrition*, 113 (9), 2015: 1384–95

Eilati, Erfan, Bahr, Janice M., and Buchanan Hales, Dale, 'Long Term Consumption of Flaxseed Enriched Diet Decreased Ovarian Cancer Incidence and Prostaglandin E2 in Hens', *Gynecologic Oncology*, 130(3), 2013: 620–28

Elwood, Peter, C., *et al.*, 'The Survival Advantage of Milk and Dairy Consumption: An Overview of Evidence from Cohort Studies of Vascular Diseases, Diabetes and Cancer', *Journal of the American College of Nutrition*, 27(6), 2008: 723S–34S

Erickson, K. L., *et al.*, 'Conjugated Linoleic Acid and Cancer', *Nutrition and Health: Bioactive Compounds and Cancer,* 2010: 235–51

Falsaperla, Mario, *et al.*, 'Support Ellagic Acid Therapy in Patients with Hormone Refractory Prostate Cancer (HRPC) on Standard Chemotherapy Using Vinorelbine and Estramustine Phosphate', *European Urology*, 47(4), 2005: 449–54; discussion 454–55

Ferruzzi, Mario, G., and Blakeslee, Joshua, 'Digestion, Absorption, and Cancer Preventative Activity of Dietary Chlorophyll Derivatives', *Nutrition Research*, 27(1), 2007: 1–12

Flower, G., *et al.*, 'Flax and Breast Cancer: A Systematic Review', *Integrative Cancer Therapies*, 2013: 1534735413502076

Freemantle, S. J., Spinella, M. J., and Dmitrovsky, E., 'Retinoids in Cancer Therapy and Chemoprevention: Promise Meets Resistance', *Oncogene*, 22(47), 2003: 7305–15

Fuhrman, Barbara J., *et al.*, 'Green Tea Intake Is Associated with Urinary Estrogen Profiles in Japanese-American Women', *Nutrition Journal*, 12, 2013: 25

Galeone, C., *et al.*, 'Onion and garlic use and human cancer', *American Journal of Clinical Nutrition*, 84 (5), 2006: 1027–32.

Ganmaa, Davaasambuu, and Sato, Akio, 'The Possible Role of Female Sex Hormones in Milk from Pregnant Cows in the Development of Breast, Ovarian and Corpus Uteri Cancers', *Medical Hypotheses*, 65(6), 2005: 1028–37

Gerber, M., 'Omega-3 Fatty Acids and Cancers: A Systematic Update Review of Epidemiological Studies', *British Journal of Nutrition*, 107, 2012: Suppl. 2, S228–39

Giacosa, A., and Rondanelli, M., 'Fish Oil and Treatment of Cancer Cachexia', *Genes and Nutrition*, 3, 2008: 25–8

Goel, Ajay, and Aggrawal, Bharat B., 'Curcumin, the Golden Spice from Indian Saffron, is a Chemosensitizer and Radiosensitizer for Tumors and Chemoprotector and Radioprotector for Normal Organs', *Nutrition and Cancer*, 62(7), 2010: 919–30

Goralczyk, Regina, 'Beta-Carotene and Lung Cancer in Smokers: Review of Hypotheses and Status of Research', *Nutrition and Cancer*, 61(6), 2009: 767–74

Gornall, J., 'Sugar: Spinning a Web of Influence', *British Medical Journal*, 350, 2015: 231

Grzanna, R., Lindmark, L., and Frondoza, C. G., 'Ginger – An Herbal Medicinal Product with Broad Anti-Inflammatory Actions', *Journal of Medicinal Food*, 8(2), 2005: 125–32

Harcombe, Z., *et al.*, 'Evidence from Randomised Controlled Trials Did Not Support the Introduction of Dietary Fat Guidelines in 1977 and 1983: A Systematic Review and Meta Analysis', *Open Heart, British Medical Journal*, 2, 2015: e000196

Hatse, S., *et al.*, 'Vitamin D Status at Breast Cancer Diagnosis: Correlation with Tumor Characteristics, Disease Outcome, and Genetic Determinants of Vitamin D Insufficiency', *Carcinogenesis*, 33(7), 2012: 1319–26

Hedelin, M., et al., 'Association of Frequent Consumption of Fatty Fish with Prostate Cancer Risk is Modified by COX-2 Polymorphism', *International Journal of Cancer*, 120(2), 2007: 398–405

Herr, I., and Buchler, M. W., 'Dietary Constituents of Broccoli and Other Cruciferous Vegetables: Implications for Prevention and Therapy of Cancer', *Cancer Treatment Reviews*, 36(5), 2010: 377–83

Hopkins, M. H., *et al.*, 'Effects of Supplemental Vitamin D and Calcium on Biomarkers of Inflammation in Colorectal Adenoma Patients: A Randomized, Controlled Clinical Trial', *Cancer Prevention Research* (Philadelphia, PA.), 4(10), 2011: 1645–54

Hu, F., *et al.*, 'Carotenoids and Breast Cancer Risk: A Meta-analysis and Meta-regression', *Breast Cancer Research and Treatment*, 131(1), 2012: 239–53

Hyunkyoung, Lee, Jong-Shu, Kim, and Euikyung, Kim, 'Fucoidan from Seaweed *Fucus versiculosus* Inhibits Migration and Invasion of Human Lung Cancer Cell via P13K-Akt-mTor Pathways', *PloS One*, 7(11), 2012: e50624

Jeong, S. C., *et al.*, 'Macrophage Immunomodulating and Anti-tumour Activities of Polysaccharides Isolated from Agaricus Bisporus White Button Mushrooms', *Journal of Medicinal Food*, 15(1), 2012: 58–65

Jones, L. W., *et al.*, 'Exercise Intolerance in Cancer and the Role of Exercise Therapy to Reverse Dysfunction', *Lancet Oncology*, 10(6), 2009: 598–605

Joseph, S. V., Edirisinghe, I., and Burton-Freeman, B. M., 'Berries: Anti-inflammatory Effects in Humans', *Journal of Agricultural and Food Chemistry*, 62(18), 2014: 3886–903

Jun, L., *et al.*, 'Consumption of Spicy Foods and Total and Cause Specific Mortality: Population Based Cohort Study', *British Medical Journal*, 2015: 351

Kaczor, T., 'Iodine and Cancer: A Summary of the Evidence To Date', *Natural Medicine Journal*, 6(6), 2014

Kang, W., *et al.*, 'Emerging Role of Vitamin D in Colorectal Cancer', *World Journal of Gastrointestinal Oncology*, 3(8), 2011: 123–7

Kensler, T. W., *et al.*, 'Modulation of the Metabolism of Airborne Pollutants by Glucoraphanin-rich and Sulforaphane-rich Broccoli Sprout Beverages in Qidong, China', *Carcinogenesis*, 33(1), 2012: 101–107.

Kharrazian, D., 'The Potential Roles of Bisphenol A (BPA) Pathogenesis in Autoimmunity', *Autoimmune Disorders*, 2014

Kidd, P. M., 'The Use of Mushroom Glucans and Proteoglycans in Cancer Treatment', *Alternative Medicine Review*, 5 (1), 2000: 4–27

Kiecolt-Glaser, Janice K., *et al.*, 'Omega-3 Supplementation Lowers Inflammation and Anxiety in Medical Students: A Randomized Controlled Trial', *Brain, Behavior, and Immunity*, 25(8), 2011: 1725–34

Knekt, P., *et al.*, 'Dietary Flavonoids and the Risk of Lung Cancer and Other Malignant Neoplasms', *American Journal of Epidemiology*, 146, 1997: 223–30

Krishnan, A. V., and Feldman, D., 'Mechanisms of the Anti-cancer and Anti-inflammatory Actions of Vitamin D', *Annual Review of Pharmacology and Toxicology*, 51, 2011: 311–36

Kristal, Alan R., *et al.*, 'Baseline Selenium Status and Effects of Selenium and Vitamin E Supplementation on Prostate Cancer Risk', *Journal of the National Cancer Institute*, 106(3), 2014: djt456

La Vecchia, C., 'Alcohol and Liver Cancer', *European Journal of Cancer Prevention*, 16(6), 2007: 495–7

Laidlaw, Maggie, Cockerline, Carla A., and Sepkovic, Daniel W., 'Effects of a Breast-Health Herbal Formula Supplement on Estrogen Metabolism in Pre- and Post-Menopausal Women Not Taking Hormonal Contraceptives or Supplements: A Randomized Controlled Trial', *Breast Cancer: Basic and Clinical Research*, 4, 2010: 85–95

Lajous, M., *et al.*, 'Carbohydrate Intake, Glycaemic Index, Glycaemic Load, and Risk of Postmenopausal Breast Cancer in a Prospective Study of French Women', *American Journal of Clinical Nutrition*, 87(5), 2008: 1384–91

Lamy, S., Gingras, D., and Béliveau, R., 'Green Tea Catechins Inhibit Vascular Endothelial Growth Factor Receptor Phosphorylation Advances in Brief', *Cancer Research*, 62, 2002: 381–85

Lappe, J. M., *et al.*, 'Vitamin D and Calcium Supplementation Reduces Cancer Risk: Results of a Randomized Trial', *American Journal of Clinical Nutrition*, 85(6), 2007: 1586–91

Lawton, C., 'A Closer Look at Phytochemicals', American Institute for Cancer Care Research, 2009: preventcancer.aicr.org

Li, Y., *et al.*, 'Sulforaphane, A Dietary Component of Broccoli/Broccoli Sprouts, Inhibits Breast Cancer Stem Cells', *Clinical Cancer Research: An Official Journal of the American Association for Cancer Research*, 16(9), 2010: 2580–90

Lippman, S. M., *et al.*, 'Effect of Selenium and Vitamin E on Risk of Prostate Cancer and Other Cancers: the Selenium and Vitamin E Cancer Prevention Trail (SELECT)', *Journal of the American Medical Association (JAMA)*, 301(1), 2013: 39–51

Liu, Haibo, *et al.*, 'Fructose Induces Transketolase Flux to Promote Pancreatic Cancer Growth', *Cancer Research*, 70(15), 2010: 6368–76

Löf, M., *et al.*, 'Dietary Fat and Breast Cancer Risk in the Swedish Women's Lifestyle and Health Cohort', *British Journal of Cancer*, 97(11), 2007: 1570–76

Manaszewicz, Rosetta, 'Theme Issue for Patients: A Picture Tells a Thousand Words. Cabbage Leaves Are a Poor Man's Poultice', *British Medical Journal (Clinical Research edn)*, 327(7412), 2003: 448

Manusirivithaya, S., *et al.*, 'Antiemetic Effect of Ginger in Gynecologic Oncology Patients Receiving Cisplatin', *International Journal of Gynecological Cancer*, 14(6), 2004: 1063–9

Mason, J. K., 'Flaxseed Oil – Trastuzumab Interaction in Breast Cancer', *Food and Chemical Toxicology*, 48(8–9), 2010: 2223–6

Menendez, J. A, *et al.*, 'Oleic Acid, the Main Monounsaturated Fatty Acid of Olive Oil, Suppresses Her-2/neu (erbB-2) Expression and Synergistically Enhances the Growth Inhibitory Effects of Trastuzumab (Herceptin) in Breast Cancer Cells with Her-2/neu Oncogene Amplification', *Annals of Oncology: Official Journal of the European Society for Medical Oncology/ESMO*, 16(3), 2005: 359–71

Mimeault, M., and Batra, S. K., 'Potential Applications of Curcumin and Its Novel Synthetic Analogs and Nanotechnology-based Formulations in Cancer Prevention and Therapy', *Chinese Medicine*, 6(1), 2011: 31

Mineva, N. D., *et al.*, 'Epigallocatechin-3-gallate Inhibits Stem-like Inflammatory Breast Cancer Cells', *PloS One*, 8(9), 2013: e73464

Mohr, S. B., *et al.*, 'Meta-analysis of Vitamin D Sufficiency for Improving Survival of Patients with Breast Cancer', *Anticancer Research*, 34(3), 2014: 1163–6

Monzavi-karbassi, Behjatolah, *et al.*, 'Fructose as a Carbon Source Induces an Aggressive Phenotype in MDA-MB-468 Breast Tumor Cells', *International Journal of Oncology*, 37, 2010: 615–22

Muti, Paola, *et al.*, 'Fasting Glucose Is a Risk Factor for Breast Cancer: A Prospective Study', *Cancer Epidemiology, Biomarkers and Prevention: A Publication of the American Association for Cancer Research, co-sponsored by the American Society of Preventive Oncology*, 11(11), 2002: 1361–68

Naseribafrouei, A., Hestad, K., and Avershina, E., 'Correlation Between the Human Fecal Microbiota and Depression', *Neurogastroenterology and Motility*, 26(8), 2014: 1155–62

Nostro, Antonia, *et al.*, 'Effects of Oregano, Carvacrol and Thymol on Staphylococcus Aureus and Staphylococcus Epidermidis Biofilms', *Journal of Medical Microbiology*, 56(4), 2007: 519–23

Osei-Hyiaman, D., 'Endocannabinoid System in Cancer Cachexia', *Current Opinion in Clinical Nutrition and Metabolic Care*, 10(4), 2007: 443–8

Oyebode, Oyinlola, *et al.*, 'Fruit and Vegetable Consumption and All-Cause, Cancer and CVD Mortality: Analysis of Health Survey for England Data', *Journal of Epidemiology & Community Health*, 2014: 1–7

Pandey, Puspa R., *et al.*, 'Resveratrol Suppresses Growth of Cancer Stem-like Cells by Inhibiting Fatty Acid Synthase', *Breast Cancer Research and Treatment*, 130(2), 2011: 387–98

Prasad, Ananda S., *et al.*, 'Zinc in Cancer Prevention', *Nutrition and Cancer*, 61(6), 2009: 879–87

Public Health England, 'Consultation on draft SACN Vitamin D and Health Report', 2015

Ravindran, Jayaraj, Prasad, Sahdeo, and Aggarwal, Bharat B., 'Curcumin and Cancer Cells: How Many Ways Can Curry Kill Tumor Cells Selectively?', *The AAPS Journal*, 11(3), 2009: 495–510

Renehan, A. G., *et al.*, 'Insulin-like Growth Factor (IGF)-1, IGF Binding Protein-3, and Cancer Risk: Systematic Review and Meta-regression Analysis', *Lancet*, 363(9418), 2004: 1346–53

Rinaldi, S., *et al.*, 'Serum Levels of IGF-1, IGFBP-3 and Colorectal Cancer Risk: Results from the EPIC Cohort, Plus a Meta-analysis of Prospective Studies', *International Journal of Cancer*, 126(7), 2010: 1702–15

Rodríguez-Ramiro, D., *et al*, 'Cocoa-rich Diet Prevents Azoxymethane-induced Colonic Preneoplastic Lesions in Rats by Restraining Oxidative Stress and Cell Proliferation and Inducing Apoptosis', *Molecular Nutrition and Food Research*, 55, 2011: 1895–9

Rooks, Michelle, G., and Garrett, Wendy, S., 'Bacteria, Food, and Cancer', *F1000 Biology Reports*, 3, June, 2011: 12

Rudel, Ruthann A., *et al.*, 'Food Packaging and Bisphenol A and Bis(2-Ethyhexyl) Phthalate Exposure: Findings from a Dietary Intervention', *Environmental Health Perspectives*, 30 March, 2011

Sears, M. E., and Genuis, S. J., 'Environmental Determinants of Chronic Disease and Medical Approaches: Recognition, Avoidance, Supportive Therapy and Detoxification', *Journal of Environmental and Public Health*, 2012, article ID: 356798

Serban, D. E., 'Gastrointestinal Cancers: Influence of Gut Microbiota, Probiotics and Prebiotics', *Cancer Letters*, 345(2), 2014: 258–70

Setchell, K. D. R., *et al.*, 'Comparing the Pharmacokinetics of Daidzein and Genestein With the Use of C-labeled Tracers in Premenopausal Women', *American Journal of Clinical Nutrition*, 77(2), 2003: 411–19

Shammas, M., 'Telomeres, Lifestyle, Cancer and Aging', *Current Opinion in Clinical Nutrition and Metabolic Care*, 14(1), 2011: 28–34

Shaw, K. A, Turner, J., and Del Mar, C., *Tryptophan and 5-Hydroxytryptophan for Depression, (Review)*, (1), The Cochrane Collaboration, John Wiley and Son, New York, 2009

Silva, A. S., *et al.*, 'The Potential Role of Systemic Buffers in Reducing Intratumoral Extracellular pH and Acid-mediated Invasion', *Cancer Research*, 69(6), 2009: 2677–84

Smith-Spangler, Crystal, *et al.*, 'Are Organic Foods Safer or Healthier Than Conventional Alternatives? A Systematic Review', *Annals of Internal Medicine*, 157(5), 2011: 348–66

Sordillo, P. P., and Helson, L., 'Curcumin and Cancer Stem Cells: Curcumin Has Asymmetrical Effects on Cancer and Normal Stem Cells', *Anticancer Research*, 35, 2015: 599–614

Stocks, T., *et al.*, 'Blood Glucose and Risk of Incident and Fatal Cancer in the Metabolic Syndrome and Cancer Project (Me-Can): Analysis of Six Prospective Cohorts', *PloS*, 6(12), 2009: e1000201

Suez, J., *et al.*, 'Non-calorific Artificial Sweeteners and the Microbiome: Findings and Challenges', *Gut Microbes* 6(2), 2015

Suzuki, R., *et al.*, 'A Prospective Analysis of the Association Between Dietary Fiber Intake and Prostate Cancer Risk', short report in *EPIC*, 249, 2009: 245–9

Tamura, M., Hoshi, C., and Hori, S., 'Xylitol Affects the Intestinal Microbiota and Metabolism of Daidzein in Adult Male Mice', *International Journal of Molecular Science*, 14(12), 2013: 23993–4007

Tang, S. N., *et al.*, 'The Dietary Bioflavonoid Quercetin Synergizes with Epigallocathechin Gallate (EGCG) to Inhibit Prostate Cancer Stem Cell Characteristics, Invasion, Migration and Epithelial-mesenchymal Transition', *Journal of Molecular Signaling*, 5(14), 2010

Tate, P. L., Bibb, R., and Larcom, L. L., 'Milk Stimulates Growth of Prostate Cancer Cells in Culture', *Nutrition and Cancer*, 63(8), 2011: 1361–6

Teegala, S. M., Willett, W. C., and Mozaffarian, D., 'Consumption and Health Effects of Trans-fatty Acids: A Review', *Journal of AOAC Int.*, 92(5), 2009: 1250–7

Thomas, R., *et al.*, 'A Double-Blind, Placebo-Controlled Randomised Trial Evaluating the Effect of a Polyphenol-Rich Whole Food Supplement on PSA Progression in Men with Prostate Cancer', The UK NCRN Pomi-T Study, *Prostate Cancer and Prostatic Diseases*, 17, 2014: 180–6

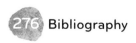

Thompson, A. K., *et al.*, 'Trans-fatty Acids and Cancer: The Evidence Reviewed', *Nutrition Research Reviews*, 21, 2008: 174–88

Thonning Olesen, *et al.*, 'Acrylamide Exposure and Incidence of Breast Cancer Among Postmenopausal Women in the Danish Diet: Cancer and Health Study', *International Journal of Cancer*, 122, 2008: 2094–100

Timmerman, G. M., and Brown, A., 'The Effect of a *Mindful Restaurant Eating* Intervention on Weight Management in Women', *Journal of Nutrition Education and Behavior*, 44(1), 2012: 22–8

Trock, B. J., Hilakivi-Clarke, L., and Clarke, R., 'Meta-analysis of Sy Intake and Breast Cancer Risk', *Journal of the National Cancer Institute*, 98(7), 2006: 459–71

Umesawa, M., *et al.*, 'Relationship Between Vegetable and Carotene Intake and Risk of Prostate Cancer: The JACC Study', *British Journal of Cancer*, 110(3), 2014: 792–6

Viñas, R., and Watson, C. S., 'Bisphenol S Disrupts Estradiol-induced Nongenomic Signaling in a Rat Pituitary Cell Line: Effects on Cell Functions', *Environmental Health Perspectives*, 121(3), 2013: 352–8

Vrieling, A., *et al.*, 'Dietary Determinants of Circulating Insulin-like Growth Factor (IGF)-1 and IGF Binding Proteins 1, -2 and -3 in Women in the Netherlands', *Cancer Causes and Control*, 15(8), 2004: 787–96

Weng, Chia Jui, and Gow, Chin Yen, 'Chemopreventive Effects of Dietary Phytochemicals Against Cancer Invasion and Metastasis: Phenolic Acids, Monophenol, Polyphenol and Their Derivatives', *Cancer Treatment Reviews*, 38(1), 2012: 76–87

Wouters, Karlijn A., *et al.*, 'Protecting Against Anthracycline-Induced Myocardial Damage: A Review of the Most Promising Strategies', *British Journal of Haematology*, 131(5), 2005: 561–78

Zhiming, Mai, Blackburn, George L., and Zhou, Jin Rong, 'Soy Phytochemicals Synergistically Enhance the Preventive Effect of Tamoxifen on the Growth of Estrogen-Dependent Human Breast Carcinoma in Mice', *Carcinogenesis* 28(6), 2007: 1217–23

Zhu, Y., *et al.*, 'Gut Microbiota and Probiotics in Colon Tumorigenesis', *Cancer Letters*, 309(2), 2011: 119–27

Zoeller, R. T *et al.*, 'Endocrine-disrupting chemicals and public health protection: A statement of principles from the Endocrine Society', *Endocrinology*, 153, 2012: pp.4097–110

4 Coping with Common Side-effects of Treatment

Choi, K., *et al.*, 'The Effect of Oral Glutamine on 5-fluorouracil/leucovorin-induced Mucositis/stomatitis Assessed by Intestinal Permeability Test', *Clinical Nutrition*, 26(1), 2007: 57–62

Gibson, Rachel J., 'Gut Microbiome and Intestinal Mucositis: A New Challenge for Researchers', *Cancer Biology and Therapy*, 8(6), 2009: 512–13

Gulletta, Norleena, and Mazurakb, V., 'Cancer Induced Cachexia', NIH Public Access, *Current Problems in Cancer*, 35(2), 2012: 1–28

Osterlund, P., *et al.*, 'Lactobacillus Supplementation for Diarrhoea Related to Chemotherapy of Colorectal Cancer: A Randomised Study', *British Journal of Cancer*, 97(8), 2007: 1028–34

Parkin, D. M., and Boyd, L., 'Cancers Attributable to Overweight and Obesity in the UK in 2010', *British Journal of Cancer*, 105 Suppl. (S2), 2011: S34–7

Prisciandaro, L. D., *et al.*, 'Evidence Supporting the Use of Probiotics for the Prevention and Treatment of Chemotherapy-Induced Intestinal Mucositis', *Critical Reviews in Food Science and Nutrition*, 51(3), 2011: 239–47

Rao, S., *et al.*, 'The Indian Spice Turmeric Delays and Mitigates Radiation-Induced Oral Mucositis in Patients Undergoing Treatment for Head and Neck Cancer: An Investigational Study', *Integrative Cancer Therapies*, 13(3), October 2013: 201–10

5 'Outside the Box' Approaches to Cancer

Abdelwahab. M. G., *et al.*, 'The Ketogenic Diet Is An Effective Adjuvant to Radiation Therapy for the Treatment of Malignant Glioma', *PloS One*, 7(5), 2012: e36197

Allen, B. G., *et al.*, 'Ketogenic Diets as an Adjuvant Cancer Therapy: History and Potential Mechanism', *Redox Biol.*, 2, 2014: 963–70

Bennett, M. H., *et al.*, 'Hyperbaric Oxygen Therapy for Late Radiation Tissue Injury', *Cochrane Database Syst. Rev.*, 2005: CD005005

Block, K. I., *et al.*, 'Impact of Antioxidant Supplementation on Chemotherapeutic Toxicity: A Systematic Review of the Evidence from Randomized Controlled Trials', *International Journal of Cancer*, 123(6), 2008: 1227–39

Bode, A. M., and Dong, Z., 'Toxic Phytochemicals and Their Potential Risks for Human Cancer', *Cancer Prevention Research*, 8, 2014: 1–8

Budwig, J., *Flax Oil as a True Aid Against Arthritis, Heart Infarction, Cancer and Other Diseases*, Apple Publishing Company, Ferndale, Washington, 1996

Champ, C. E., *et al.*, 'Targeting Metabolism with a Ketogenic Diet During the Treatment of Glioblastoma Multiforme', *Journal of Neurooncology*, 117, 2014: 125–31

Chen, M., *et al.*, 'Meta-analysis of Oxaliplatin-Based Chemotherapy Combined with Traditional Medicines for Colorectal Cancer. Contributions of Specific Plants to Tumour Response', *Integrative Cancer Therapies*, August 2015

Donahue, R. N., McLaughlin, P. J., and Zagon, I. S., 'Low-dose Naltrexone Suppresses Ovarian Cancer and Exhibits Enhanced Inhibition in Combination with Cisplatin', *Experimental Biology and Medicine*, Maywood, 236 (7), 2011: 883-95; www.ldnresearchtrust.org

Fine, E. J., *et al.* 'Targeting Insulin Inhibition as a Metabolic Therapy in Advanced Cancer: A Pilot Safety and Feasibility Dietary Trial in 10 Patients', *Nutrition*, 28, 2012: 1028–35

Frenkel, M., *et al.*, 'Integrating Dietary Supplements Into Cancer Care', *Integrative Cancer Therapies*, 12(5), 2013: 369–84

Fritz, H., *et al.*, 'Intravenous Vitamin C and Cancer: A Systematic Review', *Integrative Cancer Therapies*, 13(4), 2014: 280–300

Greenlee, H., *et al.*, 'Clinical Practice Guidelines on the Use of Integrative Therapies as Supportive Care in Patients Treated for Breast Cancer', *Journal of National Cancer Institute Monographs*, 50, 2014

Harvie, M., and Howell, A., 'Energy Restriction and the Prevention of Breast Cancer', *Proceedings of the Nutrition Society*, 71(2), 2012: 263–75

Harvie, M., Wright, *et al.*, 'The Effect of Intermittent Energy and Carbohydrate Restriction Versus Daily Energy Restriction on Weight Loss and Metabolic Disease Risk Markers in Overweight Women', *British Journal of Nutrition*, 110(8), 2013: 1534–47

Hildenbrand, G. G. L., *et al.*, 'Five-year Survival Rates of Melanoma Patients Treated by Diet Therapy After the Manner of Gerson: A Retrospective Review', *Alternative Therapies in Health and Medicine*, 1, 1995: 29–37

Hofmann, S. G., *et al.*, 'The Effect of Mindfulness-based Therapy on Anxiety and Depression: A Meta-analytic Review', *Journal of Consulting and Clinical Psychology*, 78(2), 2010: 169

Hong, G., *et al.*, 'Survey of Policies and Guidelines on Antioxidant Use for Cancer Prevention, Treatment, and Survivorship in North American Cancer Centers: What Do Institutions Perceive as Evidence?', *Integrative Cancer Therapies*, 14, 2015: 305–17

Issels, R. D., 'Hyperthermia Adds to Chemotherapy', *European Journal of Cancer*, 44(17), 2008: 2546–54

Jin, L., *et al.*, 'The Metastatic Potential of Triple-negative Breast Cancer is Decreased via Caloric Restriction-mediated Reduction of the miR-17-92 Cluster', *Breast Cancer Research and Treatment*, 146(1), 2014: 41–50

Kaefer, C. M., and Milner , J. A., 'The Role of Herbs and Spices in Cancer Prevention', *Journal of Nutritional Biochemistry*, 19(6), 2008: 347–61

Klement, R. J., and Champ, C. E., (2014). 'Calories, Carbohydrates and Cancer Therapy With Radiation: Exploiting the Five R's Through Dietary Manipulation', *Cancer Metastasis Reviews*, 2014: 217–29

Ledesma, D., and Kumano, H., 'Mindfulness-based Stress Reduction and Cancer: A Meta-analysis', *Psycho-Oncology*, 18, 2009: 571–9

Lv, M., *et al.*, 'Roles of Caloric Restriction, Ketogenic Diet and Intermittent Fasting during Initiation, Progression and Metastasis of Cancer in Animal Models: A Systematic Review and Meta-Analysis', *PLoS One*, 9, 2014: e115147

Makarević, J., *et al.*, 'Amygdalin Blocks Bladder Cancer Cell Growth In Vitro by Diminishing Cyclin A and cdk2', *PLoS One* 2014; 9(8), 2009: e105590

Massa, J., *et al.*, 'Long-term Use of Multivitamins and Risk of Colorectal Adenoma in Women', *British Journal of Cancer*, 110(1), 2014: 249–55

Moen, I., and Stuhr, L. E. B., 'Hyperbaric Oxygen Therapy and Cancer – A Review', *Targeted Oncology*, 2012: 233–42

Nebeling, L., *et al.*, 'Effects of a Ketogenic Diet on Tumour Metabolism and Nutritional Status in Pediatric Oncology Patients: Two Case Reports', *Journal of American College of Nutrition*, 1995, 14(2), 1995: 202–8

Ostermann, T., Raak, C., and Büssing, A., 'Survival of Cancer Patients Treated With Mistletoe Extract (Iscador): A Systematic Literature Review', *BMC Cancer*, 9(451), 2009

Park, S., 'The Effects of High Concentrations of Vitamin C on Cancer Cells', *Nutrients*, 5, 2013: 3496–505

Poff, A. M., *et al.*, 'The Ketogenic Diet and Hyperbaric Oxygen Therapy Prolong Survival in Mice with Systemic Metastatic Cancer', *PloS One*, 8(6), 2013: e65522

Raffaghello, L., *et al.*, 'Starvation-dependent Differential Stress Resistance Protects Normal But Not Cancer Cells Against High-dose Chemotherapy', *Proceedings of the National Academy of Sciences of the United States of America*, 105(24), 2008: 8215–20

Reed, A., James, N., Sikora, K., 'Mexico: Juices, Coffee Enemas and Cancer', *Lancet*, 336(7), 1990: 677–8

Safdie, F. M., *et al.*, 'Fasting and Cancer Treatment in Humans: A Case Series Report', *Aging*, 1, Albany, New York, 2009: 988–1007

Sarfaraz, S., *et al.*, 'Cannabinoids for Cancer Treatment: Progress and Promise', *Cancer Res.*, 68, 2008: 339–42

Seyfried, T. N., 'Is the Restricted Ketogenic Diet a Viable Alternative to the Standard of Care for Managing Malignant Brain Cancer?', *Epilepsy Research*, 100, 2012: 310–26

St Joseph's Hospital and Medical Center, Phoenix, 'Ketogenic Diet with Radiation and Chemotherapy for Newly Diagnosed Glioblastoma: Study', 2014: clinicaltrials.com NCT02046187

Stafford, P., *et al.*, 'The Ketogenic Diet Reverses Gene Expression Patterns and Reduces Reactive Oxygen Species Levels When Used As An Adjuvant Therapy for Glioma', *Nutrition and Metabolism*, 7(74), 2010

Vollbracht, C., *et al.*, 'Intravenous Vitamin C Administration Improves Quality of Life in Breast Cancer Patients During Chemo-/radiotherapy and Aftercare: Results of a Retrospective, Multicentre, Epidemiological Cohort Study in Germany', *In Vivo*, 25(6), Athens, Greece, 2011: 983–90

Zuccoli, G., *et al.*, 'Metabolic Management of Glioblastoma Multiforme Using Standard Therapy Together With A Restricted Diet: Case Report', *Nutrition and Metabolism*, 7(33), 2010

6 Life After Treatment

Bonaccio, Marialaura, *et al.*, 'Nutrition Knowledge Is Associated with Higher Adherence to Mediterranean Diet and Lower Prevalence of Obesity. Results from the Moli-Sani Study', *Appetite*, 68, 2013: 139–46

Foster, G. D., Makris, A. P., and Bailer, B. A., 'Behavioral Treatment of Obesity', *American Journal of Clinical Nutrition*, 82(suppl), 2005: 230S–5S

Parkin, D. M., and Boyd, L., 'Cancers Attributable to Overweight and Obesity in the UK in 2010', *British Journal of Cancer*, 105 Suppl. (S2), 2011: S34–7

Renehan, Andrew G., *et al.*, 'Body-Mass Index and Incidence of Cancer: A Systematic Review and Meta-Analysis of Prospective Observational Studies', *Lancet*, 371(9612), 2008: 569–7

Useful websites and resources

www.maggiescentres.org – for news, events, information and online centre

www.riverford.co.uk – provides organic boxes. Good value for money

www.bant.org.uk – British Association for Applied Nutrition & Nutritional Therapy. Provides a list of qualified practitioners

www.bodysoulnutrition.co.uk – one-to-one consultations, online programmes and webinars

www.matthewsfriends.org – Matthew's Friends charity, which specializes in ketogenic therapy for those with epilepsy and brain tumours

www.astrofund.org.uk – supports ketogenic therapy for brain tumour patients

www.soulnutrition.org – an interactive website to support mindfulness, happiness and behaviour change

www.biolab.co.uk – laboratory specializing in nutritional and environmental medicine. Requires referral from a practitioner.

www.wcrf-uk.org – World Cancer Research Fund. Provides dietary advice

www.cancernet.co.uk – information on lifestyle and cancer

www.yestolife.org.uk – provides information and funding for CAM therapies

www.canceroptions.co.uk – advice on treatments

www.drkellyturner.com – author of *Radical Remission: Surviving Cancer Against All Odds – the Nine Key Factors That Can Make a Real Difference*

www.pennybrohncancercare.org – offers online advice and residential courses for cancer patients and their carers in Bristol

www.thehaven.org.uk – offers individual complementary therapy sessions to breast cancer patients

www.foodtoglow.wordpress.com – lots of great recipes and information from Kellie, the Maggie's nutritionist in Edinburgh

www.pan-uk.org – lists the best and worst food for pesticide residues

www.canceractive.com – a helpful resource on some aspects of cancer

www.cloudstrust.org – a charity which distributes Essiac tea

www.budwigcenter.com – information on the Budwig protocol

www.theorganicholidaycompany.co.uk – a holiday company specializing in holidays where good quality organic food is the priority

www.sophiesabbage.com – read Sophie's blog and her honest and inspirational account of her cancer journey in her book *The Cancer Whisperer*

www.healthinsightuk.org – Jerome Burne's blog.

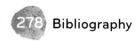

Index

Recipe pages indicated in *italics*.

2-Day Diet 108, 130
5-fluorouracil (5-FU) 102–3
5-HTP 89

acetylcholine 89
acid/alkaline balance 87–8
acid reflux 100
acrylamides 92
acupuncture 120
adjuvant therapy 272
agave syrup 77
aging 26
alcohol 28, 38, 59, 81, 84, 89, 91
alfalfa 32, 69, 117
alkaline diets 27, 30, 87–8
  see also plant-based diet
allergies 72, 80, 82
allicin 60
almonds
  almond milk *264*
  energy bombs *245*
  fragrant herb and almond chicken with quinoa *218*
  mixed fruit, seed and nut cake *246*
  nutrition 43, 90
  peaches poached in green tea with honey and almond yoghurt *238*
  quinoa salad pot *165*
aloe vera 100
alpha-linolenic acid 45–6
amaranth 79
  tabouli *175*
amino acids 42, 84, 89, 95
amygdalin 117
anaemia 55, 64, 91
anaerobic glycolysis 26
anchovies: stuffed roasted red peppers *193*
angiogenesis
  definition 272
  inflammation 27
  nutrition 32, 57, 58, 59, 61
  process 29, 122
anthocyanins 59, 100
anthracyclines 63
antibacterial agents 84
antibiotics 69, 83, 101, 113
antibodies 272
anti-inflammatory foods 28, 30, 31, 32, 67
antioxidants
  definition 272
  meditation 124–5

nutrition 27, 31, 59
organic food 69
supplements 114–16
anxiety 8, 18, 67, 89, 96, 125
apoptosis
  definition 272
  nutrition 30, 57, 58, 59, 61, 66, 68
  process 22–3
appetite loss 94, 95, 96
apples
  Bircher muesli *147*
  eight slaw *180*
  fruit and turmeric chutney *254*
  nutrition 30, 98
apricot kernels 117
apricots
  butternut and sweet potato tagine with chermoula *185*
  mixed fruit, seed and nut cake *246*
  nutrition 63
  winter dried fruit compote *149*
aromatase 81
aromatherapy 123
arsenic 78
Asian broth bowl with duck, buckwheat noodles and greens *224*
Asian power butter *230*
asparagus
  Asian broth bowl with duck, buckwheat noodles and greens *224*
  cauliflower and asparagus stir-fry *186*
  nutrition 30, 51, 52, 54
aspartame 77
ATP 25
aubergines: braised spiced aubergine *197*
autophagy 25, 31, 272
avocados
  avocado and salmon open sandwich *202*
  avocado and tofu dip *161*
  build-up smoothie *156*
  nutrition 47, 52, 89, 91
  quick cupboard salad *269*
  raw soft salad with Budwig dressing *177*
  salmon and chia cakes with dill and avocado salad *204*

bacteria 60, 65, 69, 72, 92, 97 *see also* gut microbiota; probiotics
bakeware 136–7
bananas
  banana and date loaf cake *244*

build-up smoothie *156*
  nutrition 52, 89, 91, 101
barley
  fibre 48
  gut health 98, 101
  hormones 32
  seaweed, mushroom and pearl barley risotto *194*
  types 79
  vitamins 52
basil 64, 139
beans
  alkaline diets 88
  black bean and mackerel salad *201*
  brassica and bean soup with Brazil nut pesto *171*
  budgeting 41
  cauliflower and butter bean mash *189*
  chilli con carne with beans and green and white vegetable rice *233*
  dried weight measurement 138
  nutrition 30, 32, 43, 48, 52, 54, 83, 87, 90, 98
  poached egg on spinach and pulse stir-fry *151*
  quick cupboard salad *269*
  turkey, kale and black-eyed bean broth *221*
beansprouts
  raw soft salad with Budwig dressing *177*
  Thai chicken stir-fry *220*
beef
  chilli con carne with beans and green and white vegetable rice *233*
  nutrition 43, 44, 52, 63
  simple steak with Asian power butter *230*
  turmeric beef and sweet potato pot *234*
beef stock and herb restorative soup *229*
beetroot
  beetroot and ricotta dip *163*
  nutrition 54
  roasted beetroot and goat's cheese salad *176*
  spiced beetroot and coconut milk soup (happy soup) *168*
benign, definition 272
berries
  nutrition 30, 52, 59, 100
  oats and dried berry bars *241*
beta-carotene 63, 112
beta glucans 31
beta-glucosidase 117

beta-glucuronidase 83
bicarbonate of soda 41
bile acids 48, 84, 117, 118
binge-drinking 81
bioavailability 272
biochemistry, importance of nutrition 13, 16
biologic therapy 33–4
biopsy 33
Bircher muesli *147*
biscuits: oats and dried berry bars *241*
bisphenol A 85
bitterness 117
black bean and mackerel salad 201
blackcurrants 52
black-eyed beans: turkey, kale and black-eyed bean broth 221
blenders 137
blood-sugar levels
  anaerobic glycolysis 26
  control 73–4, 75, 84, 96
  exercise 93
  fibre 48
  mood 89
  nutrition 53
  sleep 101
  spices 66, 67
  sweeteners 77
blueberries
  fresh seasonal fruit compote *150*
  grape and blueberry spread *263*
  nutrition 30, 59, 100
  oats and dried berry bars *241*
  red blast *157*
body composition 129–30
bone broth 41, 104 *see also* stock
bone health 86–7
bone marrow 53, 102
boron 87
bowel cancer 47
bowel surgery 103–4
BRAC1 gene 24
brain
  chemo brain 102–3
  dietary fat 44–5
  gut microbiota 83, 89
  herbs 65, 66
  ketogenic diet 106, 110
  nutrition 89–91
brassica and bean soup with Brazil nut pesto *171*
brassicas *see* cruciferous vegetables
Brazil nuts
  brassica and bean soup with Brazil nut pesto *171*
  nutrition 54, 63, 90

Brazil nuts (*cont.*)
oats and dried berry bars *241*
pesto *261*
bread: seeded spelt soda loaf
250
breast cancer
carotenoids 51
dietary fat 46, 47
environmental pollution 85
genes 24
indoles 57–8
insulin-like growth factor
(IGF-1) 72
iodine 60–1
mushrooms 60
phytoestrogens 80–1
quercetin 32
breastfeeding 46, 58
breathing 125
broccoli
brassica and bean soup
with Brazil nut pesto *171*
chilli con carne with beans
and green and white
vegetable rice *233*
eight slaw *180*
nutrition 51, 52, 58, 103
supplements 113, 114–15
bromelain 30, 98
brownies, chocolate walnut
242
buckwheat 79
buckwheat noodles, mixed
mushroom noodle soup
with a poached egg *173*
buddy systems 39
budgeting 41, 42, 70
Budwig dressing *177*
Budwig protocol 30, 31, 61,
109
build-up smoothie 95, *156*
burdock root 117
butter beans
brassica and bean soup
with Brazil nut pesto *171*
cauliflower and butter bean
mash *189*
butternut and sweet potato
tagine with chermoula *185*
butyrate 48

cabbage
brassica and bean soup
with Brazil nut pesto *171*
eight slaw *180*
kim-chi *253*
nutrition 52, 54, 57–8, 98
sauerkraut *252*
shepherd's pie with mash
and greens topping *226*
cacao, raw
energy bombs *245*
porridge and chia breakfast
bowl *146*

cachexia 27, 46, 95–6, 272
cadmium 69
caffeine 56, 59, 89, 91, 118
cake
banana and date loaf *244*
mixed fruit, seed and nut
246
calcium 55, 62, 72, 80, 86,
87
calorie restriction 25, 30, 31,
108, 111
CAM *see* complementary and
alternative medicines
cancer
causes 22–9
incidence rates 23
inflammation 27–8
lifestyle effects 23, 26 *see
also* epigenetics
cannabis 95–6, 119
capers
nutrition 30
oven-baked trout and kale
with millet *205*
stuffed roasted red peppers
193
capsaicin 66, 103
carbohydrates 47–8, 73, 74,
89, 92 *see also* glycaemic
index; ketogenic diet; sugar
carcinogens 85, 91, 92, 272
cardamom 66, 139
Keralan chicken liver curry
223
carminatives 65, 66, 272
carotenoids 25, 30, 51, 63, 66
carrots
eight slaw *180*
nutrition 51, 63
raw soft salad with Budwig
dressing *177*
carvacrol 65
cashew nuts
cashew cream *261*
cauliflower and asparagus
stir-fry *186*
chia strawberry and cashew
nut milk pot *144*
nutrition 43
catechins 25, 59
cauliflower
cauliflower and asparagus
stir-fry *186*
cauliflower and butter bean
mash *189*
chilli con carne with beans
and green and white
vegetable rice *233*
Indian cauliflower *188*
nutrition 54
celeriac: eight slaw *180*
celery
eight slaw *180*
juicing 68

cereals 54, 75
chamomile 65, 100
cheese
baked sweet potato stuffed
with buffalo Mozzarella
182
beetroot and ricotta dip *163*
Brazil nut pesto *261*
fridge frittata *191*
nutrition 52, 72, 82
roasted beetroot and goat's
cheese salad *176*
storage 40
stuffed roasted red peppers
193
watermelon, feta and
pomegranate salad *178*
chemical exposure 85 *see also*
environmental pollution
chemo brain 102–3
chemotherapy *see also* side-
effects
fasting 108
juicing 69
ketogenic diet 107, 111
nutrition 58, 62, 63
oxidative stress 27
process 23, 33
supplements 115
vitamins 53
chermoula *260*
cherries
nutrition 30, 89, 100
oats and dried berry bars
241
chewing 57, 67, 92, 103,
104, 180
chewing gum 97, 104
chia seeds 80
chia strawberry and cashew
nut milk pot *144*
nutrition 101
porridge and chia breakfast
bowl *146*
red blast *157*
salmon and chia cakes with
dill and avocado salad *204*
chicken
fragrant herb and almond
chicken with quinoa *218*
nutrition 43, 44, 52
shopping 137
Thai chicken stir-fry *220*
chicken liver: Keralan chicken
liver curry *223*
chickpeas
butternut and sweet potato
tagine with chermoula
185
hummus *164*
nutrition 52, 90
quick cupboard salad *269*
turmeric beef and sweet
potato pot *234*

chilli 66
chermoula *260*
harissa *262*
quinoa salad pot *165*
red blast *157*
chilli con carne with beans
and green and white
vegetable rice *233*
chlorella 52
chlorophyll 65, 68
chocolate 51, 91
walnut brownies *242*
cholesterol 45, 47, 48, 138
choline 25, 30, 52, 64
chutney, fruit and turmeric
254
cinnamon
fresh seasonal fruit
compote *150*
nutrition 32, 66–7, 101,
120
porridge and chia breakfast
bowl *146*
winter dried fruit compote
149
cleaning products 41
cling film 40
cloves 67, 139
coconut
chocolate walnut brownies
242
energy bombs *245*
pancakes with fresh fruit,
yoghurt and honey *142*
coconut milk, spiced beetroot
and coconut milk soup
(happy soup) *168*
coconut oil
flavour 138
nutrition 45
oats and dried berry bars
241
pancakes with fresh fruit,
yoghurt and honey *142*
shopping 138
coconut sugar 76
coconut water 104
smoothies *157*
cod: seed-crusted cod loin
210
coeliac disease 78
coenzyme Q10 (CoQ10) 63
coffee 92 *see also* caffeine
coffee enemas 116, 118
colon cancer 48, 51, 58, 108,
116
colonoscopy 83
colostomy 104
complementary and
alternative medicines
(CAM)
radiotherapy effects 33
research evidence
18–19, 106

compote
  fresh seasonal fruit *150*
  winter dried fruit *149*
compounds, definition 272
conjugated linoleic acid 46–7, 72
constipation 48, 61, 99, 101, 118
cooking methods 91–2
copper 54, 87
coriander
  avocado and tofu dip *161*
  braised spiced aubergine *197*
  chermoula *260*
  harissa *262*
  nutrition 67
  red lentil dhal with grated courgette *192*
  salmon and puy lentils with a coriander sauce *209*
corn oil 45
cortisol 28
costs 41, 42, 70
cottage cheese
  Budwig dressing *177*
  nutrition 43, 109
courgettes
  crab with courgette spaghetti *214*
  red lentil dhal with grated courgette *192*
crab with courgette spaghetti *214*
crackers, savoury seed *159*
cranberries
  mixed fruit, seed and nut cake *246*
  nutrition 30, 59, 88, 104
cravings 128–9
cruciferous vegetables, nutrition 25, 28–9, 51, 52, 57–8, 92, 156
cucumber 68
cumin 67
  butternut and sweet potato tagine with chermoula *185*
  chermoula *260*
  harissa *262*
cupboard food planning 38, 134–6
curcumin 23, 58 *see also* turmeric
curry
  Keralan chicken liver *223*
  red lentil dhal with grated courgette *192*
cytokines 27, 272

dairy foods
  insulin response 32
  intolerance 72, 82
  nutrition 52, 54, 72, 87, 89, 91

dates
  banana and date loaf cake *244*
  build-up smoothie *156*
  energy bombs *245*
  lamb tagine *228*
  mixed fruit, seed and nut cake *246*
Daunorubicin 63
dehydration 56
depression 83, 89, 125
detoxification
  after treatment 118
  definition 272
  exercise 30
  fibre 48, 68
  gut immunity 28
  liver health 84
  mitochondria 31
  nutrition 59, 65
  research evidence 120–1
dhal, red lentil with grated courgette *192*
diabetes 48, 66, 73–4, 77
diarrhoea 65, 99, 101, 118
diet choices 37
differentiation 22, 23, 272
digestion *see also* gut health
  mindfulness 92–3
  nutrition 58, 64–5, 67
  side-effects 97
  soups 95
digestive enzyme supplements 113
dill 65, 139
  salmon and chia cakes with dill and avocado salad *204*
DIM (3,3'-diindolylmethane) 57
dips
  avocado and tofu *161*
  beetroot and ricotta *163*
  sardine *160*
diverticulitis 48, 100
DNA (deoxyribonucleic acid) 22, 97
dopamine 73, 89
Doxorubicin 63
dried fruit
  Bircher muesli *147*
  mixed fruit, seed and nut cake *246*
  nutrition 52, 75, 76, 91
  oats and dried berry bars *241*
  winter compote *149*
drinking *see* hydration
drug resistance 57
dry mouth 97
duck: Asian broth bowl with duck, buckwheat noodles and greens *224*
dumping syndrome 104

EBM *see* evidence-based medicine
eggs
  fridge frittata *191*
  kale, mushroom and egg bake with harissa *183*
  kedgeree with leafy greens *208*
  mixed mushroom noodle soup with a poached egg *173*
  nutrition 30, 43, 52, 54, 89, 91
  pancakes with fresh fruit, yoghurt and honey *142*
  poached egg on spinach and pulse stir-fry *151*
  quick meals 138
  spiced golden tofu with vegetables *196*
  storage 142
eight slaw *180*
ellagic acid 30, 31, 59
endocrine disruptors 85
enemas 118
energy
  mitochondria 25
  mood 89
  strategies for low levels 38
  vegetables 95
  vitamins 53
energy bombs *245*
enjoyment 18
environmental pollution 25, 28, 40, 85 *see also* detoxification
epigallocatechin gallate (EGCG) 59
epigenetics 24–6, 272
Essiac tea 117–18
eugenol 67
evidence-based medicine (EBM) 18–21, 57, 106
exercise
  benefits overview 93
  blood-sugar levels 74
  digestive issues 101
  fatigue 94
  hormones 29
  lymph system 123
  metastasis 32
  mitochondria 25, 31
  mood 91
  oxygen 29, 31
  protein 96
  stress management 39, 96
extracellular matrix (ECM) 24

family support 39
farming methods 44, 45, 70, 71, 72
fasting 25, 108
fat (body) 27, 73, 129–30

fatigue
  anaemia 91
  blood-sugar levels 74
  dumping syndrome 104
  exercise 93
  ketogenic diet 110
  management 94–5
  vitamin Bs 91
fats (dietary) *see also* ketogenic diet
  Budwig protocol 109
  nutrition 43–7, 54, 75, 95, 103, 138
  shopping 138
fennel 99, 104
  fish soup *206*
fenugreek 32, 67, 69
fermentation (cellular) 25, 26
fermented foods 58, 81, 83, 101
feta: watermelon, feta and pomegranate salad *178*
fibre
  nutrition 48, 68
  prebiotics 83
  smoothies 68
  sources 48, 61, 74, 78–9, 98
figs
  mixed fruit, seed and nut cake *246*
  nutrition 54
  winter dried fruit compote *149*
fish
  avocado and salmon open sandwich *202*
  black bean and mackerel salad *201*
  fish soup *206*
  grilled fish and papaya salad *213*
  kedgeree with leafy greens *208*
  nutrition 30, 43, 45–6, 52, 54, 63, 87, 89, 91, 99
  oven-baked trout and kale with millet *205*
  salmon and chia cakes with dill and avocado salad *204*
  salmon and puy lentils with a coriander sauce *209*
  seed-crusted cod loin *210*
  shopping 41
  stuffed roasted red peppers *193*
fish oils 95, 113
flatulence 65, 103–4
flavonoids 60, 65
flaxseed oil 113
  Budwig dressing *177*
flaxseeds
  Budwig protocol 109

flaxseeds (*cont.*)
  gut health 99, 101
  nutrition 30, 32, 45, 48,
    61–2, 81
  savoury seed crackers *159*
  storage 45
  sunrise juice *157*
flour
  nutrition 73
  types 78, 79, 138
folate 52, 64, 91
food *see also* nutrition
  as medicine 11, 17
  budgeting 41, 42
  quality 40, 41, 42
  staples 38, 134–6
  to avoid 41, 47, 75, 102,
    103–4, 105, 136
  food diary 17, 37, 38, 82,
    103–4, 270–1
free radicals 26–7, 31, 122,
  272
friend support 39
frittata *191*
fructose 73, 75, 76, 84
fruit *see also specific fruit*
  alkaline diets 88
  fresh seasonal fruit
    compote *150*
  fruit and turmeric chutney
    254
  juicing 68
  nutrition 48, 52, 76
  pancakes with fresh fruit,
    yoghurt and honey *142*
  portion sizes 50–1
  rainbow 49, 51
  sugars 73
fucoidan 61
fungicides 51

GABA (gamma-aminobutyric
  acid) 89
gall bladder 118
garlic
  harissa *262*
  hummus *164*
  nutrition 54, 60, 92, 98
  poached egg on spinach
    and pulse stir-fry *151*
  quinoa salad pot *165*
  red lentil dhal with grated
    courgette *192*
gene expression 24, 111,
  124–5, 272
genes 23–4
genetically modified foods
  80
genistein, cancer stem cells
  25
Gerson therapy 108–9, 116,
  118
ginger
  chermoula *260*

Keralan chicken liver curry
  223
lamb tagine *228*
nausea 97, 100
nutrition 30, 31, 32, 67
quinoa salad pot *165*
red blast *157*
salmon and puy lentils
  with a coriander sauce
  209
glioblastoma multiforme 111
gliomas 110–11
glucoraphanin 58
glucose 26, 29, 31, 32, 72–4,
  106–7
glucose intolerance 73–4, 77
glucosinolates 57
gluten 78–80, 82
glycaemic index (GI) 73–4,
  272
glycaemic load (GL) 74
glycolysis 26
glyphosate 80
goat's cheese: roasted
  beetroot and goat's cheese
  salad *176*
Gonzalez's protocol 116
grains 78, 88
grapefruit juice 84
grapes
  grape and blueberry spread
    263
  nutrition 59, 81
  red blast *157*
green tea
  angiogenesis 29
  cancer stem cells 25, 30
  nutrition 31, 32, 51, 58–9
  peaches poached in green
    tea with honey and
    almond yoghurt *238*
  supplements 113, 114–15
guilt 18
gum disease 59
gut flora *see* microbiota
gut health *see also* digestion
  fibre 48
  juicing 68
  lycopene 63
  mood 89
  nutrition 13, 98–100
  problems 82–4
  side-effects 97
gut immunity 28, 32

habits 128–9
haemoglobin 53, 55, 91
happy soup (spiced beetroot
  and coconut milk soup) *168*
harissa, home-honed 262
heart health
  free radicals 26
  nutrition 44, 55, 63
hemp oil 113

Budwig dressing *177*
hemp seeds 95
  Bircher muesli *147*
  nutrition 30, 99
herbs *see also specific herbs*
  beef stock and herb
    restorative soup *229*
  fragrant herb and almond
    chicken with quinoa *218*
  'metallic mouth' 64, 66
  mouth coolers 139
  nutrition 32, 64–6
  storage 64
  teas 100
HIF-1 *see* hypoxia-inducible
  factor
homeopathy 119–20
honey 76–7
  oats and dried berry bars
    241
  peaches poached in green
    tea with honey and
    almond yoghurt *238*
hormones
  cancer links 28
  dairy foods 72
  definition 272
  dietary fat 45
  environmental pollution
    85
  nutrition 32, 53
  obesity 129
  pregnancy 116
  soya 80–1
hormone therapy 34, 61, 102
horseradish: sardine dip *160*
hummus *164*
hydration 38, 48, 56, 87,
  96, 101
hydrogenated fats *see*
  trans-fats
hygiene 69, 72, 102
hyperbaric oxygen therapy
  (HBOT) 29, 107, 122
hyperthermia 121
hypoxia 272
hypoxia-inducible factor
  (HIF-1) 29, 122

IGF-1 *see* insulin-like growth
  factor
ileostomy 104
immune system
  coconut oil 138
  food hygiene 69, 72
  function in cancer recovery
    23, 28
  insulin 27
  lifestyle effects 28
  Naltrexone 123
  nutrition 31, 55, 59, 60,
    63, 64, 65
  raw honey 77
  support overview 38–9

Indian cauliflower *188*
indigestion 65
indoles 57
inflammation
  acute 27
  cabbage leaves 58
  cachexia 95
  cancer treatment 23
  chronic 27–8
  dehydration 56
  free radicals 26
  gut microbiota 83
  immune system 27–8
  nutrition 30, 31, 47, 60,
    64, 65, 67, 97
  obesity 129
  sugar 73
infusions, homemade *267*
inositol hexaphosphate (IP6)
  30
insomnia 65, 101
insulin 27, 28–9, 32, 73–4,
  77, 107
insulin-like growth factor
  (IGF-1) 29, 32, 72, 74, 81,
  129
insulin response 28–9, 30,
  67, 129
integrative oncology 272
intermittent fasting 108
internal terrain 16, 24
intestinal bacteria *see* gut
  microbiota
intolerances 17, 72, 78, 79,
  82–3
intuition 71
inulin 98
iodine 54, 60–1
iron
  sources 54, 65, 67, 91
  supplements 64, 113
Iscador 116
isoflavones 80
isoleucine 95
isothiocyanates 57

Jencks, Maggie Keswick 10,
  287
Jerusalem artichokes 83, 98
juicing 68–9, 109, 137
junk food 16, 87 *see also*
  processed foods

kale
  brassica and bean soup
    with Brazil nut pesto *171*
  kale, mushroom and egg
    bake with harissa *183*
  nutrition 30, 98
  oven-baked trout and kale
    with millet *205*
  super-boost kale and
    pineapple juice smoothie
    156

turkey, kale and black-eyed bean broth *221*
Kamut 80
kedgeree with leafy greens *208*
kelp 61 *see also* seaweed
Keralan chicken liver curry *223*
ketogenic diet 30, 31, 75, 96, 106–8, 110–11
ketones 107, 272
ketosis 273
Khorasan wheat 80
kidney beans
    chilli con carne with beans and green and white vegetable rice *233*
    nutrition 43, 86, 88, 90
kidney function 42
kim-chi 83, *253*
kitchen gadgets 136–7

lactic acid 25, 26
Lactobacillus 58
lactose 72, 75, 82
Laetrile 117
lamb
    nutrition 44, 70
    shepherd's pie with mash and greens topping *226*
    tagine *228*
lavender 101
leaky gut 28, 82
leeks 83, 98
    fish soup *206*
legumes
    alkaline diets 88
    nutrition 51
lemon juice 100
lemon verbena 65, 97, 100
lentils
    budgeting 41
    lentil and spinach soup *174*
    nutrition 32, 43, 52, 54, 83, 90, 98
    poached egg on spinach and pulse stir-fry *151*
    red lentil dhal with grated courgette *192*
    salmon and puy lentils with a coriander sauce *209*
lettuce 30
leucine 95
leukaemia 115–16
lifestyle changes 8, 10, 38, 128–9
lime juice 100
linoleic acid 46
linseeds *see* flaxseeds
liquorice 32, 100
liver
    Keralan chicken liver curry *223*
    nutrition 52, 91

liver health 66, 68, 73, 81, 84
low-fibre diet 104–5
low glycaemic load diet 30, 31, 32, 73–4, 108
low-residue diet 104–5
lung cancer 51, 108, 112
lycopene 63
lymphoedema 122, 123
lymph system 29, 30, 123

macadamia nuts: simple steak with Asian power butter *230*
mackerel: black bean and mackerel salad *201*
macrophages 31, 60
magic mushrooms 119
magnesium
    nutrition 89
    sources 54, 67, 80
malignant, definition 273
manganese 54, 80, 87
mango, sunrise juice *157*
maple syrup 76
marinating 92
marjoram 65
massage 123
mastitis 58
meal sizes 95, 96
meat
    cooking methods 91–2
    fats (dietary) 44
    nutrition 44, 52, 54, 63, 87
    shopping 41, 137
meditation 124–5
Mediterranean-style diet 37, 47
melatonin 94, 101
melon 63
menopause 61, 67, 102
mental attitude 17
mercury 46, 59
metabolism 25–6, 108–9
'metallic mouth' 64, 66, 138, 139
metastasis 29, 32, 58, 61, 273
Metformin 26
Methotrexate 64
microbiome 273
microbiota 83
    dairy foods 72
    definition 273
    fermented foods 58
    fibre 48
    function 83
    nutrition 83–4, 113
    phytonutrients 51
    sweeteners 77
micro-environment 24, 26, 27, 30
    microwave cooking 40, 92

milk
    alternatives 72
    nutrition 43, 47, 52, 54, 72, 75
    pancakes with fresh fruit, yoghurt and honey *142*
    porridge and chia breakfast bowl *146*
    seeded spelt soda loaf *250*
millet 79
    oven-baked trout and kale with millet *205*
mindfulness 92–3, 125, 128
mineral supplements 113
mint
    amaranth tabouli *175*
    beef stock and herb restorative soup *229*
    braised spiced aubergine *197*
    nausea 97, 99
    nutrition 65
    super-boost kale and pineapple juice *156*
    watermelon, feta and pomegranate salad *178*
miso 81, 83, 87
miso soup *268*
mistletoe extract 116–17
mitochondria
    anaerobic glycolysis 26
    function 25, 273
    nutrition 31, 63
    obesity 129
    pH level 87
molasses
    chocolate walnut brownies *242*
    mixed fruit, seed and nut cake *246*
    nutrition 52, 76, 87
monoclonal antibodies 34
monounsaturated fats 47
mood 89
mooli: kim-chi *253*
motivation 22
mouth health *see* oral health
mouthwash 100
Mozzarella
    baked sweet potato stuffed with buffalo Mozzarella *182*
    stuffed roasted red peppers *193*
mucositis 67, 97, 100, 273
muesli, Bircher *147*
multivitamins 113
muscles 96 *see also* cachexia
mushrooms
    kale, mushroom and egg bake with harissa *183*
    mixed mushroom noodle soup with a poached egg *173*

nutrition 29, 30, 31, 32, 52, 54, 59–60, 98
raw soft salad with Budwig dressing *177*
seaweed, mushroom and pearl barley risotto *194*
mustard seeds 138
mutation, definition 273
myelin 102–3
myoglobin 55
myrosinase 57

Naltrexone 123
naringenin 84
natto 81, 87
natural killer cells 60
nausea 65, 67, 97, 99, 101
necrosis 23, 273
nervous system 53, 55, 65, 89, 102–3
neurotransmitters 83, 89, 91, 125, 273
neutropenia 97, 101–2, 273
niacin 52, 91
noodles
    Asian broth bowl with duck, buckwheat noodles and greens *224*
    mixed mushroom noodle soup with a poached egg *173*
nutraceutical
    approaches 112
    definition 273
nutrition *see also*
    biochemistry
    balanced diet 17, 18, 42–51, 57, 72, 74, 91
    cancer stem cells 25
    expert advice 36–7, 38, 112
    nutrition 75
    personalization 36–7
    research base 17, 18–19
nuts
    alkaline diets 88
    almond milk *264*
    brassica and bean soup with Brazil nut pesto *171*
    Brazil nut pesto *261*
    cashew cream *261*
    cauliflower and asparagus stir-fry *186*
    chia strawberry and cashew nut milk pot *144*
    chocolate walnut brownies *242*
    energy bombs *245*
    fragrant herb and almond chicken with quinoa *218*

nuts (*cont.*)
  mixed fruit, seed and nut
    cake *246*
  nutrition 43, 46, 47, 52,
    54, 63, 87, 90, 99
  oats and dried berry bars
    241
  peaches poached in green
    tea with honey and
    almond yoghurt *238*
  quick cupboard salad *269*
  quinoa salad pot *165*
  simple steak with Asian
    power butter *230*
  storage 45, 63

oats
  Bircher muesli *147*
  gut health 98, 101
  nutrition 32, 48, 54, 83, 90
  oats and dried berry bars
    241
  porridge and chia breakfast
    bowl *146*
obesity 27, 77, 129
oesophageal cancer 51
oestrogen
  gut microbiota 83
  hormone therapy 34
  nutrition 48, 57, 61
  obesity 129
  phytoestrogens 80–1
offal 52, 54, 63, 87, 91
off-label drugs 124
okra 86, 99
olive oil 41, 47, 138
omega fatty acids
  brain function 89
  cachexia 95
  nutrition 44, 45–6
  organic food 69
  sources 61, 72, 80, 138
  supplements 113
oncogenes 24, 122, 273
oncologists, nutritional
  knowledge 36
onions
  cooking methods 92
  eight slaw *180*
  nutrition 30, 51, 60, 83, 98
oral health 59, 60, 67, 100
oranges
  nutrition 52, 91, 101
  sunrise juice *157*
oregano 65
organic food 31, 40, 69–71,
  72, 137
organ meats *see* offal
osteoporosis 62, 123
oxidation 27, 273
oxidative stress 27, 31, 125,
  129
oxygen
  angiogenesis 29

Gerson therapy 109
haemoglobin 91
hyperbaric oxygen therapy
  122
nutrition 30, 31
respiration 25, 26
oysters 54
ozone therapy 122

packaging 40, 45, 56, 85
pak choi: Asian broth bowl
  with duck, buckwheat
  noodles and greens *224*
palliative care 130
palm oil 45
pancakes with fresh fruit,
  yoghurt and honey *142*
pancreatic enzymes 116
papaya
  grilled fish and papaya
    salad *213*
  nutrition 63, 98
  papaya drink *139*
  sunrise juice *157*
parabens 85
parsley
  amaranth tabouli *175*
  beef stock and herb
    restorative soup *229*
  nutrition 65, 104
peaches poached in green
  tea with honey and almond
  yoghurt *238*
peanuts 43, 46, 52, 91
pearl barley: seaweed,
  mushroom and pearl barley
  risotto *194*
pears
  fresh seasonal fruit
    compote *150*
  fruit and turmeric chutney
    254
peas
  nutrition 52, 54, 83, 95
  raw soft salad with Budwig
    dressing *177*
pectin 98
pepper (black) 58
peppers
  harissa *262*
  nutrition 63
  stuffed roasted red peppers
    193
  Thai chicken stir-fry *220*
periodontal disease 59
peripheral neuropathy 103,
  273
pesticides 28, 45, 49, 51,
  69–70, 79
PET (positron emission
  tomography) scans 26
pH 87
phosphates 87
phosphorus 80

phthalates 85
phytoestrogens 32, 80, 81
phytonutrients 31, 51,
  113–15
phytosterols 138
pineapple
  nutrition 30, 54, 89, 98,
    101
  super-boost kale and
    pineapple juice *156*
pine nuts: amaranth tabouli
  175
piperine 58
placebo effect 17, 21
plant-based diet 17, 30, 117
  see also Mediterranean-style
  diet
plums
  fresh seasonal fruit
    compote *150*
  nutrition 30, 54, 89
polyphenols
  definition 273
  hormones 51
  organic food 69
  sources 30, 32, 58–9
  supplements 112, 114–15
polysaccharides 60, 61
polyunsaturated fats 45
pomegranate
  supplements 113, 114–15
  watermelon, feta and
    pomegranate salad *178*
Pomi-T 36, 112, 114–15
poppy seeds: savoury seed
  crackers *159*
pork
  nutrition 43, 44, 52
  pork tenderloin with sage
    and lemon cream sauce
    235
porridge and chia breakfast
  bowl *146*
portion sizes 95, 96
positive thinking 8, 128, 129
potassium 56
potatoes
  fish soup *206*
  nutrition 52, 73, 90
  oven chips 92
  shepherd's pie with mash
    and greens topping *226*
poultry
  nutrition 30, 44, 52, 54, 91
  shopping 137
prawns
  fish soup *206*
  nutrition 43
prebiotics 32, 83, 98, 273
pregnancy 46, 116
proactivity 8
proanthocyanidins 59
probiotics 32, 83–4, 97, 101,
  113, 273

processed foods
  convenience 71
  inflammation 27
  neurotransmitters 89
  obesity 40
  protein quality 42
  salt 56
  soya 81
  sugar 75, 84
  trans-fats 44, 47
'programmed' cell death *see*
  apoptosis
prostate cancer
  capsaicin 66
  dietary fat 46
  environmental pollution 85
  exercise 93
  fibre 48
  flaxseeds 61
  insulin-like growth factor
    (IGF-1) 72
  lycopene 63
  phytoestrogens 81
  phytonutrients 51
  quercetin 30
  selenium 63, 112
  supplements 115
protein
  cachexia 95, 96
  gene mutations 24
  liver health 84
  mood 89
  nutrition 42
  sources 43, 79, 80
protein boosts 138, 139
protein shakes 42
protocols
  definition 273
  personalization 19, 36–7
prunes
  mixed fruit, seed and nut
    cake *246*
  winter dried fruit compote
    149
psilocybin 119
psyllium
  nutrition 48, 101
  savoury seed crackers *159*
Pubmed 34
pulses *see also* beans; lentils
  nutrition 48, 51, 54, 87, 91
  poached egg on spinach
    and pulse stir-fry *151*
  quick cupboard salad *269*
pumpkin seeds 138
  gut health 99
  mixed fruit, seed and nut
    cake *246*
  nutrition 30, 43, 45, 90
  savoury seed crackers *159*
  seed-crusted cod loin *210*

quark 109
quercetin 30, 32, 60

quinoa
  fragrant herb and almond chicken with quinoa *218*
  nutrition 43, 79
  salad pot *165*

radiotherapy *see also* side-effects
  hyperbaric oxygen therapy 122
  juicing 69
  ketogenic diet 107, 111
  nutrition 58, 60
  oxidative stress 27
  process 23, 33
radishes: kim-chi *253*
rancidity 45
randomized control trials (RCTs) 18, 20, 21
raspberries: fresh seasonal fruit compote *150*
rebounding 30, 32, 123
receptor, definition 273
red blast *157*
red lentil dhal with grated courgette *192*
refined carbohydrates 47, 73, 75, 89
reflexology 124
relaxation 39, 89
remission 125
research evidence 17, 51, 69, 93, 110–11, 124 *see also* evidence-based medicine
respiration 25, 31, 273
resveratrol 30, 59, 81
retinoids 63
rhodanese 117
rhubarb: fresh seasonal fruit compote *150*
rice 78
  cauliflower and asparagus stir-fry *186*
  kedgeree with leafy greens *208*
  nutrition 30, 52
  spiced golden tofu with vegetables *196*
rice milk 72
rice noodles: Asian broth bowl with duck, buckwheat noodles and greens *224*
ricotta: beetroot and ricotta dip *163*
risotto, seaweed, mushroom and pearl barley *194*
rosemary 65–6, 120, 139
rye 48

saccharin 77
safety 19, 20, 97, 102, 112
saffron
  lamb tagine *228*
  nutrition 30, 68

salads
  amaranth tabouli *175*
  black bean and mackerel *201*
  eight slaw *180*
  grilled fish and papaya *213*
  quick cupboard (pulses, nuts and avocado) *269*
  quinoa salad pot *165*
  raw soft salad with Budwig dressing *177*
  roasted beetroot and goat's cheese *176*
  salmon and chia cakes with dill and avocado *204*
  watermelon, feta and pomegranate *178*
salivary glands 97
salmon
  avocado and salmon open sandwich *202*
  nutrition 45, 87
  salmon and chia cakes with dill and avocado salad *204*
  salmon and puy lentils with a coriander sauce *209*
salt 56–7, 61, 87, 103
sandwiches, open avocado and salmon *202*
saponins 79
sardines
  nutrition 45, 46, 87
  sardine dip *160*
Sativex 119
saturated fats 44, 45
sauces
  10-vegetable tomato *255*
  chermoula *260*
  harissa *262*
sauerkraut 58, 83, 252
sea buckthorn 102
seafood 43, 52, 54, 87 *see also* prawns
sea vegetables 61
seaweed
  fish soup *206*
  miso soup *268*
  mixed mushroom noodle soup with a poached egg *173*
  nutrition 52, 54, 60–1
  seaweed, mushroom and pearl barley risotto *194*
  shopping 139
secretin 118
seeds *see also specific seeds*
  alkaline diets 88
  ground mixed-seed boost powder *258*
  mixed fruit, seed and nut cake *246*
  nutrition 30, 43, 46, 54, 75, 87
  savoury seed crackers *159*

seeded spelt soda loaf *250*
soaking 138
sprouting 52, 68–9, 139
storage 45
selenium
  safe consumption levels 63, 112
  sources 54, 63, 80
serotonin 89, 91
sesame seeds *see also* tahini
  mixed fruit, seed and nut cake 246
  nutrition 30, 32
  savoury seed crackers *159*
sex hormone binding globulin (SHBG) 48
sheep sorrel 118
shepherd's pie with mash and greens topping *226*
shopping 41
shopping lists 38, 134–6
short-chain fatty acids (SCFAs) 48
side-effects 20, 78, 94–105, 122
silicon 87
skin brushing 29, 30, 32, 123
skin cancer 62, 63
sleep 39, 89, 94–5, 101
slippery elm 99, 117–18
smoked foods 92
smoked haddock: kedgeree with leafy greens *208*
smoking 26, 92, 112
smoothies 68–9, 75, 96
  build-up smoothie 95, *156*
  red blast *157*
  sunrise juice *157*
  super-boost kale and pineapple juice *156*
sodium 56, 103
soft drinks 77, 84, 87
soups
  Asian broth bowl with duck, buckwheat noodles and greens *224*
  brassica and bean with Brazil nut pesto *171*
  fish *206*
  lentil and spinach *174*
  miso *268*
  mixed mushroom noodle with a poached egg *173*
  nutrition 56, 95, 96
  restorative beef stock and herbs *229*
  spiced beetroot and coconut milk (happy soup) *168*
soya
  cancer stem cells 25, 30
  nutrition 32, 42, 43, 46, 51, 54, 80–1

soya milk 72, 81
spelt flour
  nutrition 78–9
  pancakes with fresh fruit, yoghurt and honey *142*
  seeded spelt soda loaf *250*
spices *see also specific spices*
  alkaline diets 88
  'metallic mouth' 64, 66, 139
  nutrition 32, 64, 66–8, 92
spinach
  lentil and spinach soup *174*
  nutrition 52, 54, 91
  poached egg on spinach and pulse stir-fry *151*
  raw soft salad with Budwig dressing *177*
spirulina 52
sprouting seeds 52, 68–9, 139
squamous cell cancer 51
staple foods 38, 134–6
starchy carbohydrates 47–8, 75
steak with Asian power butter *230*
stem cells 22, 24–5, 30, 59, 273
steroids 62, 80, 86, 97, 111
stevia 77, 104
stir-fry, Thai chicken *220*
stock 95, 138, 256 *see also* bone broth
stomach ulcers 58
stomas 103–4, 273
storage 40, 45, 63, 64
strawberries
  chia strawberry and cashew nut milk pot *144*
  fresh seasonal fruit compote *150*
  nutrition 59
stress
  appetite loss 96
  farming methods 44
  gut microbiota 89
  management 38–9, 94–5, 125
  mindfulness 92–3
  protein requirement 42
sucralose 77
sucrose 73
sugar
  cachexia 95
  inflammation 31
  insulin 27, 28
  liver health 84
  nutrition 47, 72–5
sulforaphane 25, 57, 58, 92
sunflower oil 45
sunflower seeds
  Bircher muesli *147*

sunflower seeds (*cont.*)
  energy bombs *245*
  mixed fruit, seed and nut
    cake *246*
  nutrition 54, 90
  sardine dip *160*
  savoury seed crackers *159*
sunlight 62, 87, 109
sunrise juice *157*
super stocks *256*
supplements
  5-HTP 89
  antioxidants 114–16
  benefits 113
  calcium 62
  dosage 57
  expert advice 112
  low-fibre diet 104
  phytoestrogens 81
  probiotics 83–4
  research evidence 112,
    114–15
  safety 112
  vitamin Bs 64
  vitamin D 62
support network 39
surgery 33, 42, 103–4
swallowing 97, 142
sweeteners 76–7, 87
sweet potatoes
  baked sweet potato stuffed
    with buffalo Mozzarella
    182
  butternut and sweet potato
    tagine with chermoula
    185
  nutrition 63
  turmeric beef and sweet
    potato pot *234*
systemic, definition 273
tabouli, amaranth *175*
tagine
  butternut and sweet potato
    with chermoula *185*
  lamb *228*
tahini
  energy bombs *245*
  hummus *164*
  nutrition 90
Tamoxifen 58, 81
targeted therapy 33–4
tarragon 66
T-cells 60
teas *see also* caffeine; green
    tea
  cancer stem cells 25
  gut health 100
  homemade 62, 65, 67,
    267
  nausea 97
  nutrition 54, 56, 87
teeth 67
tempeh 81
temptation 128–9

terrain *see* internal terrain
testosterone 34, 48, 81
tests, personalization 37
Thai chicken stir-fry *220*
theanine 25
thyme 66
thymol 65
thyroid function 55, 60–1,
    81, 108
tiredness *see* fatigue
tofu
  avocado and tofu dip *161*
  miso soup *268*
  nutrition 43
  spiced golden tofu with
    vegetables *196*
tomatoes
  10-vegetable tomato sauce
    255
  amaranth tabouli *175*
  avocado and tofu dip *161*
  braised spiced aubergine
    197
  chilli con carne with beans
    and green and white
    vegetable rice *233*
  fish soup *206*
  lamb tagine *228*
  nutrition 52, 63, 89, 104
  red lentil dhal with grated
    courgette *192*
  stuffed roasted red peppers
    193
  turmeric beef and sweet
    potato pot *234*
trans-fats 31, 44, 47, 89–91,
    109
treatment methods 33–4 *see
  also* protocols
trigger avoidance 128–9
trophoblasts 116
trout: oven-baked trout and
    kale with millet *205*
tryptophan
  mood 89
  sources 89, 90, 138
tumours
  definition 273
  grades 23
tumour-suppressor genes 24,
    30, 273
tuna 45, 46
turkey
  nutrition 43, 89
  turkey, kale and black-eyed
    bean broth *221*
turkey rhubarb 118
turmeric
  cancer treatment 23
  chermoula *260*
  detoxification 120
  fruit and turmeric chutney
    254
  mouthwash 100

nutrition 25, 30, 31, 32,
    58, 101, 103
  supplements 113, 114–15
  turmeric beef and sweet
    potato pot *234*

vaccines 34
valine 95
vascular endothelial growth
  factor (VEGF) 29, 59, 273
vegetable oils 45
vegetables *see also specific
  vegetables*
  10-vegetable tomato sauce
    255
  alkaline diets 88
  cancer stem cells 25, 30
  cooking methods 92
  fridge frittata 191
  juicing 68–9
  kedgeree with leafy greens
    208
  nutrition 30–2, 48, 51, 52,
    63, 75, 87, 91
  portion sizes 50–1
  rainbow 49, 51
  shepherd's pie with mash
    and greens topping
    226
  spiced golden tofu with
    vegetables 196
  Thai chicken stir-fry 220
vegetarians
  protein 42, 79
  zinc 63
VEGF *see* vascular endothelial
  growth factor
vinegar 41, 88, 102
visceral fat 130
vitamin A 25, 32, 52, 63
vitamin Bs 52, 64, 89, 91,
    103
vitamin C
  intravenous 122–3
  iron absorption 91
  sources 52, 65, 67
  supplements 115–16
vitamin D
  Budwig protocol 109
  cancer stem cells 25
  nutrition 62, 87
  sources 54, 62, 87, 98
  supplements 113
  tests 37, 62
vitamin E 54, 102
vitamin K 54, 67, 87
vitamins (generally) *see also*
  antioxidants
  function 52–5
  immune system 31
  sources 52–5, 139
  supplements 113
volume modulated ablative
  therapy (VMAT) 33

waist to hip ratio 130
walnuts
  build-up smoothie *156*
  chocolate walnut brownies
    242
  mixed fruit, seed and nut
    cake *246*
  nutrition 30, 45, 52, 89,
    90, 99
Warburg effect 25–6, 31,
    106, 109
water 38, 48, 56, 85, 96, 101
watercress
  beef stock and herb
    restorative soup *229*
  raw soft salad with Budwig
    dressing *177*
watermelon: red blast *157*
watermelon, feta and
    pomegranate salad *178*
weight gain 96
weight loss 27, 95–6 *see also*
  cachexia
weight management 31, 32,
    48, 108, 129–30
wheatgrass 68
wheat intolerance 78, 79
whey 95, 100
white cell counts 60, 97, 98,
    101–2
wholegrain products 48, 52,
    74–5, 89, 91
wine 59, 81
World Cancer Research Fund
    (WCRF) 17

xenoestrogens 85
xylitol 77, 104

yeast 52
yoghurt
  build-up smoothie *156*
  gut health 99, 101, 104
  nutrition 43, 82, 83
  pancakes with fresh fruit,
    yoghurt and honey *142*
  peaches poached in green
    tea with honey and
    almond yoghurt *238*
  salmon and puy lentils
    with a coriander sauce
    209

zinc
  nutrition 63–4, 89, 91
  sources 54, 63, 80, 87, 138

MAGGIE'S CENTRES

MAGGIE'S OFFERS FREE PRACTICAL, emotional and social support to people with cancer and their family and friends, offering a programme of support that has been shown to strengthen physical and emotional wellbeing. Built in the grounds of specialist NHS cancer hospitals, Maggie's Centres are warm and welcoming places with professional staff on hand to offer the support people need to find their way through cancer. The Centres provide a place to find practical support about benefits and eating well; a place where qualified experts provide emotional support; a place to meet other people or simply sit quietly with a cup of tea.

The charity's philosophy about cancer care was originally laid out by its founder, Maggie Keswick Jencks, who was determined that people should not 'lose the joy of living in the fear of dying'. Maggie was a landscape architect and writer who lived with advanced cancer for two years, and during that time she worked with her husband, Charles Jencks, and her medical team, using her knowledge and experience, to create a blueprint for a new type of cancer care. She believed you needed information that would allow you to be an informed participant in your medical treatment, stress-reducing strategies, psychological support and the opportunity to meet other people in similar circumstances in a relaxed domestic atmosphere.

The first Maggie's Centre was built in Edinburgh at the Western General Hospital where Maggie was treated. Maggie and her husband found a disused stable building in the grounds of the hospital that was just the homely shape and size she was looking for. They wanted a building that was non-institutional, comforting, uplifting and stimulating and it seemed to fit the bill for conversion perfectly. Maggie died in 1995 but her ideas live on today in the charity and Centres that bear her name. The following year, in November 1996, the first Maggie's Centre opened in Edinburgh and what Maggie had planned became real.

What began as one person's idea has become a network of eighteen Centres across the UK, online and abroad, providing a unique model of cancer support that is alive, respected and growing, with the ability to reach more people with more types of cancer. As design and architecture are a vital part of the care offered, Maggie's works with great architects like Norman Foster and Richard Rogers, who give their time for little to nothing to create each Centre. Their skills deliver the calm environments that make the people who visit and work in the Centres feel safe, valued and comfortable, in an atmosphere that lifts their spirits.

Despite many breakthroughs in cancer treatment, there are two million people in the UK living with or after cancer today, and this figure is steadily rising, with over 300,000 new diagnoses each year. As cancer will touch even more of us in our lifetime, the aim is for everyone who needs it to have access to the support Maggie's offers.

Visiting Maggie's

There is no need to make an appointment at any Maggie's Centre; no referral is required, and it's completely free. You can simply drop in whenever you want for as long as you need. Our small team of professionally trained staff are on hand to provide practical and emotional support for people with cancer and their family and friends.

Find your nearest Centre at **www.maggiescentres.org**.

Supporting Maggie's

There are many ways in which you can show your support for Maggie's. Any help you give is valued and ensures we can continue to support more people affected by cancer and their families and friends across the UK.

You can make a donation of any amount, no matter how big or small, either as a one-off or a regular payment. You can join one of the many fundraising events that we organize each year throughout the country, or create your own event to raise money – and we'll help you every step of the way.

You could ask your company for support by forming a charity partnership, donating their time or skills, offering payroll giving or matching employee fundraising. Or when you come to think about your will, you might like to consider leaving a small percentage as a legacy to Maggie's.

You can also support Maggie's in a very direct way by helping us as a volunteer. Our regular fundraising events and projects always need 'hands on deck' to make everything run smoothly, or you can get involved at our Centres or in one of our offices.

If you would like to find out more about how you can help or donate, please visit **www.maggiescentres.org/howyoucanhelp**

Or contact us on:

Email: **enquiries@maggiescentres.org**

Tel: **0300 123 1801**

Share and text MAGG13 £3 to 70070 to donate to Maggie's Centres and make a difference today.

Whatever you choose to do, thank you for supporting Maggie's.

You can download Maggie Keswick Jencks' book, *A View from the Frontline*, in the publications section at **www.maggiescentres.org**